T0344660

Impacted Third Molars

Impacted Third Molars

Edited by

John Wayland
San Francisco Bay Area, California, USA

Second Edition

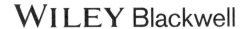

Library of Congress Cataloging-in-Publication Data

Names: Wayland, John, editor.
Title: Impacted third molars / edited by John Wayland.
Description: Second edition. | Hoboken, NJ : Wiley Blackwell, 2024. | Preceded by Impacted third molars / John Wayland. 2018. | Includes bibliographical references and index.
Identifiers: LCCN 2023003653 (print) | LCCN 2023003654 (ebook) | ISBN 9781119930303 (hardback) | ISBN 9781119930310 (ebook) | ISBN 9781119930327 (epub) | ISBN 9781119930334 (oBook)
Subjects: MESH: Molar, Third--surgery | Tooth, Impacted--surgery | Tooth Extraction--methods
Classification: LCC RK521 (print) | LCC RK521 (ebook) | NLM WU 605 | DDC 617.6/43--dc23/eng/20230620
LC record available at https://lccn.loc.gov/2023003653
LC ebook record available at https://lccn.loc.gov/2023003654

Cover Image: Courtesy of John Wayland
Cover Design: Wiley

Set in 9.5/12.5pt STIXTwoText by Integra Software Services Pvt. Ltd, Pondicherry, India

SKY10052475_080323

To my wife and best friend, Betty Yee

Contents

List of Contributors

Jamieson Brady, DDS

Faculty, Bay Area IV Wisdom
Private Practice, Chicago, IL.
SUNY Buffalo School of Dental Medicine, 2016
University at Buffalo summa cum laude Dental
Degree in 2016
Oral & Maxillofacial Surgery internship at
Chicago Cook County Hospital
Member of the American Dental Association

Matthew Diercks, DDS

Faculty, Bay Area IV Wisdom
Private Practice, University of the Pacific
School of Dentistry
Private Practice, Los Gatos, CA
Faculty, Bay Area IV Wisdom
University of the Pacific Dental Degree in 1998
Member of the American Dental Association

Andy Le, DDS

Faculty, Bay Area IV Wisdom
Private Practice, San Leandro, CA
Faculty, Bay Area IV Wisdom
Marquette University Dental Degree in 2001
Diplomat of the American Board of Oral
Implantology and Implant Dentistry
Fellow of the International Congress of Oral
Implantology
Member of the American Dental Association.

Preface

Most dentists receive minimal exodontia training in dental school. All difficult extractions and surgical procedures are referred to specialty programs: OMFS, AEGD, and GPR. Exodontia courses are hard to find after dental school, especially courses for the removal of impacted third molars. Most oral surgeons are reluctant to share their third molar knowledge. Very few general dentists have the third molar experience or training to pass on to their colleagues.

The removal of third molars is one of the most common procedures in dentistry. The majority of impacted third molars are removed by oral surgeons who also do hospital procedures, including orthognathic, cleft palate, TMJ, reconstructive, and other complex surgical procedures. Compared to complex oral surgery, the removal of third molars is a relatively simple procedure that can be done safely by most general practitioners.

Why Should YOU Remove Third Molars?

The removal of impacted third molars is a predictable and profitable procedure that benefits your practice and patients. Proper case selection and surgical procedure will minimize complications and can be learned by any dentist. The author has removed more than 25,000 wisdom teeth with no significant complications (i.e., no permanent paresthesia).

Fear of the unknown is a common barrier preventing dentists from removing third molars. They often ask themselves, "Is this third molar too close to the inferior alveolar nerve? How much bleeding is normal? What should I do if there's infection?" You probably asked similar questions with your first injection, filling, root canal, or crown. Now those procedures are routine. The removal of third molars, including impactions, will also become routine.

It's estimated that 10 million wisdom teeth are removed in the United States every year. Imagine a dentist who refers only one third molar patient per month for the removal of four third molars. If the cost per patient averaged $1500, including sedation, this dentist would refer $360,000 in 20 years! Conversely, the dentist could have treated his own patients and used the $360,000 to fund a retirement plan, pay off a mortgage, or send his or her children to college.

Your patients don't want to be referred out of your office. They prefer to stay with a doctor and staff that they know and trust.

Prophylatic Removal of Third Molars Controversy

There is no debate about the removal of third molars when pain or pathology is present. However, the prophylactic removal of third molars is controversial. There are many studies published to support either side of this controversy. However, the author believes common sense would support prophylactic removal.

Most patients with retained third molars will develop pathology. Third molars are difficult to keep clean. Every hygienist routinely records deep pockets near retained third molars. Caries are commonly found on third molars or the distal of second molars.

It is well documented that early removal of wisdom teeth results in fewer surgical complications. The incidence of postoperative infections and dry socket is also reduced.

Intended Audience

This book is intended for general dentists who would like to predictably, safely, and efficiently remove impacted third molars. It can be read cover to cover or by selected areas of interest. Emphasis has been placed on practical and useful information that can be readily applied in the general dentistry office.

1

Anatomy

Third molar surgical complications can be minimized or eliminated with proper case selection, surgical protocol, and a thorough knowledge of oral anatomy. Removal of third molars, including impactions, can become routine. A brief review of oral anatomy related to third molars is the first step in your journey to become proficient in the safe removal of impacted third molars. The structures relevant in the safe removal of third molars are:

1) Nerves
2) Blood vessels
3) Buccal fat pad
4) Submandibular fossa
5) Maxillary sinus
6) Infratemporal fossa

Nerves

In classical anatomy there are 12 paired cranial nerves (I–XII) providing sensory and motor innervation to the head and neck. (See Figure 1.1.)

The **trigeminal nerve (V)**, the fifth cranial nerve, is responsible for sensations of the face and motor functions of the muscles of mastication. This cranial nerves derives its name from the fact that each trigeminal nerve (one on each side of the pons) has three major branches: the ophthalmic nerve (V_1), the maxillary nerve (V_2), and the mandibular nerve (V_3). (See Figure 1.2.) The ophthalmic and maxillary nerves are purely sensory, while the mandibular nerve has sensory and motor functions. (See Figure 1.3.)

The **mandibular nerve** (V_3) is the largest of the three branches or divisions of the trigeminal nerve, the fifth (V) cranial nerve. (See Figure 1.4.) It is made up of a large sensory root and a small motor root. The mandibular nerve exits the cranium through the foramen ovale and divides into an anterior and posterior trunk in the infratemporal fossa. The mandibular nerve divides further into 9 main branches, 5 sensory and 4 motor.

The infratemporal fossa also contains many blood vessels in addition to nerves. This becomes important during the removal of high, palatally placed, maxillary third molars. These teeth may be displaced into the infratemporal fossa which contains these vital structures.

The five sensory branches of the mandibular nerve control sensation to teeth, tongue, mucosa, skin, and dura.

Impacted Third Molars, Second Edition. Edited by John Wayland.
© 2024 John Wiley & Sons, Inc. Published 2024 by John Wiley & Sons, Inc.

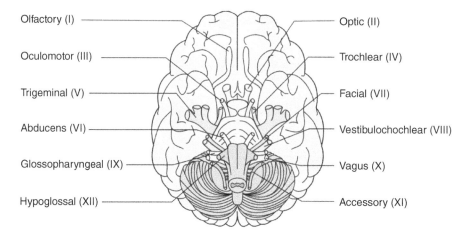

Olfactory (I) — Optic (II)

Oculomotor (III) — Trochlear (IV)

Trigeminal (V) — Facial (VII)

Abducens (VI) — Vestibulochochlear (VIII)

Glossopharyngeal (IX) — Vagus (X)

Hypoglossal (XII) — Accessory (XI)

Figure 1.1 The 12 cranial nerves emerge from the ventral side of the brain. (Drawing by Michael Brooks).

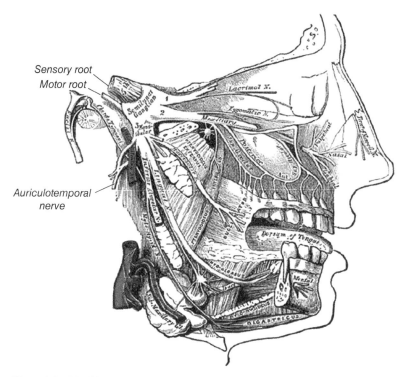

Sensory root
Motor root

Auriculotemporal
nerve

Figure 1.2 The fifth cranial nerve and three branches of the trigeminal nerve: (1) the ophthalmic nerve, (2) the maxillary nerve, and (3) the mandibular nerve. (by Henry Vandyke Carter / Wikimedia commons / Public Domain).

1) Inferior Alveolar – exits the mental foramen as the mental nerve and continues as the incisive nerve.
   - The nerve to mylohyoid is a motor and sensory branch of the inferior alveolar nerve
   - The nerve to anterior belly of the digastric muscle is a motor branch of the inferior alveolar nerve
   - Mean inferior alveolar nerve diameter is 4.7 mm.[1]
2) Lingual – lies under the lateral pterygoid muscle, medial to and in front of the inferior alveolar nerve.
   - Carries the chorda tympani nerve affecting taste and salivary flow.
   - May be round, oval, or flat and varies in size from 1.53 mm to 4.5 mm.[2]

- Average diameter of the main trunk of the lingual nerve is 3.5 mm.[3]

3) Auriculotemporal – innervation to the skin on the side of the head.
4) Buccal or long buccal – innervation to the cheek and second and third molar mucosa.
5) Meningeal – innervation to dura mater.

The four motor branches of the mandibular nerve control the movement of eight muscles, including the four muscles of mastication: the masseter, the temporal, and the medial and lateral pterygoids. The other four muscles are the tensor veli palatini, tensor tympani, mylohyoid, and the anterior belly of the digastric. Nerves to the tensor veli tympani and tensor palatini are branches of the medial pterygoid nerve. Nerves to the mylohyoid and anterior belly of the digastric muscles are branches of the inferior alveolar nerve.

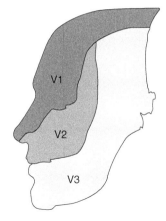

Figure 1.3 Sensory innervation of the three branches of the trigeminal nerve. (by Madhero88 / Wikimedia commons / CC BY 3.0).

6) Masseteric
7) Deep temporal
8) Lateral pterygoid
9) Medial pterygoid

Nerve Complications Following the Removal of Impacted Third Molars

Injury to the inferior alveolar, lingual, mylohyoid, and buccal nerves may cause altered or complete loss of sensation of the lower 1/3 of the face on the affected side.

The majority of serious nerve complications result from inferior alveolar or lingual nerve injuries. Most surgical injuries to the inferior alveolar nerve and lingual nerve cause temporary sensory change, but in some cases they can be permanent. Injury to these nerves can cause anesthesia (loss of sensation), paresthesia (abnormal sensation), hypoesthesia (reduced sensation), or dysesthesia (unpleasant abnormal sensation). Injury to the lingual nerve and associated chorda tympani nerve can also cause loss of taste of the anterior 2/3 of the tongue.

Damage to the mylohyoid nerve has been reported to be as high as 1.5% following lower third molar removal, but this is probably due to the use of lingual retraction.[4] Most third molars can be

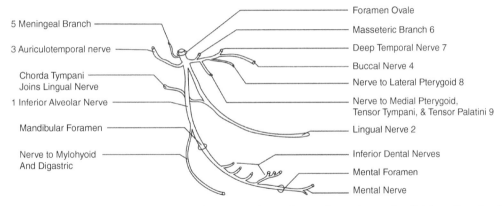

Figure 1.4 Mandibular nerve branches from the main trunk; anterior, and posterior divisions. (Drawing by Michael Brooks).

removed by utilizing a purely buccal technique. Utilizing this technique, it is not necessary to encroach on the lingual tissues or to remove distal, distolingual, or lingual bone.[5]

A search of the literature found no specific reports of long buccal nerve involvement (AAOMS white paper, March 2007), although one article did note long buccal involvement when the anatomical position was aberrant. In this case, the long buccal nerve was coming off the inferior alveolar nerve once it was already in the canal and coming out through a separate foramen on the buccal side of the mandible.[6] Long buccal nerve branches are probably frequently cut during the incision process, but the effects are generally not noted.[7]

Blood Vessels

Life-threatening hemorrhage resulting from the surgical removal of third molars is rare. However, copious bleeding from soft tissue is relatively common. One source of bleeding during the surgical removal of third molars is the inferior alveolar artery and/or vein. These central vessels can be cut during sectioning of third molars leading to profuse bleeding. The path of vessels leading to the inferior alveolar neurovascular bundle begins with the common carotid arteries and the heart.

The common carotid arteries originate close to the heart and divide to form the internal and external carotid arteries. The left and right external carotid arteries provide oxygenated blood to the areas of the head and neck outside the cranium. These arteries divide within the parotid gland into the superficial temporal artery and the maxillary artery. The maxillary artery has three portions; maxillary, pterygoid, and pterygomaxillary. (See Figures 1.5a and 1.5b.)

The first portion of the maxillary artery divides into five branches. The inferior alveolar artery is one of the five branches of the first part of the maxillary artery. The inferior alveolar artery joins the inferior alveolar nerve and vein to form the inferior alveolar neurovascular bundle within the mandible. Three studies confirm that the inferior alveolar vein lies superior to the nerve and that there are often multiple veins. The artery appears to be solitary and lies on the lingual side of the nerve, slightly above the horizontal position.[8]

Bleeding during and after third molar impaction surgery is expected. Local factors resulting from soft-tissue and vessel injury represent the most common cause of postoperative bleeding.[9] Systemic causes of bleeding are not common, and routine preoperative blood testing of patients, without a relevant medical history, is not recommended.[10]

Hemorrhage from mandibular molars is more common than bleeding from maxillary molars (80% and 20%, respectively),[11] because the floor of the mouth is highly vascular. The distal lingual aspect of mandibular third molars is especially vascular and an accessory artery in this area can be cut leading to profuse bleeding.[12,13] The most immediate danger for a healthy patient with severe post-extraction hemorrhage is airway compromise.[14]

Most bleeding following third molar impaction surgery can be controlled with pressure. Methods for hemostasis will be discussed further in Chapter 3.

Buccal Fat Pad

The buccal fat pad is a structure that may be encountered when removing impacted third molars. It is most often seen when flap incisions are made too far distal to maxillary second molars. It is a deep fat pad located on either side of the face and is surrounded by the following structures. (See Figure 1.6.)

- Anterior – angle of the mouth
- Posterior – masseter muscle

(a)

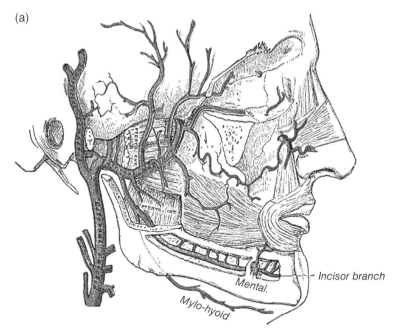

Incisor branch

Mental.

Mylo-hyoid

Figure 1.5a   The Maxillary Artery. (Henry Gray / Wikimedia commons / Public Domain).

(b)

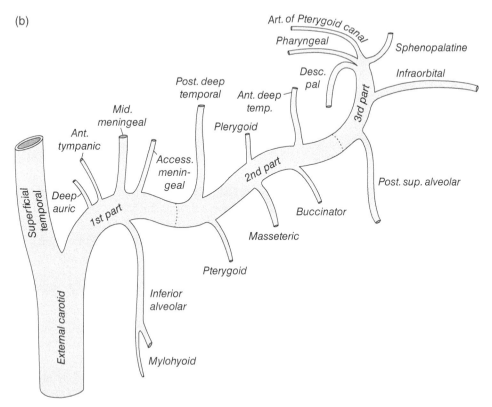

Art. of Pterygoid canal

Pharyngeal

Sphenopalatine

Desc. pal

Infraorbital

Post. deep temporal

Ant. deep temp.

3rd part

Mid. meningeal

Ant. tympanic

Pterygoid

Access. menin-geal

2nd part

Superficial temporal

Deep auric

1st part

Post. sup. alveolar

Buccinator

Masseteric

Pterygoid

Inferior alveolar

External carotid

Mylohyoid

Figure 1.5b   Branches of the maxillary artery depicting maxillary, pterygoid, and pterygomaxillary portions. (by Henry Vandyke Carter / Wikimedia commons / Public Domain).

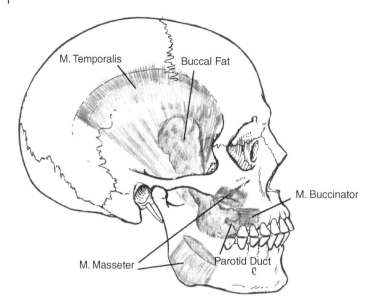

Figure 1.6   Buccal fat pad. (By Otto Placik / Wikimedia commons / CC BY 3.0).

- Medial – buccinator muscle
- Lateral – platysma muscle, subcutaneous tissue, and skin
- Superior – zygomaticus muscles
- Inferior – depressor anguli oris muscle and the attachment of the deep fascia to the mandible

Zhang, Yan, Wi, Wang, and Liu reviewed the anatomical structures of the buccal fat pad in 11 head specimens (i.e., 22 sides of the face).

> The enveloping, fixed tissues and the source of the nutritional vessels to the buccal fat pad and its relationship with surrounding structures were observed in detail. Dissections showed that the buccal fat pad can be divided into three lobes – anterior, intermediate, and posterior, according to the structure of the lobar envelopes, the formation of the ligaments, and the source of the nutritional vessels. Buccal, pterygoid, pterygopalatine, and temporal extensions are derived from the posterior lobe. The buccal fat pad is fixed by six ligaments to the maxilla, posterior zygoma, and inner and outer rim of the infraorbital fissure, temporalis tendon, or buccinator membrane. Several nutritional vessels exist in each lobe and in the subcapsular vascular plexus forms. The buccal fat pads function to fill the deep tissue spaces, to act as gliding pads when masticatory and mimetic muscles contract, and to cushion important structures from the extrusion of muscle contraction or outer force impulsion. The volume of the buccal fat pad may change throughout a person's life.[15]

Submandibular Fossa

The submandibular fossa is a bilateral space located in the mandible, medial to the body of the mandible, and below the mylohyoid line. (See Figure 1.7.) It contains the submandibular salivary gland which produces 65–70% of our saliva.

Third molar roots are often located in close proximity to the submandibular space. (See Figure 1.8.) The lingual cortex in this area may be thin or missing entirely. Therefore, excessive or

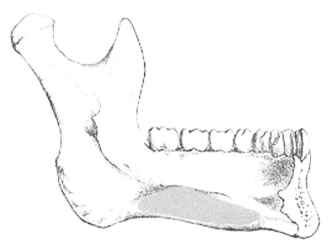

Figure 1.7 Submandibular fossa. (Adapted from Henry Vandyke Carter, via Wikimedia Commons).

misplaced force can dislodge root fragments or even an entire tooth into the adjacent submandibular space.[16]

Patients presenting with partially impacted third molars can develop pericoronitis. This localized infection can spread to the submandibular, sublingual, and submental spaces. Bilateral infection of these spaces is known as Ludwig's angina.[17] Prior to the advent of antibiotics this infection was often fatal due to concomitant swelling and compromised airway.

Maxillary Sinus

The maxillary sinus is a bilateral empty space located within the maxilla, above the maxillary posterior teeth. It is pyramidal in shape consisting of an apex, base, and four walls. (See Figure 1.9 and Box 1.1.)

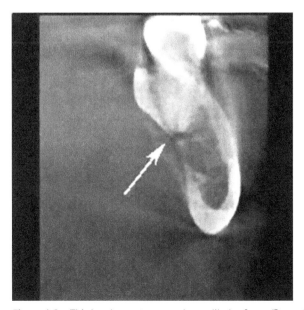

Figure 1.8 Third molar roots near submandibular fossa. (Reproduced with permission of Dr. Jason J. Hales, DDS).

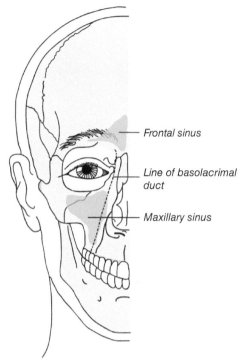

Frontal sinus

Line of basolacrimal duct

Maxillary sinus

Figure 1.9   Maxillary sinus coronal view. (by Henry Vandyke Carter / Wikimedia commons / Public Domain).

Box 1.1   Boundaries of the maxillary sinus.
Apex – pointing towards the zygomatic process Anterior wall – facial surface of the maxilla Posterior wall – infratemporal surface of the maxilla Superior – floor of the orbit Inferior – alveolar process of the maxilla Base – cartilaginous lateral wall of the nasal cavity

The size and shape of the maxillary sinus varies widely among individuals and within the same individual. The average volume of a sinus is about 15 ml (range between 4.5 and 35.2 ml).[18]

Maxillary third molar teeth and roots are often in close proximity to the maxillary sinus. The distance between the root apices of the maxillary posterior teeth and the sinus is sometimes less than 1 mm.[19] Complications related to the removal of maxillary third molars include sinus openings, displacement of roots or teeth into the sinus, and postoperative sinus infections.

Infratemporal Fossa

The infratemporal fossa is an irregularly shaped space located inferior to the zygomatic arch and posterior to the maxilla. Six structures form its boundaries. (See Figure 1.10 and Box 1.2.)

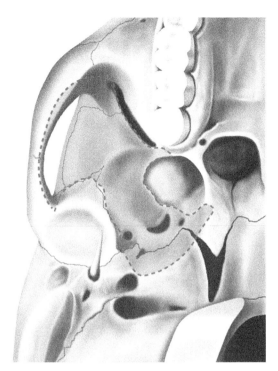

Figure 1.10   Boundaries of the infratemporal fossa. (Reproduced with permission from Joanna Culley BA(hons) IMI, MMAA, RMIP).

Box 1.2 Boundaries of the infratemporal fossa.

Anterior: posterior maxilla
Posterior: tympanic plate and temporal bone
Medial: lateral pterygoid plate
Lateral: ramus of the mandible
Superior: greater wing of the sphenoid bone
Inferior: medial pterygoid muscle

Although rare, there are documented cases of maxillary third molars displaced into the infratemporal fossa. Unlike the maxillary sinus, the infratemporal fossa is not an empty space. It contains many vital structures including nerves, arteries, and veins. A third molar displaced into the infratemporal fossa is considered a major complication. Dentists removing impacted maxillary third molars should understand the anatomy of the infratemporal fossa.

This chapter is not intended to be a comprehensive review of oral anatomy, but instead is a review of structures relevant to third molars. This knowledge is essential to avoid surgical complications. Although no surgical procedure is without risk, most impacted third molars can be removed safely and predictably.

An important key to avoid complications is deciding when to refer to an oral surgeon. This will be different for each dentist depending on experience and training. "When to refer" may be the most important factor to consider prior to treating your patients. Case selection, including surgical risk and difficulty, is discussed in the next chapter.

References

1 Svane TJ. Vascular Characteristics of the Human Inferior Alveolar Nerve, *J Oral Maxillofacl Surg*. 1986;44:431.

2 Graff-Radford SB, Evans RW. Disclosures. *Headache*. 2003;43(9): 9.

3 Zur KB, Mu L, Sanders I. Distribution pattern of the human lingual nerve. *Clin Anat*. 2004 Mar;17(2):88–92.

4 Carmichael FA, McGowan DA. Incidence of nerve damage following third molar removal: a West of Scotland Surgery Research Group study. *Brit J Oral Maxillofac Surg*. 1992;30:78.

5 Gargallo-Albiol J, Buenechea-Imaz R, Gay-Escoda C. Lingual nerve protection during surgical removal of lower third molars. *J Oral Maxillofac Surg*. 2000;29:268.

6 Singh S. Aberrant buccal nerve encountered at third molar surgery. *Oral Surg Oral Med Oral Pathol*. 1981;52:142.

7 Merrill RG. Prevention, treatment, and prognosis for nerve injury related to the difficult impaction. *Dent Clin North Am*. 1979;23:471.

8 Pogrel MA, Dorfman D, Fallah H. The anatomic structure of the inferior alveolar neurovascular bundle in the third molar region. *J Oral Maxillofac Surg*. 2009 Nov;67(11):2452–4.

9 Allen FJ. Postextraction hemorrhage. A study of 50 consecutive cases. *Br Dent J*. 1967;122(4):139–43.

10 Suchman AL, Mushlin AI. How well does activated partial thromboplastin time predict postoperative hemorrhage? *JAMA*. 1986;256(6):750–3.

11 Jensen S. Hemorrhage after oral surgery. An analysis of 103 cases. *Oral Surg Oral Med Oral Pathol*. 1974;37(1):2–16.

12 Funayama M, Kumagai T, Saito K, Watanabe T. Asphyxial death caused by post extraction hematoma. *Am J Forensic Med Pathol*. 1994;15(1):87–90.

13 Goldstein BH. Acute dissecting hematoma: a complication of an oral and maxillofacial surgery. *J Oral Surg*. 1981;39(1):40–3.

14 Moghadam HG, Caminiti MF. Life-threatening hemorrhage after extraction of third molars: case report and management protocol. *J Can Dent Assoc*. 2002;68(11):670–5.

15 Zhang HM, Yan YP, Qi KM, Wang JQ, Liu ZF. Anatomical structure of the buccal fat pad and its clinical adaptations. *Plast Reconst Surg*. 2002;109(7):2509–18; discussion 2519–20.

16 Aznar-Arasa L, Figueiredo R, Gay-Escoda C. Iatrogenic displacement of lower third molar roots into the sublingual space: report of 6 cases. *Int J Oral Maxillofac Surg*. 2012;70:e107–15.

17 Vijayan A, et al. Ludwigs angina: report of a case with extensive discussion on its management. *URJD*. 2015;5(2):82–86.

18 Kim JH. *A review of the maxillary sinus*. Sinus, OK: Perio Implant Advisory.

19 Hargreaves KM, Cohen S, web editor, Berman LH, editor. *Cohen's pathways of the pulp*, 10th edition. St. Louis, MO: Mosby Elsevier, 2010, 590,592.

2

Case Selection

The best way to avoid complications when removing impacted third molars is to select patients and surgeries that are commensurate with your level of training and experience. Will you treat medically compromised patients? Or, will you only remove impacted third molars for healthy teens? Have you removed thousands of impactions? Or, are you about to remove your first maxillary soft tissue impaction? This chapter will help you decide which third molar surgery patients should be referred to a maxillofacial surgeon or kept in your office. It will also help you know when you are ready to move to the next level of difficulty.

Medical Evaluation

The medical evaluation includes a complete health history/patient interview, physical assessment, clinical exam, and psychological evaluation of the patient. The removal of impacted third molars is an invasive surgical procedure with risk of complications higher than most dental procedures. Furthermore, patients are often apprehensive and have anxiety about the procedure.

Health History and Patient Interview

A thorough health history and patient interview should be completed prior to treatment. The primary purpose of a patient's health history is to attempt to find out as much about each patient as possible, so that the patient can be treated safely and knowledgeably. A health history form, completed by the patient, should be reviewed before interviewing the patient. The American Dental Association's 2014 Health History form is provided as an example. (See Figures 2.1a, 2.1b, and 2.1c.)

The patient's health history can be subpoenaed in court cases, such as a malpractice suit, or when disciplinary action is taken against a dental professional by a regulatory board. Medical evaluation documents can be used as legal evidence and must be thorough and comprehensive.

The patient interview is an essential part of a medical evaluation. It's not uncommon to have an unremarkable health history, only to learn during the interview that the patient has a history of health issues and medication. Good interview technique requires open-ended questions and active listening. Open-ended questions always begin with What, How, When, or Where. These questions cannot be answered with a simple yes or no answer. Yes or no questions should be limited to the health history form.

Impacted Third Molars, Second Edition. Edited by John Wayland.
© 2024 John Wiley & Sons, Inc. Published 2024 by John Wiley & Sons, Inc.

CAMP is a useful mnemonic to remember key interview questions.

Chief complaint – What brings you to the office?

Allergies – What are you allergic to? What else?

Medications – What medications do you take? What medications have you taken previously?

Past Medical History – What medical problems have you had in the past and when did you have them?

Confidential Health History

Patient Name: _____ Date of Birth: _____

I. CIRCLE APPROPRIATE ANSWER (Leave blank if you do not understand the question)

1. Yes / No Is your general health good?
    If NO, explain: _____

2. Yes / No Has there been a change in your health within the last year?
    If YES, explain: _____

3. Yes / No Have you gone to the hospital or emergency room or had a serious illness in the last three years?
    If YES, explain: _____

4. Yes / No Are you being treated by a physician now? If YES, explain: _____
    Date of last medical exam? _____ Reason for exam: _____

5. Yes / No Have you had problems with prior dental treatment?
    If YES, explain: _____
    Date of last dental exam: _____ Name of last treating dentist: _____

6. Yes / No Are you in pain now?
    If YES, explain: _____

II. HAVE YOU EVER EXPERIENCED ANY OF THE FOLLOWING? (Please circle Yes or No for each)

Yes / No Chest pain (angina)	Yes / No Blood in stools	Yes / No Frequent vomiting
Yes / No Fainting spells	Yes / No Diarrhea or constipation	Yes / No Jaundice
Yes / No Recent significant weight loss	Yes / No Frequent urination	Yes / No Dry mouth
Yes / No Fever	Yes / No Difficulty urinating	Yes / No Excessive thirst
Yes / No Night sweats	Yes / No Ringing in ears	Yes / No Difficulty swallowing
Yes / No Persistent cough	Yes / No Headaches	Yes / No Swollen ankles
Yes / No Coughing up blood	Yes / No Dizziness	Yes / No Joint pain or stiffness
Yes / No Bleeding problems	Yes / No Blurred vision	Yes / No Shortness of breath
Yes / No Blood in urine	Yes / No Bruise easily	Yes / No Sinus problems

Other: _____

III. HAVE YOU EVER HAD OR DO YOU HAVE ANY OF THE FOLLOWING? (Please circle Yes or No for each)

Yes / No Heart disease	Yes / No AIDS/HIV	Yes / No Psychiatric care
Yes / No Family history of heart disease	Yes / No Surgeries	Yes / No Osteoporosis
Yes / No Heart attack	Yes / No Hospitalization	Yes / No Thyroid disease
Yes / No Artificial joint	Yes / No Diabetes	Yes / No Asthma
Yes / No Stomach problems or ulcers	Yes / No Family history of diabetes	Yes / No Hepatitis
Yes / No Heart defects	Yes / No Tumors or cancer	Yes / No Sexual transmitted disease
Yes / No Heart murmurs	Yes / No Chemotherapy	Yes / No Herpes
Yes / No Rheumatic fever	Yes / No Radiation	Yes / No Canker or cold sores
Yes / No Skin disease	Yes / No Arthritis, rheumatism	Yes / No Anemia
Yes / No Hardening of arteries	Yes / No Emphysema or other lung disease	Yes / No Liver disease
Yes / No High blood pressure	Yes / No Kidney or bladder disease	Yes / No Eye disease
Yes / No Seizures	Yes / No Stroke	Yes / No Transplants
Yes / No Cosmetic surgery	Yes / No Eating disorders	Yes / No Tuberculosis

Other: _____

Figure 2.1a   Health History (Reproduced by permission of ADA).

IV. ARE YOU ALLERGIC TO OR HAVE YOU HAD A REACTION TO ANY OF THE FOLLOWING?

(Please circle Yes or No for each)

Yes / No Aspirin	Yes / No Valium or other sedatives	Yes / No Codeine or other narcotics
Yes / No Penicillin or other antibiotics	Yes / No Latex	Yes / No Food
Yes / No Nitrous oxide	Yes / No Local anesthetic	Yes / No Metal

Others: _____

V. ARE YOU TAKING OR HAVE YOU TAKEN ANY OF THE FOLLOWING IN THE LAST THREE MONTHS?

(Please circle Yes or No for each)

Yes / No Recreational drugs	Yes / No Tobacco in any form	Yes / No Antibiotics
Yes / No Over-the-counter medicines	Yes / No Alcohol	Yes / No Supplements
Yes / No Weight loss medications	Yes / No Bisphosphonate (Fosamax)	Yes / No Aspirin
Yes / No Anti-Depressants	Yes / No Herbal Supplements	

Please list all prescription medications: _____

VI. WOMEN ONLY (Please circle Yes or No for each)

Yes / No   Are you or could you be pregnant? If YES, what month? _____

Yes / No   Are you nursing?

Yes / No   Are you taking birth control pills?

VII. ALL PATIENTS (Please circle Yes or No for each)

Yes / No   Do you have or have you had any other diseases or medical problems NOT listed on this form?

If YES, please explain: _____

_____

Yes / No   Have you ever been pre-medicated for dental treatment? If YES, why: _____

Yes / No   Have you ever taken Fen-Phen? If YES, when: _____

Yes / No   **Is there any issue or condition that you would like to discuss with the dentist in private?**

The practice of dentistry involves treating the whole person. If the dentist determines that there may be a potentially medically compromised situation, medical consultation may be needed prior to commencement of dental treatment.

I authorize the dentist to contact my physician.

Patient's Signature: _____   Date: _____

Physician's Name: _____   Phone Number: _____

Whom would you like us to contact in case of an emergency?

Name: _____   **Relationship**: _____   **Phone Number**: _____

I certify that I have read and understand this form. To the best of my knowledge, I have answered every question completely and accurately. I will inform my dentist of any change in my health and/or medication. Further, I will not hold my dentist, or any other member of his/her staff, responsible for any errors or omissions that I may have made in the completion of this form.

_____   _____   _____   _____

Signature of Patient (Parent or Guardian)   Date   Signature of Dentist   Date

Figure 2.1b   Health History Update (Reproduced by permission of ADA).

MEDICAL UPDATES

I have reviewed my Health History and confirm that it accurately states past and present conditions.

DATE	PATIENT SIGNATURE	CHANGES TO HEALTH HISTORY	DENTIST INITIALS

(AS 10/2014)

Figure 2.1c   Patient Interview (Reproduced by permission of ADA).

Physical Assessment

The American Society of Anesthesiologist's (ASA) physical classification system is a useful guide when deciding to refer third molar surgical patients.[1] (See Table 2.1.)

A study published in the *Journal of Public Health Dentistry* in 1993 evaluated the general health of dental patients on the basis of the physical status classification system of the American Society of Anesthesiologists. A total of 4,087 patients completed a risk-related, patient-administered

Table 2.1   ASA physical status classification system.

Classification	Description
ASA 1	Normal healthy
ASA 2	Mild systemic disease
ASA 3	Severe systemic disease
ASA 4	Disease is a constant threat to life
ASA 5	Not expected to survive without operation
ASA 6	Declared brain dead patient donating organs

questionnaire. On the basis of their medical data, a computerized ASA classification was determined for each patient: 63.3% were in ASA class I, 25.7% in class II, 8.9% in class III, and 2.1% in class IV. Eighty-nine percent of patients in this study were ASA Class I or II.[2]

Another study measured the medical problems of 29,424 dental patients (age 18 years and over) from 50 dental practices in the Netherlands. This study found that the number of patients seen with hypertension, cardiovascular, neurological, endocrinological, infectious, and blood disease increased with age.[3]

Kaminishi states that the number of patients over age 40 requiring third molar removal is increasing. Over a five-year period, 1997–2002, the incidence almost doubled to 17.9%. This age category is known to be high risk for third molar surgery. At equal or higher risk is the rapidly growing number of patients seeking third molar surgery that are moderately or severely medically compromised.[4]

There are no absolute case selection recommendations based on these studies. However, most experts agree that ASA I and II patients can be treated safely in a dental office setting. Medically compromised ASA III patients are taking medications that do not adequately control their disease. The author recommends referral of medically compromised ASA III patients and the elderly. Alternatively, an anesthesiologist can sedate these patients. Fortunately, the majority of patients seen for third molar impaction surgery are relatively young, healthy, ASA I and II patients.

The physical assessment begins at first contact with the patient.

● Overall appearance – What is their overall appearance? Is the patient obese, elderly, frail?
● Lifestyle – Do they use drugs or alcohol in excess? Do they have an active lifestyle?
● Vital signs – multiple blood pressure readings are recommended.

Every patient considering the removal of impacted third molars should have their vital signs checked at the surgery consultation and on the day of surgery. Patients with hypertension are more prone to cardiovascular complications. Hypertension can be diagnosed with simple blood pressure readings. This is especially important if the patient will be sedated because a baseline recording is needed to compare with readings during the procedure. According to the US Department of Health and Human Services, desired systolic pressure ranges from 90 to 119. The desired diastolic range is 60–79.[5] (See Table 2.2.)

As of 2000, nearly one billion people, approximately 26% of the adult population of the world, had hypertension.[6] Forty-four percent of African American adults have hypertension.[7]

Table 2.2   Classification of blood pressure for adults.

Category	Systolic, mm Hg	Diastolic, mm Hg
Hypotension	< 90	< 60
Normal	90–119	60–79
Prehypertension	120–139	80–89
Stage 1 hypertension	140–159	90–99
Stage 2 hypertension	160–179	100–109
Hypertensive emergency	>180	>110

Clinical Exam

Access is particularly important during the removal of impacted third molars. Poor access can make the procedure much more difficult. Patients with orthodontics in progress, small mouths, short anterior posterior distance, large tongues, and limited opening can make the removal of impacted third molars nearly impossible. A useful guide to evaluate access is the Mallampati airway classification. See Figure 2.2.

Class IV patients are typically patients with square faces, short necks, and large tongues. The coronoid process will move close to maxillary third molars during translation, severely limiting access. In addition, these patients may have small arch size and limited soft tissue opening. A prudent dentist would consider referring these patients to a maxillofacial surgeon.

Psychological Evaluation

The psychological and emotional status of impacted third molar patients is an important factor in their successful treatment. Dr. Milus House has been credited with developing a system to classify the psychology of denture patients. Although this system was devised in 1937 to evaluate denture

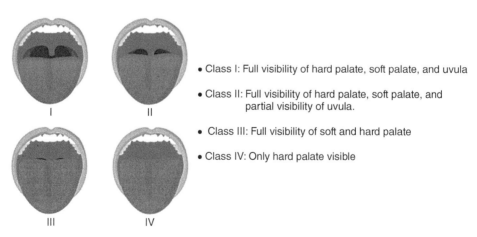

- Class I: Full visibility of hard palate, soft palate, and uvula
- Class II: Full visibility of hard palate, soft palate, and partial visibility of uvula.
- Class III: Full visibility of soft and hard palate
- Class IV: Only hard palate visible

Figure 2.2   Mallampati classification can be used to predict airway management and oral access. (By Jmarchn / Wikimedia commons / CC BY 3.0).

patients, it is still applicable today for third molar patients. Class I and II patients are most likely to have a positive treatment result. (See Box 2.1.)

Box 2.1 House's emotional and psychological patient classification.

Class 1: Philosophical – Accepts dentist's judgement and instructions, best prognosis.
Class 2: Exacting – Methodical and demanding, asks a lot of questions, good prognosis.
Class 3: Indifferent – Doesn't care about dental treatment and gives up easily, fair prognosis.
Class 4: Critical – Emotionally unfit, never happy, worst prognosis.

In a study conducted in 2007, National Institute of Mental Health researchers examined data to determine how common personality disorders are in the United States. 5,692 adults, ages 18 and older, answered screening questions from the International Personality Disorder Examination (IPDE).

The researchers found that the prevalence for personality disorders in the United States is 9.1%.[8] Nearly 10% of dental patients ages 18 and older may have some form of personality disorder!

Patients who have psychological and emotional challenges may be less compliant and unable to cope with the stress of surgical procedures.(See Figure 2.3.) The author recommends referral of these patients to a maxillofacial surgeon or treatment with an anesthesiologist

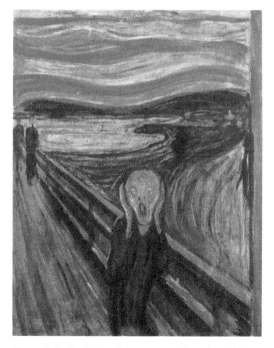

Figure 2.3   Patients with severe anxiety should be treated with GA. (Edvard Munch / Wikimedia Commons / Public domain).

Radiographic Assessment

A thorough evaluation of radiographs is essential to avoid surgical complications. Resolution, contrast, and clarity should not be compromised. Panoramic radiographs are ideal for viewing structural relationships. They allow for visualization of the third molar's relationship to the following structures: inferior alveolar nerve canal, maxillary sinus, ramus, and second molar. Intraoral films further delineate the third molar periodontal ligament, root structure, and position. Most third molar surgeries can be completed safely with high-quality panoramic and intraoral films.

Cone beam CT scans have yet to become the standard of care in outpatient oral surgery. However, a CT scan may be appropriate for patients with fully developed roots near vital structures. For example, CT imaging may be appropriate when intimate contact with the inferior alveolar nerve is suspected after reviewing panoramic films or when a third molar is located near the palate.

The following factors are important when assessing radiographs.

1) Position
2) Depth
3) Angulation
4) Combined root width
5) Root length, size, and shape
6) Periodontal ligament and follicle
7) Bone elasticity and density
8) Position relative to the inferior alveolar canal

Position

The anterior posterior position of impacted third molars is always a significant factor. Third molars positioned in or near the ramus will have limited access. The position of mandibular third molars can be classified in relation to the second molar and ascending ramus. (See Figure 2.4.) Mandibular

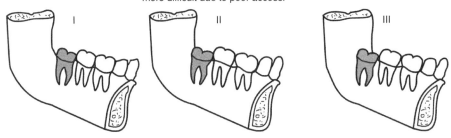

Position - 2nd Molar to Ramus

Class I - EASY - Sufficient room for third molar eruption

Class II - MODERATE - Some of the third molar is in the ramus

Class III - DIFFICULT - Most or all of the third molar is in the ramus

* This assessment is related to AP distance.
Class III maxillary impactions are usually
more difficult due to poor access.

Figure 2.4 Surgical difficulty based on AP distance, second molar, and ramus. (Reproduced by permission of Robert J. Whitacre).

third molars are classified as Class I position when there is sufficient room for eruption between the second molar and ascending ramus. The tooth should have no tissue covering the distal aspect. Class II mandibular third molars do not have sufficient room for normal eruption. Some of the third molar is in the ramus. Mandibular third molars are Class III when the majority of the third molar is in the ramus.

A Class III position, short anterior posterior distance, will severely limit access to maxillary impactions.

Depth

The depth of mandibular third molars can be classified relative to the occlusal surface and CEJ of the adjacent second molar. A mandibular third molar is Depth A when it is even with or above the occlusal surface of the second molar. It is Depth B when it is located between the occlusal surface and CEJ of the second molar. It is Depth C when it is located below the second molar CEJ. Surgical difficulty increases in direct proportion to depth for both mandibular and maxillary third molars. (See Figure 2.5.)

This classification system produces 9 possible outcomes when position and depth are combined. IA would be considered the easiest position and depth while IIIC would be the most difficult position and depth. This system is often attributed to Gregory and Pell. It is a modification of the classification developed by George B. Winter.

Angulation

Angulation refers to the mandibular third molar longitudinal axis relative to its adjacent second molar longitudinal axis. Mandibular impaction angulations can be mesioangular (43%), horizontal (3%), vertical (38%), or distoangular (6%).[9]

The long axis of mesioangular impactions is tilted toward the second molar. The mesioangular impacted third molar is notorious for third molar pain. Its crown is often partially erupted leading to localized infection and pericoronitis. They represent 43% of all impactions and are

Depth - 2nd Molar Occlusal Surface & CEJ

Class A - Easy - Third Molar is even with second molar occlusal surface

Class B - Moderate - Third molar is between second molar occlusal surface and CEJ

Class C - Difficult - Third molar is between second molar apex and CEJ

* A deep maxillary third molar will be very difficult due to access

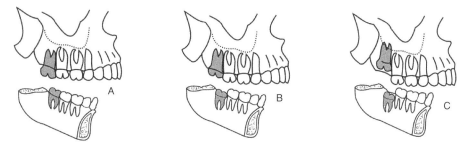

Figure 2.5 Surgical difficulty based on depth relative to second molar. (Reproduced by permission of Robert J. Whitacre).

usually the easiest to remove with a straight surgical handpiece. The long axis of horizontal impactions is perpendicular or nearly perpendicular to the second molar long axis. Horizontal impactions are the second easiest surgical angulation after the mesioangular. Inexperienced surgeons often mistake this angulation for the most difficult surgical angulation. Horizontal impactions represent 3% of all impactions. The vertical impaction long axis parallels the long axis of the second molar. Vertical impactions are considered to be more difficult than horizontal impactions due to access. This is especially true for deep vertical impactions. The vertical impaction represents 38% of impacted third molars. Finally, the distoangular mandibular impaction is tilted toward the ramus. The path of removal is toward the ramus. (See Figure 2.6.) This is the reason why this angulation is considered the most difficult of all mandibular third molar impactions. Fortunately, they only account for 6% of mandibular third molar impactions. All of these impactions can be in buccal version or lingual version. The remaining 10% of mandibular impactions are transverse or inverted. A transverse impaction is growing toward the cheek or tongue. Inverted impactions are "upside down."

The surgical difficulty when removing maxillary impactions is opposite of mandibular impactions. Mesioangular impactions are normally more difficult than distoangular impactions.

Combined Root Width

Combined root width is always a significant factor. A tooth with a conical root will be easier to remove than one with divergent roots. The roots of teeth with multiple roots are often divergent. The removal of these teeth will be more difficult when the combined root width is greater than the tooth width at the CEJ. Third molars with divergent roots may require sectioning. (See Figures 2.7a and 2.7b.)

Root Length, Size, and Shape

Root length, size, and shape are always significant factors, but are often overlooked. Third molar roots that are long, thin, or curved may fracture leaving root fragments that are difficult to remove. The root fragments may be near vital structures such as the inferior alveolar nerve, maxillary sinus, infratemporal fossa, or submandibular fossa. It's always prudent to carefully assess quality radiographs to avoid root fracture. Sectioning may be required. (See Figures 2.8a and 2.8b.)

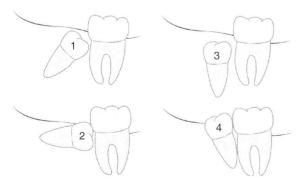

Figure 2.6   Surgical difficulty by angulation – 4 most difficult.

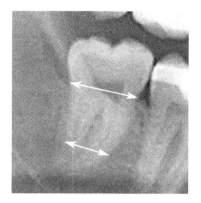

Figure 2.7a   Conical.

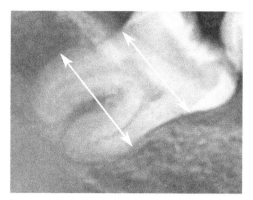

Figure 2.7b   Divergent.

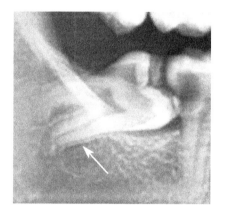

Figure 2.8a   Long, thin, curved.

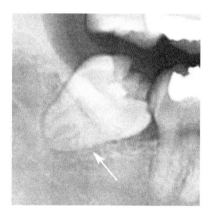

Figure 2.8b   Short, thick, straight.

Periodontal Ligament and Follicle

The periodontal ligament and follicle are always significant factors. A periodontal ligament space or follicle visible on a radiograph is a positive sign. These spaces allow for movement of the tooth with elevators and forceps. Periotomes, luxators, and proximators can be wedged into this space to luxate a tooth or root. (See Figure 2.9a.)

A dental follicle is always present with developing third molars. This structure differentiates into the periodontal ligament as the tooth develops.[10] The dental follicle provides a space larger than the periodontal ligament space. (See Figure 2.9b.) The follicular space is one reason oral surgeons recommend removing third molars early, usually in the teenage years

Tooth ankylosis can be defined as the fusion of bone to cementum resulting in partial or total elimination of the periodontal ligament. An ankylosed tooth, or one with a narrow periodontal ligament, has no space for the insertion of instruments. This condition is in dramatic contrast to a developing third molar with follicular space. (See Figure 2.9c.)

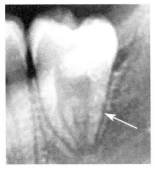

Figure 2.9a Wide periodontal ligament.

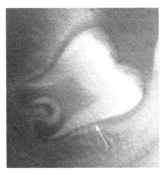

Figure 2.9b Third molar follicle.

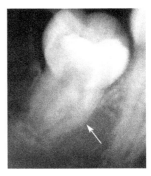

Figure 2.9c Narrow periodontal ligament.

Bone Density and Elasticity

Density is defined as the degree of compactness of a substance. Elasticity is the ability of an object or material to resume its normal shape after being stretched or compressed. Both of these characteristics play a profound role in the removal of impacted third molars. Compact bone is very dense, strong, and stiff bone. Cancellous bone is softer and weaker than compact bone, but is more elastic. Radiographs can provide indications of bone density. (See Figures 2.10a and 2.10b.) Age-related weakening of bony elasticity makes extractions more difficult and mandibular fracture more likely.[11]

Position Relative to the Inferior Alveolar Canal

Superimposition

Proper interpretation of a quality panoramic radiograph can significantly reduce inferior alveolar nerve injuries. Many, if not most, general dentists assume that any third molar with roots extending to or beyond the radiographic inferior alveolar canal is at high risk of paresthesia. However, most third molar roots that appear to be near or beyond the canal are actually buccal or lingual to the nerve. This condition, known as superimposition, is indicated on a panoramic radiograph by continuous white

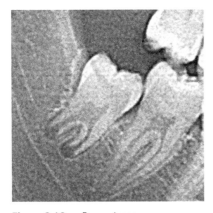

Figure 2.10a Dense bone.

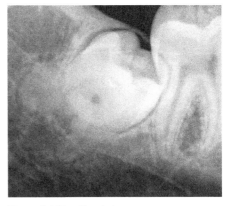

Figure 2.10b Elastic bone.

lines created by the inferior alveolar canal bone. Superimposed tooth roots are buccal or lingual to the canal and IAN injury is unlikely. (See Figure 2.11.)

Grooving

The inferior alveolar canal develops before third molar roots. Grooving of the third molar root is caused by a third molar root developing in close proximity to the IAN. Thinning of the developing root is caused by contact with the inferior alveolar canal. This condition, known as grooving, is indicated on radiographs by a radiolucent band where the canal crosses over the third molar root. The canal's radiographic white lines are not visible on the radiograph. Grooving increases the possibility of IAN paresthesia. (See Figure 2.12.)

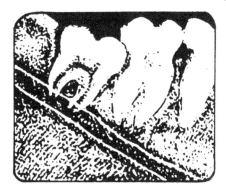

Figure 2.11 Continuous white lines indicate superimposition. (Drawing by Michael Brooks).

Notching

Notching, like grooving, is caused by the developing tooth contacting the inferior alveolar canal. In this case, the tooth root develops directly above the canal. This is seen on a radiograph as a radiolucent third molar apex and loss of the top white line as the canal passes over the root. The dark apex may also indicate an open apex for young patients whose third molar roots are still developing. Notching increases the possibility of IAN paresthesia. (See Figure 2.13.)

Perforation

In rare cases, the developing third molar root completely encircles the inferior alveolar canal. This is seen on the radiograph as a narrowing, radiolucent band where the canal crosses over the third molar root. The top and bottom white lines are not visible on the radiograph. (See Figure 2.14.)

Other radiographic signs of intimate root contact with the inferior alveolar canal include canal deflection, root deflection, bifid roots, and root narrowing. A detailed discussion of these radiographic signs, including several studies, can be found in Chapter 3, "Complications."

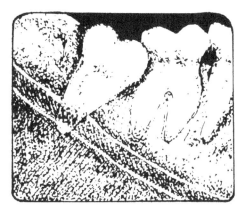
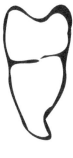

Figure 2.12 A radiolucent band and loss of white lines indicates grooving. (Drawing by Michael Brooks).

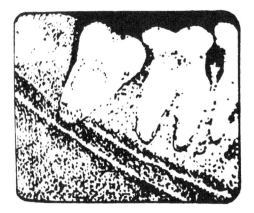 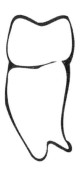

Figure 2.13 A radiolucent apex and loss of the top white line indicates notching. (Drawing by Michael Brooks).

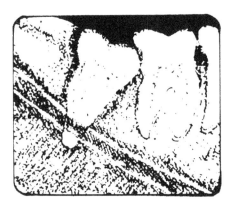 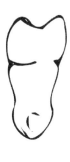 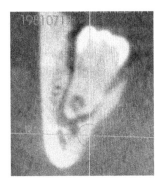

Figure 2.14 Narrowing of the IAN canal and loss of white lines indicates perforation. (Drawing by Michael Brooks).

Early Third Molar Removal

Age may be the most significant factor in case selection. Several studies have shown that teenage patients have fewer surgical and postoperative complications.

A prospective study evaluated the surgical and postsurgical complications of 9,574 patients who had 16,127 third molars removed. It was concluded that removal of mandibular third molar teeth during the teenage years resulted in decreased operative and postoperative morbidity.

The study showed that increased numbers of complications (alveolar osteitis, infection, and dysesthesias) occur in the removal of impacted third molars of older patients. This study suggests that, when indicated, third molars should be removed during the teenage years, thereby decreasing the incidence of postoperative morbidity.[12]

Another study estimated the frequency of complications after mandibular third molar surgery as related to patient age. 4,004 subjects had a total of 8,748 mandibular third molars removed. The mean age was 39.8 =/−13.6 years, with 245 subjects (6.1%) age 25 and younger. The study concluded that increased age (>25 years) appears to be associated with a higher complication rate for mandibular third molar extractions.[13]

The American Association of Oral and Maxillofacial Surgeons published a white paper in 2007. They reviewed 205 publications related to various aspects of third molars. The effects of age on various parameters relating to third molars are so important that the AAMOS findings related to age are included verbatim in this chapter by permission of AAMOS (Reproduced by permission of the American Association of Oral and Maxillofacial Surgeons).

The Effects of Age on Various Parameters Relating to Third Molars[14]

Symptomatology and Age: "A study of 1,151 patients from 13–69 years of age with third molars showed that of those who had symptoms, pain was the most common symptom (35.3%), followed by swelling (21.7%), discomfort from food impaction (3.6%), and purulent discharge (3%). The frequency of each increased generally with age. Slade also noted that 37% of patients presenting with wisdom tooth problems reported pain and swelling as the indication for seeking treatment. Additionally, this study noted that Health Related Quality of Life indicators were reported more frequently as patients got older."

Periodontal Pathology and Age: "Asymptomatic periodontal defects associated with third molars are more common in patients older than 25 (33%) than those under 25 (17%). Inflammatory mediators and periodontal pathogens were similarly correlated with the periodontal defects. On two year follow-up, 24% of the periodontal defects deteriorated by a further 2 mm. A study of 6,793 persons 52 to 74-years old, found that they had 1.5 times the odds of having a periodontal defect > 5 mm on the adjacent second molar if the third molar was visible. A comparison of 5,831 patients aged 25 to 34 with a group aged 18 to 24 showed a 30% greater chance of having a periodontal defect on the adjacent second molar when a third molar was present in the older age group versus the younger age group. In a study of 342 subjects with a mean age of 73 who had at least one third molar present at three year follow-up, attachment losses ≥ 2 mm were detected on the third molars in 45% of subjects."

Caries and Age: "Caries prevalence in 342 subjects with a mean age of 73 years with at least one third molar present showed an increased caries prevalence in the third molars over time. Another study of 22 to 32-year-old cohorts followed for three years, showed that caries prevalence in the third molars also increased with time in this younger age group. Caries were also correlated in third molars with the experience in non-third molars. Shugars suggested that a 40% risk of caries in erupted third molars exists before the end of the third decade. Patients over 25 years of age have a greater caries experience compared to patients under 25 years of age."

Postoperative Risks and Age: "A critical review showed lower postoperative morbidity in a younger age group of patients. All risks associated with third molar removal increased from age under 25, to 25 to 35, to over 35. Health Related Quality of Life indicators similarly deteriorated for recovery as correlated with age following third molar removal. A study of 4,004 patients showed a 1.5 times likelihood of a complication if the patient having third molars removed at over 25 years of age with generalized increasing risks with age through age 65. Similarly, in a study of 583 patients, age was correlated with risk. Other studies also show that postoperative risks increase with increasing age. A consensus of the literature supports the concept that postoperative risks from third molar removal increase with age.

The risk of postoperative fracture following third molar removal may be age related, and one study shows a mean age at fracture to be 45 years. The incidence of oroantral perforation from upper third molar removal may also increase with age past 21 years. Postoperative periodontal defects occur twice as commonly (51%) in patients over 26 years of age, than those under 25 following third molar removal. Significant postoperative defects in 215 second molars were three times more common when removing impacted third molars over the age of 25 than under the age of 25. Pockets on the second molars in 215 cases were studied two years postoperatively. Persistence of postoperative periodontal defects compared to preoperative defects in these patients were shown to be age related. Postoperative periodontal defects after third molar extraction are two to three times more common over the age of 25, and persistence of defects was age related."

Germectomy or Lateral Trepanation: "For the purposes of this document, germectomy is defined as the removal of a tooth that has one third or less of root formation and also has a radiographically discernible periodontal ligament. A study of 15 cases of early third molar removal in patients aged between 13 and 16 years of age showed no postoperative periodontal pocketing and no pocketing developing one year later. In a study of 500 lower wisdom teeth removed in patients aged 9 to 16, there were no cases of alveolar osteitis, nerve involvement, or second molar damage, and a 2% infection rate was reported. In a study where germectomy was performed in 300 teeth in patients aged 12 to 19 years of age, there were no lingual nerve injuries. A study of 149 germectomies reported a 2% infection rate and no case of nerve involvement. A study of 86 patients aged 8 to 17 years, having 172 germectomies, reported that three patients developed infection, and no cases of nerve involvement or alveolitis were encountered. It does appear that early third molar removal may be associated with a lower incidence of morbidity and also less economic hardship from time off work for the patient."

The Presence of Third Molars and Age: "One study noted that between 1997 and 2002 there was an increase in patients over the age of 40 requiring third molar removal. The number increased from 10.5% to 17.3% of all third molars removed. This was felt to be due to changing demographics in the geographical areas served by this study. It does appear that the eruption of third molars in older patients is more frequent than may be thought, but in some cases, rather than the third molar erupting, it may become visible due to periodontal bone loss and subsequent gingival recession and exposure. Many of these late erupting teeth have pathology, including caries and periodontal disease. A study of 14 to 45 year olds found that 51% of 312 late erupting third molars had periodontal disease in a 2.2 year follow-up." (Nance 2006)

Conclusions

Periodontal defects, as assessed by pocket depths, deteriorate with increasing age in the presence of retained third molars. Caries in erupted third molars increases in prevalence with increasing age. The incidence of postoperative morbidity following third molar removal is higher in patients > 25 years.

The selection of patients is critical to success when removing impacted third molars. Most teenage patients can be treated with confidence when proper surgical protocol is followed. Caution is advised when treating patients of ages 20–25 with fully developed roots. Patients over age 25 will have more surgical and postoperative complications. All factors, including age, must be considered before selecting patients for impacted third molar surgery. Referral to a maxillofacial surgeon may be prudent for many patients older than age 25.

Prophylactic Removal of Third Molars

Studies presented in this chapter support the early removal of third molars. Surgical and postoperative complications are minimized when third molars are removed in the teenage years. Early removal of third molars includes germectomy, the removal of a third molar with 1/3 or less root development. Germectomy is always prophylactic because the teeth are full bony impactions with little or no root development. Advocates of early removal of third molars believe that it is better to intercept and prevent potential issues than to simply react and deal with the consequences. Opponents believe that there is no reliable evidence to support the prophylactic removal of disease-free impacted third molars.

The prophylactic removal of asymptomatic third molars is controversial. Many studies have been published supporting both sides of the argument. The UK-based National Health Service and the "National Institute for Clinical Excellence" (NICE) published guidelines in 2000 citing a "lack of evidence for prophylactic removal of asymptomatic wisdom teeth."[15] The American Association of Maxillofacial Surgeons 2007 white paper concluded that early third molar removal may be associated with lower incidence of morbidity and less economic hardship from time off work for the patient.[14] Each side has been criticized for bias.

Cochrane reviews are systematic reviews of research in healthcare and health policy. Cochrane reviews authors apply methods which reduce the impact of bias. Cochrane is an independent network of researchers, professionals, patients, caregivers, and people interested in health. Their work is recognized as representing an international gold standard for high-quality, trusted information.

A 2016 Cochrane review looked at prophylactic removal of asymptomatic impacted third molars versus retention in adolescents and adults. The electronic database search found insufficient evidence to support or refute routine prophylactic removal of asymptomatic disease-free impacted wisdom teeth. Cochrane concluded that patient values and clinical expertise should guide shared decision making with patients who have asymptomatic disease-free impacted wisdom teeth.[16]

Patients are responsible for the final decision regarding the prophylactic removal of asymptomatic disease-free third molars. The dentist and oral surgeon are responsible for informing the patient of the risks and benefits of retention or prophylactic removal.

The author is an advocate for the early prophylactic removal of third molars in most cases. This advocacy stems from evidence-based research and 40 years of experience removing impacted third molars. The author has removed more than 35,000 third molars with no permanent paresthesia or significant complication. Most of these patients were younger than age 25.

In rare cases, when patients have sufficient room for eruption and hygiene, retention is recommended. These patients should be closely monitored since the ability to erupt does not guarantee third molar health. Sufficient access is required to ensure adequate oral hygiene.

Summary

Case selection is vitally important to ensure a good surgical result for patients. Dentists who are just beginning to remove impacted third molars are advised to carefully select appropriate patients. Special attention should be given to the age of patients undergoing third molar removal. Research shows that teenagers will experience fewer complications and will have better recovery. Third molar removal when roots are undeveloped is more predictable than when roots are fully formed and may be near vital structures. Difficult cases should be referred to an oral and maxillofacial surgeon. More challenging cases can be done as skills improve.

References

1 ASA physical status classification system. American Society of Anesthesiologists. Retrieved 2007 Jul 09.

2 de Jong KJ, Oosting J, Abraham-Inpijn L. Medical risk classification of dental patients in The Netherlands. *J Public Health Dent*. 1993 Fall; 53(4):219–22.

3 Smeets EC, de Jong KJ, Abraham-Inpijn L. Detecting the medically compromised patient in dentistry by means of the medical risk-related history. A survey of 29,424 dental patients in The Netherlands. *Prev Med*. 1998 Jul-Aug;27(4):530–5.

4 Kaminishi RM, Kaminishi KS. New considerations in the treatment of compromised third molars. *J Calif Dent Assoc*. 2004 Oct;32(10):823–5.

5 US Department of Health and Human Services, National High Blood Pressure Educational Program. NIH publication No. 3-5233, 2003 Dec.

6 Awino BO, et al. Awareness status and associated risk factors for hypertension among adult patients attending Yala sub-county hospital, Siaya County, Kenya. *Public Health Res*. 2016;6(4):99–105.

7 Lloyd-Jones D, Adams RJ, Brown TM, et al. Heart disease and stroke statistics–2010 update: a report from the American Heart Association. Circulation. 2010 Feb 23;121(7):e46–215.

8 Lenzenweger MF, Lane MC, Loranger AW, Kessler RC. DSM-IV personality disorders in the National Comorbidity Survey Replication. *Biol Psychiatry*. 2007 Sep 15;62(6):553–64.

9 Peterson LJ. *Principles of management of impacted teeth in contemporary oral and maxillofacial surgery*, 2nd edition. Missouri: Mosby Publications, 1993, 237–9.

10 Nanci A. *Ten Cate's Oral Histology: development, structure, and function*. St. Louis: Elsevier, 2013, 220.

11 Cankaya AB, et al. Iatrogenic mandibular fracture associated with third molar removal. *Int J Med Sci*. 2011;8(7):547–53.

12 Osborn TP, et al. A prospective study of complications related to mandibular third molar surgery. *J Oral Maxlllofac Surg*. 1965;43:767–9.

13 Chuang SK, Perrott DH, Susarla SM, Dodson TB. Age as a risk factor for third molar surgery complications., *J Oral Maxillofac Surg*. 2007 Sep;65(9):1685–92. doi: 10.1016/j.joms.2007.04.019. PMID: 17719384.

14 American Association of Maxillofacial Surgeons, White Paper on Third Molar Data. The effects of age on various parameters relating to third molars. 2007.

15 Eng R. Third molar surgery: a review of current controversies in prophylactic removal of wisdom teeth. *Oral Health*. 2009 Jun 1.

16 Ghaeminia H, Perry J, Nienhuijs ME, Toedtling V, Tummers M, Hoppenreijs TJ, Van der Sanden WJ, Mettes TG. Surgical removal versus retention for the management of asymptomatic impacted wisdom teeth. *Cochrane Database Syst Rev*. 2020 May 4;5(8):CD003879.

3

Complications

The expected postoperative healing following the removal of impacted third molars includes pain, swelling, bleeding, and muscle trismus. Complications are uncommon and usually avoidable when proper case selection and surgical protocol are followed. The purpose of this chapter is to discuss potential third molar surgical complications.

A retrospective cohort study by Bui, Seldin, and Dodson found the overall complication rate for the removal of mandibular third molars is 4.6%. The risks of complications are lower for maxillary third molars than for mandibular third molars. Risk increases with age, position of third molars relative to the inferior alveolar nerve, and positive medical histories.[1]

Possible complications include paresthesia, alveolar osteitis, infections, bleeding and hemorrhage, jaw fracture, osteomyelitis, damage to proximal teeth, buccal fat pad exposure, oral-antral communication, displacement of third molars, aspiration, periodontal defects, and temporomandibular joint injury. The four most common postoperative complications of third molar extraction reported in the literature are paresthesia, alveolar osteitis, infection, and bleeding/hemorrhage.[2]

Paresthesia

Impacted mandibular third molar teeth are in close proximity to the lingual, inferior alveolar, mylohyoid, and buccal nerves.[3] (See Figure 3.1.)

The possibility of paresthesia is a common reason for referral to maxillofacial surgeons by general dentists. The referral is usually made after viewing a panoramic radiograph showing a third molar root near the inferior alveolar canal. However, as we learned in Chapter 2, mandibular third molar roots, seen on radiographs are often superimposed on the inferior alveolar canal. Radiographic superimposition indicates that the roots are either buccal or lingual to the canal.

Many studies have been published on the risk of nerve injury following the removal of third molars. A sample of those studies is presented here.

Buccal and Mylohyoid Nerve Studies

Although the buccal and mylohyoid nerves may be near third molars, they are rarely affected. Alves studied 10 cadaver heads and found that the buccal nerve crossed the anterior border of the

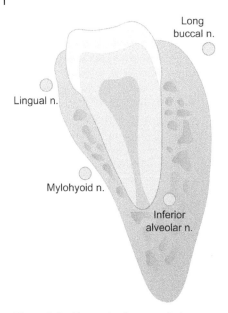

Figure 3.1   Nerves in close proximity to mandibular third molars.

ramus at a point far above the retromolar region. He concluded that the risk of injury to the buccal nerve was low.[4]

Merril and MacGregor postulated that the buccal nerve was frequently cut during incisions for the removal of mandibular third molars, but sensory changes go unnoticed.[5,6] The author found one study of mylohyoid injuries. The study, published in 1992 by Carmichael, found injury to the mylohyoid nerve to be as high as 1.5%, probably due to lingual retraction.[7]

There is very little evidence in the literature demonstrating injury to the buccal and mylohyoid nerves following the removal of impacted mandibular third molars. The nerves most commonly affected are the inferior alveolar and lingual nerves. Many studies have been conducted in an attempt to estimate the possibility of inferior alveolar and lingual nerve injury when removing third molars. A summary of selected studies follows.

IAN Studies

Sarikov et al. conducted a systematic review of 14 studies.[8] He found IAN injury ranged from 0.35% to 8.4%. 96% of IAN injuries recovered within 8 weeks. Sarikov concluded that injury of the IAN can be predicted by various panoramic radiological signs. These signs included narrowing of the canal, dark root apexes, bifid root apexes, narrowing of the root, loss of the canal "white line" on radiographs, deflection of the canal, and deflection of the root. When panoramic radiological signs indicate intimate contact between a third molar and the inferior alveolar canal, 3D imaging with computed tomography is recommended. (See Figure 3.2.)

The IAN is normally buccal or lingual to third molar roots. The radiographic roots are superimposed on the canal. Superimposition is indicated on radiographs when there is no interruption of radiographic white lines (See Figure 3.3.) Superimposition indicates no intimate contact with the IAN canal and a low probability of nerve injury; especially, for patients under age 25.

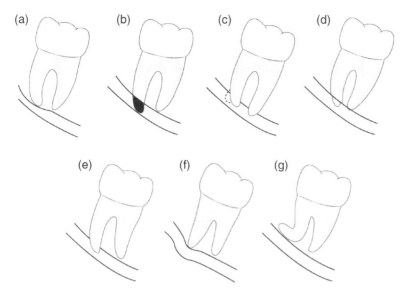

Figure 3.2 Radiographic indications of root contact with IAN. a) Narrowing of canal, b) Dark root apex, c) Bifid root apex, d) Narrowing of root, e) Loss of "white line," f) Deflection of canal, g) Deflection of root.

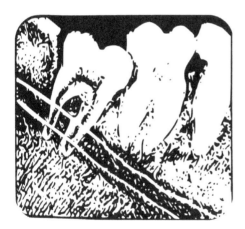

Figure 3.3 Superimposition of roots on IAN canal, the white line is continuous and uninterrupted. (Drawing by Michael Brooks).

Levine et al. studied the IAN canal position within the body of the mandible.[9] The average IAN canal position was 4.9 mm from the lateral surface of the mandible and 17.4 mm apical from the alveolar crest. (See Figure 3.4.) It's important to note that the IAN may be lingual to third molar roots for two reasons:

1. Third molars are often in a linguoversion position with roots near or touching buccal bone.
2. The 17.4 mm and 4.9 mm distances are average distances. Variable positions are very common.

The buccal lingual IAN canal position was associated with age and race. Older patients and white patients had less distance between the buccal aspect of the canal and the buccal surface of the

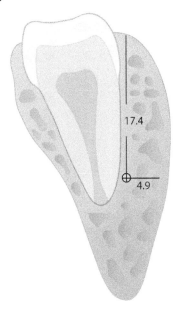

Figure 3.4 One study's average IAN position – IAN position is highly variable.

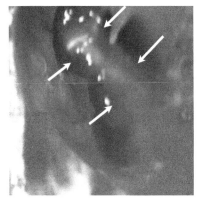

Figure 3.5 IAN "true relationship" following third molar removal.

mandible. To minimize the risk of IAN injury, these variables should be considered when removing impacted mandibular third molars.

In a landmark inferior alveolar nerve article by Howe and Poyton in 1960 it was determined after evaluating 1,355 impacted mandibular molars clinically and radiographically at the time of extraction that a true relationship existed in only 7.5% of cases.[10] A "true relationship" was defined as the visualization of the neurovascular bundle at the time of tooth removal. (See Figure 3.5.)

An "apparent" relationship was defined by radiographs when the roots of the teeth appeared to be in an intimate relationship to the IAN. This occurred in 61.7% of the mandibular third molars.

Of the 70 cases that developed nerve impairment over 50% of them had a true relationship with the IAN. This was a 13 times greater incidence than that occurring with those teeth exhibiting an apparent one. The study found that permanent nerve injury is much more likely to occur if there is a true relationship between the IAN and the roots of mandibular third molar teeth. Permanent IAN injury occurred in less than 1% of all patients even though an apparent relationship existed in 61.7% of all radiographs. The results of this study seem to indicate that the radiographic appearance of third molar roots close to the IAN is not a good predictor of IAN injury.

The Howe-Poyton study further noted an increased incidence in older patients, teeth that were deeply impacted, those which exhibited grooving, notching, or perforation, as well as a threefold and fourfold increase in mesial and horizontally impacted teeth with linguoversion.

Valmeseda-Castellon et al. had similar findings in their study published in 2000.[11] They found the location of impacted teeth and a person's age contributed to the incidence of injury. There is a greater incidence of injury as persons become older. Wisdom teeth that are lingually oriented, or those where there is direct contact with the inferior alveolar canal, are more likely to be associated with injury. Injury seems to adversely affect females more often than males. Surgical duration is another variable that may contribute to nerve injury.

Lingual Nerve Studies

The incidence of lingual nerve injury following mandibular third molar removal may depend on the surgical technique. Raising and retracting a lingual mucoperiosteal flap with a Howarth periosteal elevator may result in more frequent injury, but this is usually temporary.[12]

In a study of 1117 consecutive surgical procedures to remove a lower third molar by a variety of operators, the incidence of lingual nerve damage was determined to be 11%. Lingual flaps were implicated in this study. The percentage of nerve injury varied among surgeons. Permanent damage arose when distal bone was removed with a bur.[13]

Karakas et al. studied the relationship of the lingual nerve to third molars using radiographic images. A literature search found the incidence of lingual nerve damage during mandibular region surgery varies between 0.6% and 2.0%.[14]

Combined Inferior Alveolar and Lingual Nerve Studies

The incidence of reported postoperative dysesthesia of the inferior alveolar and the lingual nerve varies widely in published studies. Bui and colleagues studied 583 patients who had third molars removed by an experienced oral surgeon between 1996 and 2001. The majority of subjects in this study were healthy college students. Approximately 75% of the mandibular third molars were in close proximity to the inferior alveolar canal. IAN and lingual nerve injuries were 0.4% and 0% respectively.[1]

In a study published in 2000 by Gargallo-Albiol et al., the incidence of temporary disturbances affecting the IAN or the LN was found to range from 0.278% to 13%.[15]

Zuniga et al. found the incidence of injury to the IAN to range from 0.4% to 25%. Lingual nerve injury ranged from 0.04% to .6%. In this study the incidence of permanent nerve damage varied between 0.5% and 2%.[16]

Cheung et al. carried out a study in which lower third molar extractions were performed by surgeons with different levels of skill. In this study, 0.35% developed IAN deficit and 0.69% developed LN deficit. Inexperienced surgeons caused more lingual nerve injuries. He concluded that distoangular impactions increased the risk of LN deficit significantly. Deep impactions increased the risk of IAN sensory deficit.[17]

Anwar Bataineh found lingual nerve paresthesia in 2.6% of patients. There was a highly significant increase in the incidence associated with the use of lingual flaps. The incidence of inferior alveolar nerve paresthesia was 3.9%. The study concluded that the elevation of lingual flaps and the experience of the operator are significant factors contributing to lingual and inferior alveolar nerve paresthesia, respectively.[18]

Meshram et al. studied 147 patients, three of which reported paresthesia.[3] Two patients reported lingual nerve paresthesia (1.36%) and one patient reported inferior alveolar nerve paresthesia (.68%). One of the lingual paresthesia third molars was a horizontal Gregory-Pell class IIC; a deep impaction partially in the ramus. The second lingual paresthesia was a distoangular Gregory-Pell class IIA, a minimally deep impaction partially in the ramus. The third molar with inferior alveolar nerve paresthesia was a Gregory-Pell class IIA mesioangular impaction (a minimally deep impaction partially in the ramus). In this study, incidence of injury to IAN and LN was comparatively very low, and all cases were of transient paresthesia. Various factors are responsible for the injury to the inferior alveolar nerve and lingual nerve in third molar surgery. Most studies have shown that when paresthesia follows extraction, it is likely to be temporary and to resolve within the first 6 months.

The combined findings of IAN and LN studies are presented in Table 3.1.

These studies found IAN and LN paresthesia ranging from .28% to 13.0% and 0% to 13% respectively. Some studies found a very low percentage of nerve injury while others found a relatively high incidence. These inconsistencies are probably due to variability in study design. For example, studies completed with an expert surgeon, patients under age 25, or without lingual flap found a lower incidence of nerve injury than studies with less experienced surgeons,

Table 3.1 Combined findings of IAN and LN studies.

Study	IAN %	Risk Factors	LN %	Risk Factors
Bui	.4		0	
Gargallo-Albiol	.278–13		.278–13	
Zuniga	.4–25 .5–2 permanent		.04–.6 .5–2 permanent	
Cheung	.35	Depth	.69	Distoangular position Lingual flap Lingual version Vertical sectioning Surgeon experience
Bataineh	3.9	Surgeon experience	2.6	Lingual flap
Meshram	.68		1.36	
Sarikov	.35–8.4	Root deflection Root narrowing Root dark/bifid Canal narrowing Canal diversion		
Blackburn			11.0	Lingual flap Surgeon experience Distal bone removed
P. Karakas			.6–2.0	
Howe J.	< 1.0	Age Depth Grooving Notching Perforation Linguoversion		

Box 3.1 Factors affecting nerve injury.

Surgical skill	Roots near IAN on X-ray
Age of patient	Distal bone removal
Fully developed roots	Sectioning multiple times
Depth of impaction	Mesial/horizontal impactions
Surgical access	Long procedure time
Lingoversion	

---

older patients, or with lingual flap technique. Factors affecting the risk of nerve damage are shown in Box 3.1.

IAN and LN paresthesia can profoundly affect patients both psychologically and physically. Speech and chewing can be impaired following nerve injury and lead to litigation. Therefore, it's important to thoroughly document nerve injury in the patient's chart.

An evaluation of the extent of IAN injury should be conducted as soon as an altered sensation is reported by the patient. The patient's subjective assessment of change is important. The surgeon should ask the patient if there is any change in sensation since the teeth were removed. Any change in sensation is a positive sign and indicates probable recovery of normal sensation. The patient should be informed that recovery is likely, but full recovery may take a few weeks or more than a year. Mapping is used to record the areas affected when no change is reported.

Mapping is accomplished using sophisticated tests such as Semmes Weinstein monofilament or simple cotton fibers. A sharp instrument such as an explorer is commonly used for mapping. Light touch fibers or explorer are applied to the affected area and slowly moved until the patient reports sensation. The point where the patient is aware of stimulus is recorded in the patient's chart. Photographic documentation can be recorded by marking points of sensation on the patient's face with an erasable marker. Recovery of normal sensation is often slow and patients may not be aware of progress. Mapping provides a semi-objective measurement of change. If no change is found after three months, the patient should be referred to an appropriate maxillofacial surgeon for evaluation and possible nerve repair. The extent of nerve injury can be documented using systems for classification. Seddon described three classes of peripheral nerve injury.[19]

Class I – Neurapraxia

Class I nerve injury is the mildest form of nerve injury and full recovery is expected. There is a temporary loss of conduction without loss of axonal continuity. In neurapraxia, there is a physiologic block of nerve conduction in the affected axons. Full recovery takes days to weeks. The axon portion distal to the injury does not degenerate.

Class II – Axonotmesis

Class II injuries involve the loss of the relative continuity of the axon and it's covering of myelin, but preservation of the connective tissue framework of the nerve (the encapsulating tissue, the epineurium and perineurium, are preserved). Axon degeneration occurs distal to the site of injury. Axonal regeneration occurs and recovery is possible without surgical treatment.

Class III – Neurotmesis

Class III injuries are the most severe and involve total severance or disruption of the entire nerve. Degeneration occurs distal to the site of injury and sensory problems are severe. There is no nerve conduction distal to the site of injury. Surgical intervention is necessary. Seddon's peripheral nerve classification was expanded by Sunderland to include five degrees of nerve injury.[20]

For purposes of documentation following nerve injury, it is recommended to document Class I–II (recovering) injury vs Class III (requires surgical repair).

Paresthesia Conclusions

The risk of paresthesia following the removal of third molars is low when certain guidelines are followed. Risk factors to avoid have been identified in many studies. Most of these factors can be eliminated with proper case selection and good surgical protocol.

The author has removed more than 35,000 third molars with no permanent nerve injury. Thirteen patients had temporary paresthesia. Most of the treated patients were teenagers with 1/3 to 2/3 root development. Early third molar removal appears to be a vital key to avoid paresthesia. In the opinion of the author, virtually all risk factors can be eliminated when third molars are removed prior to full root development using a buccal approach. Dentists with

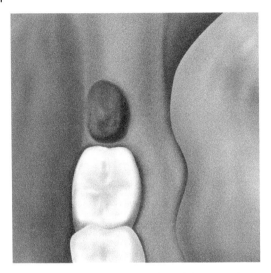

Figure 3.6 Post extraction socket with exposed bone. (Reproduced by permission of Joanna Culley BA(hons) IMI, MMAA, RMIP)

minimal experience should begin by removing soft tissue impactions for teenagers with partial root development.

Radiographic superimposition of third molar roots on the inferior alveolar canal is not an absolute contraindication for treatment. A cone beam CT scan can confirm the relationship between third molar and inferior alveolar canal when intimate contact is suspected. Patients should be referred to a maxillofacial surgeon when significant risk of paresthesia exists.

Alveolar Osteitis

Alveolar osteitis (AO) is the most common complication following the removal of third molars. (See Figure 3.6.) Alveolar osteitis is commonly called "dry socket." It's also known as alveolitis, localized osteitis, fibrinolytic alveolitis, septic socket, necrotic socket, alveolalgia, and fibrinolytic alveolitis. Symptoms typically develop 4 to 5 days following surgery. AO is self-limiting and will resolve spontaneously if left untreated. Treatment is palliative.

AO is characterized by extreme pain radiating to the ear or temporal region, empty socket, and foul odor/taste. The condition is significant because it causes extreme pain and usually requires several visits to treat. The exact cause of AO is not well known and many concepts about the condition are controversial.

Possible Causes

Antonia Kolokythas et al. completed a comprehensive review of AO literature and published an article in 2010. Sixteen possible causes were found in their literature search.[21]

1. **Surgical Trauma and Difficulty of Surgery**
   Most authors agree that surgical trauma and difficulty of surgery play a significant role in the development of AO. This could be due to more liberation of direct tissue activators secondary to bone marrow inflammation following the more difficult, hence, more traumatic extractions. Surgical extractions, in comparison to nonsurgical extractions, result in a tenfold increased incidence of AO. Lilly et al. found that surgical extractions involving reflection of a flap and removal of bone are more likely to cause AO.

2. **Lack of Operator Experience**
   Many studies claim that operator's experience is a risk factor for the development of AO. Larsen concluded that surgeon's inexperience could be related to a bigger trauma during the extraction, especially surgical extraction of mandibular third molars. Alexander and Oginni et al. both reported a higher incidence of AO following extractions performed by the less experienced operators. Therefore, the skill and experience of the operator should be taken into consideration.

3. **Mandibular Third Molars**

   It has been shown that alveolar osteitis is more common following the extraction of mandibular third molars. Some authors believe that increased bone density, decreased vascularity, and a reduced capacity of producing granulation tissue are responsible for the site specificity. However, there is no evidence suggesting a link between AO and insufficient blood supply. The area specificity is probably due to the large percentage of surgically extracted mandibular third molars and may reflect the effect of surgical trauma rather than the anatomical site.

4. **Systemic Disease**

   Some researchers have suggested that systemic disease could be associated with alveolar osteitis. One article proposed immunocompromised or diabetic patients being prone to development of alveolar osteitis due to altered healing. But no scientific evidence exists to prove a relationship between systemic diseases and AO.

5. **Oral Contraceptives**

   Oral contraceptive is the only medication associated with developing AO. Oral contraceptives became popular in 1960s and studies conducted after 1970s (as opposed to studies prior to 1960s) show a significant higher incidence of AO in females. Sweet and Butler found that this increase in the use of oral contraceptives positively correlates with the incidence of AO. Estrogen has been proposed to play a significant role in the fibrinolytic process. It is believed to indirectly activate the fibrinolytic system (increasing factors II, VII, VIII, X, and plasminogen) and therefore increase lysis of the blood clot. Catellani et al. further concluded that the probability of developing AO increases with increased estrogen dose in the oral contraceptives. One author even suggested that in order to reduce the risk of AO, hormonal cycles should be considered when scheduling elective exodontia.

6. **Patient's Gender**

   Many authors claim that female gender, regardless of oral contraceptive use, is a predisposition for development of AO. MacGregor reported a 50% greater incidence of AO in women than that in men in a series of 4000 extractions, while Colby reported no difference in the incidence of AO associated with gender.

7. **Smoking**

   Multiple studies demonstrated a link between smoking and AO. A dose dependent relationship between smoking and the occurrence of alveolar osteitis has been reported. Among a total of 4000 surgically removed mandibular third molars, patients who smoked a half-pack of cigarettes a day had a four- to five-fold increase in AO (12% versus 2.6%) when compared to nonsmokers. The incidence of AO increased to more than 20% among patients who smoked a pack per day and 40% among patients who smoked on the day of surgery. Whether a systemic mechanism or a direct local affect (heat or suction) at the extraction site is responsible for this increase is unclear. Blum speculated that this phenomenon could be due to the introduction of foreign substance that could act as a contaminant in the surgical site.

8. **Physical Dislodgement of the Clot**

   Although a very commonly discussed theory, no evidence exists in the literature verifying that physical dislodgement of the blood clot caused by manipulation or negative pressure created via sucking on a straw would be a major contributor to AO.

9. Bacterial Infection

Most studies support the claim that bacterial infections are a major risk for the development of AO. It has been shown that the frequency of AO increases in patients with poor OH, preexisting local infection such as periocoronitis and advanced periodontal disease. Attempts have been made to isolate specific causative organisms. A possible association of *Actinomyces viscosus* and *Streptococcus mutans* in AO was studied by Rozantis et al., where they demonstrated delayed healing of extraction sites after inoculation of these microorganisms in animal models. Nitzan et al. observed high plasmin-like fibrinolytic activities from cultures of *Treponema denticola*, a microorganism present in periodontal disease. Catenalli studied bacterial pyrogens in vivo and postulated that they are indirect activators of fibrinolysis.

10. Excessive Irrigation or Curettage of Alveolus

It has been postulated that excessive repeated irrigation of alveolus might interfere with clot formation and that violent curettage might injure the alveolar bone. However, the literature lacks evidence to confirm these allegations in the development of AO.

11. Age of the Patient

Little agreement can be found as to whether age is associated with peak incidence of AO. The literature supports the general axiom that the older the patient, the greater the risk. Blondeau et al. concluded that surgical removal of impacted mandibular third molars should be carried out well before age of 24 years, especially for female patients since older patients are at greater risk of postoperative complications in general.

12. Single Extraction versus Multiple Extractions

Limited evidence exists indicating higher prevalence of AO after single extractions versus multiple extractions. In one study, AO prevalence was 7.3% following single extractions and 3.4% following multiple extractions. This difference could possibly be due to less pain tolerance in patients with single extractions compared to patients with multiple extractions whose teeth have deteriorated to such an extent that multiple extractions are needed. Moreover, multiple extractions involving periodontally diseased teeth may be less traumatic.

13. Local Anesthetic with Vasoconstrictor

It has been suggested that the use of local anesthesia with vasoconstrictors increases the incidence of AO. Lehner found that AO frequency increases with infiltration anesthesia because the temporary ischemia leads to poor blood supply. However, the studies that followed indicated that ischemia lasts for one to two hours and is followed by reactive hyperemia, which makes it irrelevant in the disintegration of the blood clot. One study reported no significant difference in AO prevalence following extraction of teeth requiring infiltration anesthesia versus regional block anesthesia with vasoconstrictor. It is currently accepted that local ischemia due to vasoconstrictor in local anesthesia has no role in the development of AO.

14. Saliva

A few authors have argued that saliva is a risk factor in the development of AO. However, no firm scientific evidence exists to support this claim. Birn found no evidence that saliva plays a role in AO.

15. Bone/Root Fragments Remaining in the Wound

Some authors have suggested that bone/root fragments and debris remnants could lead to disturbed healing and contribute to development of AO. Simpson, in his study, showed that small bone/root fragments are commonly present after extractions and these fragments do not necessarily cause complications as they are often externalized by the oral epithelium.

16. Flap Design/Use of Sutures

Some previous literature claims that flap design and the use of sutures affect the development of AO. However, more recent studies found little evidence to prove such relationship. In the absence of any significant evidence, it is reasonable to assume that these are not major contributing factors.

A summary of possible causes of AO, and their significance, is presented in Table 3.2.

Mandibular third molars have the highest incidence of AO following removal. One possible explanation for this is the difficulty and trauma related to the removal of impacted third molars. It has been reported that the incidence of AO is ten times greater following surgical extractions (impacted third molar) than non-surgical extractions.[22]

Table 3.2 Contributing factors in the development of alveolar osteitis.

Proposed AO Causes	Major	Minor or Unproven
Smoking	X	
Age	X	
Surgeon experience	X	
Surgical difficulty/trauma	X	
Oral contraceptives	X	
Female gender	X	
Bacterial infection		X
Systemic disease		X
Physical dislodgement of clot		X
Excessive irrigation/curettage		X
Multiple vs single extraction		X
Anesthetic and vasoconstrictor		X
Saliva		X
Bone/root fragments in wound		X
Flap design and sutures		X
Systemic disease		X
Compromised blood supply		X
Radiotherapy		X
Mandibular third molars		X

Prevention

Many studies have been conducted regarding the prevention of AO. The results of these studies are often controversial and inconsistent. However, the literature provides some insight into the clinical management of AO.

A study done in 2017 assessed the effect of platelet-rich fibrin (PRF) on postoperative pain, analgesic consumption, soft tissue healing, and socket complications following the extraction of mandibular third molars. Fifty impacted third molars were surgically removed from 47 patients. PRF was placed in the extraction sockets, while the sockets remained empty in the control group. One of the variables studied was socket complications encountered during the first postoperative week. The study found that PRF could reduce alveolar osteitis following removal of impacted mandibular third molars. For more on PRF please see Chapter 13.[23]

There is evidence to support the use of a 0.12% and .2% chlorhexidine rinse prior to the extraction and one week post extraction to prevent the occurrence of dry socket following tooth extraction. (See Figure 3.7.)

In a prospective, randomized, double-blind placebo-controlled study, this regime was associated with a 50% reduction in alveolar osteitis compared to the control group.[23] In 2007 Shepard analyzed five randomized controlled trials studying prevention of alveolar osteitis (dry socket). The analysis indicated that 0.12% chlorhexidine gluconate rinsing preoperatively and 7 days postoperatively reduces the frequency of alveolar osteitis following surgical removal of lower third molars.[24]

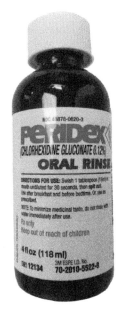

Figure 3.7 Chlorhexidine rinse.

Renton et al. reviewed the literature and concluded that prophylactic antibiotics reduce the risk of AO following the removal of mandibular third molars.[25] However, the potential for anaphylaxis, the development of resistant bacterial strains, and other adverse side effects preclude the routine use of antibiotics. Patients with a known risk for AO such as smokers and females on birth control may benefit from prophylactic antibiotics. Among the many antibiotics studied, topical tetracycline has shown promising results. The reported method of delivery includes powder, aqueous suspension, gauze drain, and Gelfoam sponges (preferred). However, side-effects including foreign body reactions have been reported with the application of topical tetracycline.[26] There is also evidence that antifibrinolytic agents applied to the socket after the extraction may reduce the risk of dry socket.[27]

Treatment

Treatment of AO is focused on medications to alleviate pain since the condition is self-limiting. Systemic pain medications may be used, but are rarely sufficient without topical dressings. The most common treatment involves irrigation of the extraction site with chlorhexidine and the placement of medicated dressings in the socket. (See Figures 3.8a, 3.8b, and Box 3.2.) Many different medicaments and carrier systems are commercially available.

The author has had success using iodoform gauze strips coated with dry socket paste. Dry socket paste containing guaiacol balsam Peru, eugenol, and 1.6% chlorobutanol (Sultan Healthcare, York, PA) can be placed with iodoform gauze. Another common medicament used in the management of AO is Alvogyl containing butamben (anesthetic), eugenol (analgesic), and iodoform (antimicrobial). All AO topical dressings contain varying amounts of similar ingredients designed to control pain and bacterial growth.

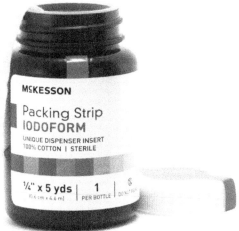
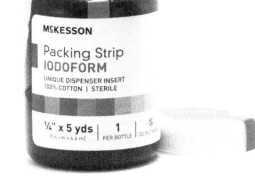

Figure 3.8a   Iodoform gauze.

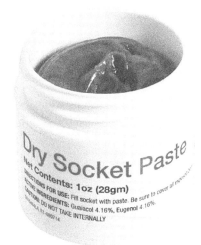

Figure 3.8b   Dry socket paste.

Box 3.2 A typical regimen used in the treatment of AO.

1) Remove debris from socket and irrigate with chlorhexidine
2) Fill socket with dressing – dry socket paste/eugenol with iodoform gauze
3) Replacement of gauze and/or dressing at 48 hours is recommended

---

Alveolar Osteitis Conclusions

Alveolar osteitis is the most common complication following the removal of impacted third molars. AO etiology is unknown, but many contributing factors have been suggested. Major factors include smoking, surgeon's experience, difficult extractions, female gender, oral contraceptives, bacterial infection, and age. Pre-operative and postoperative rinsing with chlorhexidene has been shown to reduce AO by 50%. Treatment of AO is focused on the management of pain. Irrigation and dressing of the socket will usually eliminate pain within minutes.

Infection

Most third molar infections occur in the mandible. The most common third molar infection is pericoronitis. A study in the United Kingdom assessed 25,001 third molars. Pericoronitis was the most common indication for extraction and was found in 39.5% of all extractions.[28] Third molar related infections can present prior to surgery or at varying times following surgery. Postoperative infections have been reported to range from 0.8% to 4.2%.[29] Peterson stated that almost all postoperative infections are minor. About 50% of all postoperative infections are localized subperiosteal abscess infections related to the surgical flap. The remaining 50% of postoperative infections rarely require hospitalization.[2] Although hospitalization is rare, serious life-threatening space infections are possible.

Pericoronitis

Pericoronitis is a localized infection around the crown of an erupting or partially impacted third molar. The infection can be chronic or acute. Chronic pericoronitis may exist with mild or no symptoms. Acute pericoronitis is always associated with pain and red, inflamed tissue surrounding the third molar. Both chronic and acute pericoronitis can present with exudate. Patients present with some or all of the symptoms and signs in Table 3.3.

The fundamental cause of pericoronitis is bacteria. Oral hygiene access is limited near third molars. Food accumulates under tissue overlying a partially erupted third molar and provides a substrate for bacterial growth. (See Figure 3.9.)

Localized infection can be exacerbated by a super erupted opposing maxillary third molar irritating the area when chewing. Chronic pericoronitis can lead to bone loss. (See Figure 3.10.) The arrow indicates the position of the tissue covering the distal half of tooth #17.

Acute pericoronitis usually develops endogenous microorganisms during a period of poor oral hygiene or when the immune system is challenged by diabetes, HIV, stress, or infections such as colds, flu, and respiratory tract infections. Meurman et al. collected data from 14,500 male patients to determine if a relationship exists between pericoronitis and respiratory tract infection.[30] The incidence of respiratory tract infection was significantly higher during the two weeks before acute pericoronitis was diagnosed compared with that in controls. The study concluded that a cause and effect relationship exists between pericoronitis and respiratory tract infections. Respiratory tract infection may precipitate acute pericoronitis. Conversely, third molar removal for pericoronitis can trigger respiratory tract infection.[31]

Pericoronitis is usually found in patients under the age of 25 with erupting mandibular third molars. Patients with good oral hygiene and adequate room for eruption can be treated conservatively by irrigation, ultrasonic debridement, and removal of overlying tissue (operculum). Antibiotics are usually not indicated for healthy patients when swelling is absent.

Removal of infected third molars is recommended when patients have poor oral hygiene and inadequate room for eruption. Antibiotics are indicated prior to surgical intervention when patients exhibit significant swelling, lymphadenopathy, fever, or complain of malaise. These signs and symptoms may indicate cellulitis.

It is important to distinguish between cellulitis and abscess. Cellulitis is a diffuse infection spreading through soft tissue fascia. It is a firm, non-fluctuant, painful, indurated area (i.e., warm, red, swollen) of the face or neck. Antibiotics are indicated for cellulitis to reduce infection prior to

Table 3.3 Symptoms and signs consistent with a diagnosis of pericoronitis.

Symptoms	Signs
Increasing pain for 3–4 days	Red, inflamed tissue overlying third molar
Bad odor or taste	Tissue tender to palpation with or without pus
Difficulty chewing, opening, closing, swallowing	Limited opening
Sore throat	Lymph nodes tender to palpation
General feeling of ill health	Increased temperature
Recent or concurrent respiratory infection	Partial eruption – usually vertical or distoangular
Pain when biting teeth together	Super erupted opposing maxillary third molar

surgery. Streptococcus is the most common cause of early-stage cellulitis. As the infection progresses, a mixed streptococcal/anaerobic infection develops. As the local tissue condition changes to a more hypoxic state, the predominant bacteria become anaerobic species, such as bacteroides or fusobacterium.[30] An abscess is a localized area of pus that is fluctuant. Incision and drainage is indicated for an abscess.

Surgical Site Infections (SSI)

Third molar SSIs are usually caused by normal endogenous microorganisms. Risk factors for SSIs are similar to those for pericoronitis and include the following:

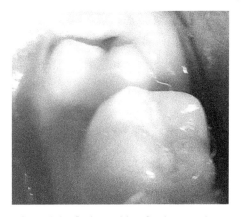

Figure 3.9   Pericoronitis – food accumulates under tissue overlying the third molar.

- Medical problems or diseases
- Elderly adults
- Overweight adults
- Smoking
- Cancer
- Weakened immune system
- Diabetes
- Surgery that lasts more than two hours
- Pre-existing infection

The most common third molar SSI is a localized subperiosteal abscess-type infection that occurs 2–4 weeks after a previously uneventful postoperative course. These are usually attributed to debris or food

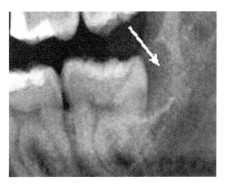

Figure 3.10   Pericoronitis bone loss.

left under the mucoperiosteal flap. The definitive treatment is surgical debridement and drainage.[32] Odontogenic infections are typically polymicrobial; however, anaerobes generally outnumber aerobes by at least four -fold. Metronidazole is a bactericidal agent that is highly active against most anaerobes. In serious infections, metronidazole works well with penicillin or amoxicillin.[30]

The author has treated six patients for subperiosteal infection over 40 years of clinical practice. Each of these patients called the office about one month after an uneventful recovery and complained of unilateral swelling of the lower face. Clinically, intraoral healing appeared normal with no evidence of surgery. However, significant unilateral swelling was noted. One patient was treated by reopening the mucoperiosteal flap, debridement, and irrigation followed by antibiotics. The remaining patients were successfully treated with a combination of amoxicillin 500 mg and metronidazole 500 mg, tid, for 10 days. Although most postoperative infections are minor, a small percentage can be life threatening. Early intervention and treatment is very important to prevent the spread of infection to deep spaces.

Space Infections

Surgical site infections (SSI) that progress to deep space infections are rare. However, general knowledge of space infections is needed for accurate diagnosis. SSI infections can spread via blood vessels, lymphatics, or fascial planes. Head and neck spaces can be classified as primary, secondary, and deep neck. Infections involving spaces of the head and neck may give varying signs and symptoms depending upon the space(s) involved. Trismus (difficulty opening the mouth) is a sign that the muscles of mastication are involved. Dysphagia (difficulty swallowing) and dyspnea (difficulty breathing) may be signs that the airway is being compressed by the swelling.[33]

Pus and cellulitis from odontogenic infections move by hydrostatic pressure and will follow the path of least resistance. Most untreated intraoral infections drain through sinus tracts and fistulas. Some infections spread to fascial spaces. Fascial spaces are either pathological spaces (clefts), potential spaces between facial layers, or normal spaces (compartments) containing salivary glands, lymph nodes, blood vessels, nerves, or muscles. The fascia surrounding these spaces is strong and inflexible. Fascial planes offer anatomic highways for infection to spread from superficial to deep planes.[34] Clefts between fascia and structures of head and neck are created by the pathological spread of infection and do not exist in health. Spaces and planes are defined by bone, fascia, and muscle attachments, especially the mylohyoid, buccinator, masseter, medial pterygoid, superior constrictor, and orbicularis oris muscles.

Spaces of the head and neck can be divided into primary and secondary spaces. Primary spaces are located close to the source of infection. Odontogenic infections spread directly from teeth and bone to primary spaces. The primary spaces are the canine, buccal, vestibular, submandibular, sublingual, and submental. Secondary spaces are located away from the source of infection. Secondary space infections are created by the spread of infection from primary spaces. The secondary spaces are the masticator, pterygomandibular, masseteric, temporal (superficial and deep), infratemporal, prevertebral, lateral pharyngeal, and retropharyngeal. Space infections are summarized in Table 3.4.

Canine space infections originate almost exclusively from a maxillary canine tooth. Canine space infections result in significant swelling lateral to the nose and upper lip that may cause eye closure and drooling. Infections of the canine space can spread hematogenously into the cavernous sinus. This can result in a life-threatening condition known as cavernous sinus thrombosis. Although rare, death from cavernous sinus thrombosis has been reported as a result of third molar removal.[35]

Infections spread to the buccal or vestibular spaces directly from maxillary or mandibular molars. The initial spread of infection is dependent on the attachment of the buccinator muscle in relation to the roots of the molars. Infections from roots inside the buccinator attachment will spread to the vestibular space. Infections outside the buccinator attachment will spread to the buccal space. Infections can spread from these spaces to the pterygomandibular space, submasseteric space, deep and superficial temporal spaces, and the lateral pharyngeal space.

Submandibular space infections originate directly from mandibular third molars and second molars that have roots located below the mylohyoid line. Sublingual space infections originate from mandibular first molars, second molars, and premolars that have roots located above the mylohyoid line. Submental space infections arise from mandibular incisors. The three spaces collectively (submandibular, sublingual, and submental) are sometimes called the submandibular spaces. The submandibular spaces communicate with each other, the masticator space, and deep neck secondary spaces.

Ludwig's angina is a rapidly spreading cellulitis of the submandibular, sublingual, and submental spaces.

It produces pronounce swelling, displacement of the tongue, and induration of the submandibular region. Signs and symptoms include trismus, drooling, and dyspnea. Upper airway

Table 3.4   Summary of space infection: origin, signs, and symptoms.

Primary Spaces	Origin of Infection	Signs/Symptoms
Canine	Maxillary canine or first premolar	Painful swelling lateral to the nose including loss of the nasolabial fold
Buccal	Maxillary or mandibular 1st, 2nd, and 3rd molars, roots outside buccinator muscle attachment	Painful swelling is ovoid, below the zygomatic arch and above the inferior border of the mandible
Vestibular	Maxillary or mandibular 1st, 2nd, and 3rd molars, roots inside buccinator muscle attachment	Painful swelling of vestibular tissue overlying affected tooth
Submandibular	Mandibular 2nd/3rd molars below mylohyoid muscle	Painful swelling under posterior mandible
Sublingual	Mandibular 1st/2nd molars, premolars above mylohyoid	Painful, firm swelling of the anterior floor of the mouth, difficult to swallow
Submental	Mandibular incisors	Painful swelling under anterior mandible or chin
Secondary Spaces		
Masticator		
● Pterygomandibular	Mandibular 2nd/3rd molars	Significant trismus, pain with no visible swelling
● Masseteric	Mandibular 3rd molars via buccal space	Mild to moderate trismus, swelling of the posterior inferior portion of the mandible
● Temporal (deep and superficial)	Mandibular 3rd molars	Rare infection, trismus, pain, swelling, possible deviation of mandible on opening
Deep Neck Spaces		
Parapharyngeal (lateral pharyngeal)	Mandibular 3rd molars	Trismus, fever, sore throat, dysphagia, swollen neck, mediastinitis, airway obstruction
Retropharyngeal	Mandibular 3rd molars	Trismus, fever, sore throat, dysphagia, swollen neck, mediastinitis, airway obstruction
Prevertebral ("Danger space")	Mandibular 3rd molars	Trismus, fever, sore throat, dysphagia, swollen neck, mediastinitis, airway obstruction

obstruction can lead to death. The usual cause of Ludwig's angina is an odontogenic infection from a mandibular second or third molar.[30]

   There are three secondary spaces of the mandible located near the ramus and angle of the mandible; the masseteric, pterygomandibular, and temporalis secondary spaces. These three spaces are collectively known as the masticator space, because they are bounded by the muscles of mastication: masseter, medial pterygoid, and temporalis. Infections can spread to the masticator spaces from infected mandibular third molars via the buccal, submandibular, and sublingual primary spaces. The masticator spaces communicate with one another and the parapharyngeal, sublingual and submandibular spaces.[36]

The pterygomandibular space may become infected when infection spreads from the submandibular and sublingual spaces or from an infected mandibular third molar (pericoronitis). A key diagnostic feature of pterygomandibular space infections is significant trismus and pain with no swelling.

Masseteric space infections are relatively rare. Infection may spread to this space from the buccal space or an infected mandibular third molar (pericoronitis).[37] Infection is characterized by significant trismus and swelling at the inferior posterior portion of the mandible.

The third compartment found in the masticator space is the temporal space. The temporal space is posterior and superior to the masseteric and pterygomandibular spaces. It is divided into a superficial and deep portion by the temporalis muscle. The inferior portion of the deep temporal space is the infratemporal space. Infection can spread to the temporal space from adjacent masticator spaces or the infratemporal space. The signs and symptoms of temporal space infections are swelling and trismus.

Deep Neck Spaces

Authors disagree regarding the number and nomenclature of deep neck spaces. As many as eleven deep neck spaces have been reported in the literature.[38] Three major deep neck spaces are discussed in this section; the parapharyngeal, retropharyngeal, and vertebral. These three deep neck spaces communicate with each other allowing infection to spread. The parapharyngeal and vertebral spaces are sometimes known as the lateral pharyngeal and "danger space" respectively. Spread within the danger space tends to occur rapidly (hence the name danger space) because of the loose areolar tissue that occupies this region.

1. **Paraphayngeal (lateral pharyngeal)**
    The parapharyngeal space connects with the masticator, retropharyngeal, submandibular spaces and all other deep neck spaces. Parapharyngeal space infections may occlude the airway due to swelling of the posterior pharyngeal wall. Medial displacement of the lateral pharyngeal wall and tonsil is a hallmark of parapharyngeal space infections. Trismus, drooling, and difficulty swallowing are commonly observed.
2. **Retropharyngeal**
    Retropharyngeal infections can extend down to the superior mediastinum resulting in infections of the pleural cavity and heart. If the infection perforates the posterior border of the retropharyngeal space, it enters the danger space.[38]
3. **Vertebral (danger space)**
    The vertebral space lies posterior to the retropharyngeal space. The danger space is so called because its loose areolar tissue offers a potential route for the downward spread of infection. The vertebral space extends down the entire mediastinum to the level of the diaphragm. Infections of the danger space most commonly occur when an abscess in the retropharyngeal space ruptures through the retropharyngeal fascia
    Odontogenic origin is the most common etiology of deep space infections in adults.[39] Dentists removing third molars should be aware that deep space infections can be caused by oral surgical procedures. Once diagnosed, deep space and resistant infections should be referred to a maxillofacial surgeon for treatment.

Bleeding and Hemorrhage

Bleeding is normal following the removal of impacted third molars. Oozing of blood may continue throughout the first day following surgery. It is vital that patients are informed that bleeding should be expected. Patients may have experienced the removal of a single permanent or deciduous tooth and will be unprepared for the amount of blood seen after the removal of four impacted third molars.

Normal postoperative bleeding can be controlled by biting on gauze. The author prefers 4×4, filled, gauze. Filled gauze is very absorbent and easier to manage than multiple, unfilled, 2 × 2 gauze. The patient is instructed to avoid talking or moving their mouth for ½ hour. Patients should remain inactive for the entire day following the procedure. This protocol is sufficient to control bleeding for most patients.

Significant bleeding is most often found in the mandible (80%). Risk factors include older patients, distoangular impactions, and deep impactions near the inferior alveolar neurovascular canal.[40]

Persistent intraoperative bleeding can often be controlled with a vasoconstrictor such as epinephrine 1:50,000. Other alternatives include additional sutures, Gelfoam, Surgicel, ActCel, BloodSTOP, Collaplug, tranexamic acid, and bone wax. (See Box 3.3.) Arterial, nutrient canal, bleeding may require electrocautery or ligation.

Bleeding beyond that expected for the procedure or bleeding that persists beyond the normal time for clot formation, 6–12 hours, is considered excessive.[41] The author has experienced one case of excessive bleeding.

A 16-year-old male patient, presented for the removal of impacted third molars. His medical and dental history was unremarkable, and the procedure was uneventful. The patient's father was given postoperative instructions, verbal and written, and the patient was dismissed. The patient's father called that evening and stated that his son was still bleeding. Postoperative instructions were reviewed and biting on a tea bag was recommended. The patient's father was instructed to call again if there was no improvement within two hours. A phone call was received at 11:30 pm stating that there was no improvement and that the patient was still bleeding. The patient was instructed to drink lots of water, continue to bite on gauze or tea bag, and come to the office in the morning at 8 am.

The patient was still bleeding when he arrived at the office. 4 × 4 gauze was changed every ½ hour for two hours with no improvement. The patient was referred to the local emergency room and was later admitted to the hospital to conduct bleeding tests. The patient was diagnosed with Von Willebrand's disease, an abnormality of the coagulation cascade. Von Willebrand's factor (vWF) promotes normal platelet function and stabilizes factor VIII.

Box 3.3 Options to control postoperative bleeding.

Positive pressure on gauze – 4 × 4 filled	BloodSTOP (LifeScience PLUS)
Vasoconstrictor – epinephrine 1:50,000	ActCel (Coreva Health Sciences)
Tranexamic acid (Pharmacia & Upjohn Company)	Additional sutures
Gelfoam (Pfizer)	CollaPlug (Integra LifeSciences)
Surgicel (Johnson & Johnson)	Bone Wax (Ethicon)

It was later discovered that the patient had a history of hematoma in his thigh sustained while playing soccer. This was unreported on his medical history and preoperative assessment. This case clearly illustrates the importance of a thorough preoperative medical history and assessment to rule out bleeding disorders. Patients with coagulation disorders may be identified by questions regarding personal or familial history of bleeding and bruising. Preoperative assessment of intrinsic coagulation disorders and the use of anticoagulant and antiplatelet medications (Coumadin, Plavix) is essential.[41]

Tranexamic acid is an antifibrinolytic chemical that has been used successfully to treat and prevent excessive bleeding following surgical procedures for patients on anticoagulants. Ramstrom G. et al. studied the hemostatic effect of tranexamic acid solution (4.8%) used as a mouthwash compared with a placebo solution in 93 patients on continuous, unchanged, oral anticoagulant treatment undergoing oral surgery. In the placebo group, 10 patients developed bleeding requiring treatment, while none of the patients treated with tranexamic acid solution had bleeding. It was concluded that most patients on oral anticoagulants can undergo oral surgery within the therapeutic range (INR 2.10–4.00) without reducing the dosage of anticoagulants, provided that local antifibrinolytic treatment with tranexamic acid solution is instituted.[42] Patients should be instructed to rinse with 10 ml four times daily for 7 days following surgery.[43]

The level of the impaction and its proximity to the neurovascular bundle are the most important risk factors for excessive bleeding. Excessive bleeding has been reported to occur more frequently with the extraction of mandibular third molars versus their maxillary counterparts. Excessive bleeding is more frequent, regardless of the type of impaction, for inexperienced surgeons. It is also more commonly reported in older patients, probably because of vascular fragility and less effective coagulation mechanisms. It is reported that men are as much as 60% more likely to suffer from excessive bleeding than women.[44] Hypovolemia and deep space hematomas are potentially fatal. Symptoms of hypovolemic hemorrhagic shock may appear with blood loss near 1000 ml. (See Box 3.4.)

Most studies have found that blood loss from dental surgeries is less than 200 ml. To put this in perspective, a blood donation of one pint is 473 ml.[45] Dentists removing impacted third molars should keep in mind that long procedures increase the possibility of excessive blood loss. Uncontrollable intraoral hemorrhage can quickly lead to airway compromise either because of an expanding hematoma in the neck or from blood pooling in the airway.[46]

The possibility of uncontrolled hemorrhage when treating healthy patients is remote. However, dentists removing impacted third molars should be aware that excessive bleeding can be fatal.

Box 3.4 Signs and symptoms of hypovolemia and hemorrhagic shock.

Anxiety or agitation	Cool, clammy skin
Confusion	Decreased or no urine output
General weakness	Unconsciousness
Pale skin color (pallor)	Sweating, moist skin
Rapid breathing	

Jaw Fracture

One of the most severe complications from third molar surgery is mandibular fracture. (See Figure 3.11.)

Mandibular fractures resulting from third molar removal are extremely rare. Fractures can occur at the time of surgery or can be delayed. Libersa et al. found mandibular fractures during or after the removal of third molar to occur in 0.00049% of cases.[47] This complication is very serious; especially, when it includes nerve injury. Uncontrolled force and deep impactions are the common denominators in surgically related jaw fractures. Experienced surgeons can usually remove deeply impacted third molars without fracture (see Figures 3.12a and 3.12b), but even the most experienced oral surgeons may experience this complication when removing deep impactions. Mandibular fracture is a serious complication that can lead to litigation. It should be included in consent forms and discussed with all patients presenting with deep third molar impactions near the inferior border of the mandible

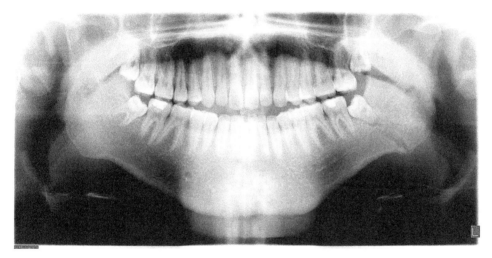

Figure 3.11   Fracture of the mandible near a third molar. (Reproduced with permission of Dr. Joanne Toy).

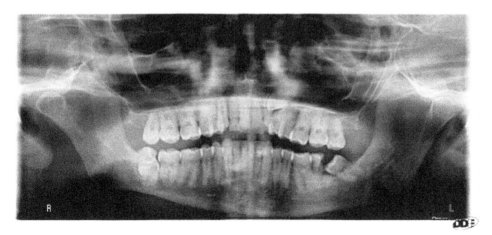

Figure 3.12a   #32 Deep Impaction Pre-operative Panograph (Dr. Vincent Vella).

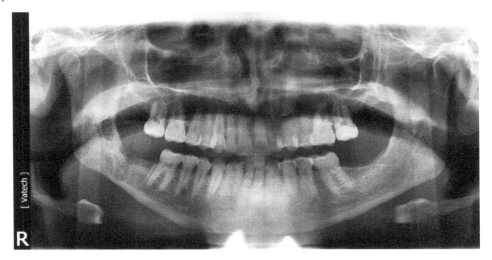

Figure 3.12b   #32 Deep Impaction Postoperative Panograph (Dr. Vincent Vella).

Some studies have shown older patients as a risk factor for jaw fracture.[48] Mandibular fractures may be stabilized with open reduction, closed reduction, or soft diet depending on the severity of the fracture and the direction of muscle pull.

The most common jaw fracture is maxillary tuberosity fracture. The distal aspect of maxillary third molars has no support and the bone is soft osteoporotic bone. The maxillary sinus may compromise bone support. These factors combined with excessive force make this area subject to fracture. A fractured tuberosity with good blood supply, attached to periosteum, can be repositioned and monitored. Tuberosity fracture may be accompanied by mucosal tears. In this case, sutures are required to hold the fractured bone in place.

Several options are available to prevent tuberosity fracture. (See Box 3.5.) Preoperative radiographs can be used to evaluate bone thickness, periodontal ligament space, and proximity of the maxillary sinus. A periosteal elevator can be placed distal to the third molar to separate it from the periodontal ligament and tuberosity. A "pinch grip," grasping the alveolus between thumb and index finger of the non-dominant hand, can be used while applying force. This technique provides tactile feedback to the operator regarding tooth movement and bone fracture. Finally, the tooth can be sectioned and bone judiciously removed to prevent fracture.

Tuberosity fracture may be unavoidable when removing impacted maxillary third molars. However, in most cases, the mobile fractured bone has a good blood supply and remains attached to periosteum.

Box 3.5 Options to prevent tuberosity fracture.

Preoperative radiographs	Periosteal elevator dissection
Pinch grip feedback	Tooth sectioning
Bone removal	Elevator and forceps combination

Osteomyelitis

Osteomyelitis (OM) is an inflammatory condition of bone marrow which may be classified as acute, chronic, or suppurative. Acute osteomyelitis is OM which has been present for less than one month. The infection is considered chronic when the condition lasts for more than a month.[49] Osteomyelitis infections with the formation of pus may be classified as suppurative.

Suppurative osteomyelitis of the jaws is uncommon in developed countries. There have been many reported cases occurring in Africa which are coexistent with acute necrotizing ulcerative gingivitis. In the pre-antibiotic era, acute OM of the jaws was more extensive. Massive, diffuse infections commonly involved the whole side of the mandible. Before antibiotics, OM was a common complication of odontogenic infections frequently ending in death.

Osteomyelitis of the jaws occurs in the bones of the maxilla and mandible, but is most common in the mandible due to limited blood supply from the inferior alveolar neurovascular bundle. In Europe and the United States, most cases follow dental infections, extractions, or mandibular fractures in patients with compromised host defenses. OM may occur as a result of contamination of a surgical site.

Diabetes, alcoholism, autoimmune disease, radiation therapy, chemotherapy, steroid use, osteoporosis, myeloproliferative diseases, and malnutrition can contribute to the development of osteomyelitis. Patients with acute osteomyelitis often present with dull deep pain, fever, malaise, swelling, fistula, and trismus. In contrast, patients with chronic osteomyelitis often present without the symptoms of acute osteomyelitis. Radiographs may have a "moth eaten" pattern of bony sequestrum.[50]

Damage to Proximal Teeth

Clinical and radiographic evaluation of the patient is essential to avoid damage to proximal teeth when removing third molars. Patients should be informed prior to the procedure of possible injury to adjacent teeth. Second molar teeth with large restorations, crowns, or caries may be damaged during the removal of third molars. Complications include displacement of restorations and crowns, fractured restorations and crowns, and fracture of adjacent teeth weakened by large restorations or caries. Judicious bone removal and meticulous technique that avoids contact with these structures is necessary. Fortunately, displaced or fractured restorations and crowns can normally be replaced.

Second molar teeth with short, conical roots may be accidentally loosened or avulsed. Teeth that are minimally loosened can often be repositioned and left alone. Seriously loosened or avulsed teeth should be repositioned and stabilized for 10–14 days with the least rigid fixation possible to prevent ankylosis and root resorption.[51]

Buccal Fat Pad Exposure

The buccal fat pad is located bilaterally between the buccinator muscle, masseter muscle, and ramus. It consists of a central body and four extensions; buccal, pterygoid, superficial, and deep temporal. The buccal extension is located superficially within the cheek. Deep incisions distal to the maxillary tuberosity may cause herniation of the buccal extension. (See Figure 3.13.)

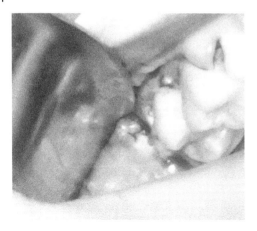

Figure 3.13 Buccal fat pad herniation.

The unexpected herniation of the buccal fat pad is alarming. However, this complication is typically innocuous. The buccal fat pad is frequently used to repair small and medium intraoral defects such as oral antral fistulas. Exposed buccal fat is epithelialized within 2–3 weeks.[52]

The exposed fat should be repositioned if possible; although this is analogous to replacing toothpaste back into the toothpaste tube. The procedure should be terminated and the patient rescheduled for removal of the third molar. Experienced surgeons may be able to work around the defect and complete the procedure.

Oral-antral Communication

The most common molar involved with a sinus communication is the first molar, followed by the second molar, and third molar. Removal of maxillary third molars with roots near the maxillary sinus can result in an oral-antral communication (OAC) between the oral cavity and sinus. An opening into the maxillary sinus that does not epithelialize may become a permanent communication known as an oral antral fistula.

OAC is diagnosed by applying the Valsalva maneuver used by divers to "clear their ears." The patient's nose is pinched shut and the patient is instructed to gently blow their nose. Air passing through an opening can be heard and seen as bubbles of blood and fluid are expressed. This is diagnostic for an OAC. Alternatively, a mouth mirror can be held next to the extraction site and the Valsalva maneuver performed. The mirror will fog if an opening is present.

Openings less than 2 mm in diameter usually close spontaneously.[53] Furthermore, impacted maxillary third molar flaps usually cover the extraction site and aid in closure. Intermediate size openings of 2 mm–7 mm may be treated with a collagen plug or Gelfoam placed in the socket. A figure 8 suture will help to stabilize socket dressings and the clot. Openings greater than 7 mm and OAFs generally require surgical repair by an oral and maxillofacial surgeon.

Postoperative instructions, written and oral, should be given to any patient diagnosed with OAC. The condition should be explained to patients in terms that are easy to understand. Patients are instructed to not blow their nose and to sneeze with their mouths open for two weeks. Medications include antibiotics, nasal decongestants, and an antihistamine. Amoxicillin is recommended for five days to prevent the development of sinusitis. Sudafed, a nasal decongestant, is used for two weeks to open nasal passages. An antihistamine nasal spray such as Neo-Synephrine or Afrin should be used for two weeks to reduce sneezing and nose blowing. (See Box 3.6.)

Box 3.6 Oral-antral communication postoperative instructions.

Amoxicillin 500 mg, tid, until gone, #30
Decongestant (Sudafed) – for two weeks
Antihistamine (Neo-Synephrine or Afrin)
Do not blow your nose for two weeks
Sneeze with your mouth open for two weeks
Avoid smoking and straws

Careful assessment of radiographs can reduce the incidence of OAC when removing impacted third molars. Older patients with dense bone, divergent roots, and sinus pneumatization around roots are red flags. These teeth should be carefully luxated and sectioned to minimize the chance of an OAC.

Displacement of Third Molars

Third molars and their roots can be displaced into adjacent spaces during removal. This is a rare complication associated with deep impactions, poor access and visualization, and uncontrolled forces. Maxillary third molars or their roots can be displaced into the maxillary sinus or infratemporal fossa. (See Figures 3.14a and 3.14b.) These teeth may develop palatal to the maxillary arch. This position predisposes displacement into the maxillary sinus and infratemporal fossa. Access and visualization of third molars in this position are often restricted. Poor access, excessive apical force, and poor technique increase the chance of displacement into the maxillary sinus or infratemporal fossa.

The maxillary sinus is an empty space that contains no vital structures. Pogrel has recommended suction through the oral antral communication to retrieve teeth displaced into the maxillary sinus. A second attempt can be made with irrigation of the sinus followed by suction. Pogrel states that a third attempt should not be made and the patient should be placed on antibiotics and nasal decongestant.[53] The patient should be referred to a maxillofacial surgeon and the tooth retrieved via Caldwell-Luc approach. The oral antral communication can be closed at the same appointment.

The infratemporal fossa is located posterior to the maxilla, lateral to the lateral pterygoid plate, and inferior to the lateral pterygoid muscle. Displacement of maxillary third molars into the infratemporal fossa is a rarely reported complication with an unknown incidence. This complication is far more serious than displacement into the maxillary sinus. In contrast to the maxillary sinus, the infratemporal

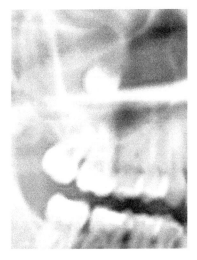

Figure 3.14a   Third molar in maxillary sinus. (Jaime Aparecido Cury et al. 2005 / The Scientific Electronic Library Online (SciELO) / CC BY-NC 4.0.)

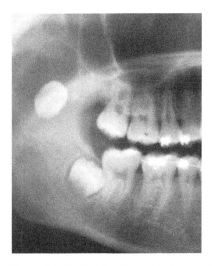

Figure 3.14b   Third molar in infratemporal fossa.

fossa is not an empty space. It contains vital structures including the pterygoid plexus, maxillary artery, and mandibular nerve (the third branch of the trigeminal nerve). Treatment of this complication is varied and depends on the position of the tooth, experience of the surgeon, and patient's wishes. Treatment choices include intraoral retrieval, extraoral retrieval, and observation. A CT scan is ordered to localize the exact position of the tooth. Retrieval is hindered by poor visualization and bleeding from the pterygoid plexus.[54] Treatment may be immediate to avoid infection or delayed to allow for development of fibrous tissue around the tooth. Fibrous tissue may aid in retrieval of the tooth.

The author has had one accidental displacement of a right maxillary third molar into the infratemporal fossa. The patient, a 15-year-old male with orthodontic arch wires in place, was referred by his orthodontist for removal of developing (germectomy) third molars. In addition to the orthodontic appliances, the patient had a small mouth with limited opening. The right maxillary third molar was located and visualized near the apex of the second molar and in a palatal position. Gentle force was applied to the tooth when it suddenly disappeared.

A panographic X-ray was taken which confirmed location of the third molar in the infratemporal fossa. The patient was referred to the UCSF Department of Maxillofacial Surgery where he was seen several times over a period of three months. Cone beam CT images were taken and the patient was monitored for symptoms of pain or signs of infection. Fortunately, the patient was asymptomatic and no treatment was recommended.

Factors increasing the potential for maxillary third molar displacement include deep (high) impactions with the crown near the apex of the second molar, palatal location, distoangular position, and poor access and visualization. (See Box 3.7.)

A good axiom to remember when removing maxillary impacted third molars is, "A difficult maxillary third molar will be much more difficult than a difficult mandibular third molar."

Mandibular third molars or their roots can also be displaced into the submandibular, sublingual, and pterygomandibular spaces. (See Figure 3.15.) In addition, the roots of mandibular third molars can be displaced into the inferior alveolar canal. The lingual cortical plate is often thin or nonexistent in the posterior region of the mandible. Fenestrations of the lingual plate can be found on the lingual aspect of some impacted mandibular third molars.[55]

The submandibular space is located below the mylohyoid muscle. The sublingual space is located above the mylohyoid muscle. Displacement of third molar teeth or roots into these spaces can sometimes be prevented by finger pressure on the lingual periosteum, inferior to the third molar roots, prior to applying force. The procedure should be stopped whenever access and direct vision is impaired. Open flaps and bone removal may be needed to improve visibility when third molar teeth are moving in an apical, lingual direction. Care should be taken to not displace the tooth or roots deeper into the space. Displaced roots can sometimes be manipulated back into their socket with lingual finger pressure. Patients should be referred to a maxillofacial surgeon when these attempts are unsuccessful.

Box 3.7 Factors affecting the potential for maxillary third molar displacement.

Deep impactions
Palatal location
Distoangular position
Poor access
Poor visualization

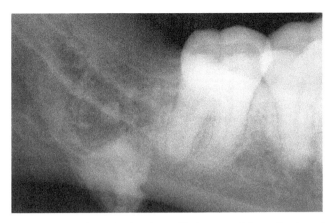

Figure 3.15 Third molar in submandibular space. (Kivanc Kamburoglu et al.2010 / Springer Nature / CC BY 2.0.).

A root tip or tooth fragment can be left in the tooth socket if it is less than 5 mm in length and is not infected or palpable. Baseline X-rays should be taken and the patient should be informed of the possibility of infection. The patient should be monitored for deep space infection or foreign body reaction.[56]

Aspiration and Ingestion

Aspiration and ingestion is probably under reported. Approximately 92.5% of objects are ingested while 7.5% are aspirated.[57] This complication can be prevented by using 4 × 4 gauze throat packs. A pharyngeal curtain can be created by gently rolling this gauze into a soft ball and placing it above the patient's oropharyngeal airway. A Weider retractor can be used to hold the gauze in position and create a clean surgical field. (See Figure 3.16.)

The 4 × 4 gauze will completely block openings to the pharynx and patients airway. Filled gauze is more absorbent than non-filled gauze. The assistant should be trained to suction close to the

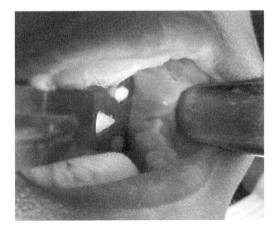

Figure 3.16 Weider retractor and 4 × 4 filled gauze pharyngeal screen.

surgical site and to alert you if openings are visible around the gauze. A large bore surgical suction is recommended to increase suction and rapidly remove fluid, pieces of tooth, or entire teeth after removal. Additionally a gauze "handle" (protruding gauze) around the Weider retractor is recommended for easy and rapid removal if needed.

Cough and gag reflexes of sedated patients are obtunded. These patients are more likely to aspirate or ingest objects. The pharyngeal curtain is especially important for sedated patients. A decrease in oxygen saturation without coughing or gag reflex may indicate aspiration or ingestion. HVE suction should be used in an attempt to remove the object and ACLS protocol initiated. The Heimlich maneuver should be used to dislodge the object. If this is unsuccessful, EMS should be called. If the patient becomes cyanotic and unconscious, advanced airways or cricothyrotomy should be considered. Patients should be transported to the emergency room to remove objects that have passed through the vocal cords.

Temporomandibular Joint Injury

Temporomandibular joint (TMJ) injury as a result of third molar surgery is not supported by the literature. Threlfall et al. found that patients diagnosed with anterior disc displacement with reduction were no more likely to have undergone third molar removal than controls. The data did not exclude the possibility that long, traumatic procedures or procedures with general anesthesia could be at risk for developing TMJ symptoms.[2]

Normal surgical protocol requires the use of a bite block and support of the patient's jaw during the removal of mandibular third molars. Unusual apical force with elevators without supporting the patient's jaw is not recommended.

Complications Summary

The possibility of surgical complications during and after the removal of impacted third molars can be intimidating for the untrained dentist. However, it should be emphasized that the majority of complications discussed in this chapter are rare. The four most common postoperative complications of third molar extraction reported in the literature are alveolar osteitis, paresthesia, infection, and bleeding/hemorrhage. These four complications can be virtually eliminated with proper case selection and good surgical technique.

The author has removed more than 40,000 impacted third molars including thousands of germectomies. Approximately 90% of these patients were teenagers. The remaining 10% included a variety of ages and surgical risk. Complications included 13 temporary inferior alveolar nerve injuries, 6 subperiosteal infections, 2 alveolar osteitis infections, and 2 displaced teeth. These complications represent a percentage that is much lower than what is found in the literature. All of the nerve injury patients were more than 20 years old. Age is a major factor in case selection and avoiding surgical complications.

References

1 Bui C, et al. Types, frequencies, and risk factors for complications after third molar removal, American Association of Oral and Maxillofacial Surgeons. *J Oral Maxillofac Surg*. 2003;61:1379–89.

2 Bouloux GF, Steed MB, Perciaccante VJ. Complications of third molar surgery. *Oral Maxillofac Surg Clin North Am*. 2007 Feb;19(1):117–28, vii.

3 Meshram VS, Meshram PV, Lambade P. Assessment of nerve injuries after surgical removal of mandibular third molar: a prospective study. *Asian J Neurosci.* 2013;2013, Article ID 291926:6 pages.

4 Alves N. Study of descendent course of buccal nerve in adults individuals. *Int J Morphol.* 2009;27(2):295–8.

5 MacGregor AJ. *The impacted lower wisdom tooth.* New York: Oxford University Press, 1985.

6 Merrill RG. Prevention, treatment, and prognosis for nerve injury related to the difficult impaction. *Dent Clin North Am.* 1979;23:471–88.

7 Carmichael FA, McGowan DA. Incidence of nerve damage following third molar removal: a West of Scotland Surgery Research Group study. *Br J Oral Maxillofac Surg.* 1992;30:78.

8 Sarikov R, Juodzbalys G. Inferior alveolar nerve injury after mandibular third molar extraction: a literature review. *J Oral Maxillofac Res.* 2014;5(4):e1.

9 Levine MH, Goddard AL, Dodson TB. Inferior alveolar nerve canal position: a clinical and radiographic study. *J Oral Maxillofac Surg.* 2007 Mar;65(3):470–4.

10 Howe J, Poyton H. Prevention of damage to the inferior alveolar dental nerve during the extraction of mandibular third molars. *Br Dent J.* 1960;109:355.

11 Valmeseda-Castellon E, Berini-Aytes L, Gay-Escoda C. Lingual nerve damage after third molar extraction. *Oral Surg Oral Med Oral Pathol Oral Radiol Endod.* 2000;90:567–73.

12 Graff-Radford SB, Evans RW. Disclosures. *Headache.* 2003;43(9):188–92.

13 Blackburn CW, Bramley PA. Lingual nerve damage associated with the removal of lower third molars. *Br Dent J.* 1989 Aug 5;167(3):103–7.

14 Karakas P, Üzel M, Koebke J. The relationship of the lingual nerve to the third molar region using radiographic imaging. *Br Dent J.* 2007;203:29–31.

15 Gargallo-Albiol J, Buenechea-Imaz R, Gay-Escoda C. Lingual nerve protection during surgical removal of lower third molars: a prospective randomised study. *Int J Oral Maxillofac Surg.* 2000;29(4):268–71.

16 Zuniga JR. Management of third molar-related nerve injuries: observe or treat? *Alpha Omegan.* 2009;102(2):79–84.

17 Cheung LK, Leung YY, Chow LK, Wong MCM, Chan EKK, Fok YH. Incidence of neurosensory deficits and recovery after lower third molar surgery: a prospective clinical study of 4338 cases. *Int J Oral Maxillofac Surg.* 2010;39(4):320–6.

18 Bataineh AB. Sensory nerve impairment following mandibular third molar surgery. *J Oral Maxillofac Surg.* 2001;59(9):1012–17.

19 Seddon HJ. Classification of nerve injuries. *Br Med J.* 1942;2:237.

20 Sunderland S. A classification of peripheral nerve injuries producing loss of function. *Brain.* 1951;74(4):491–516.

21 Kolokythas A, Olech E, Miloro M. Alveolar osteitis: a comprehensive review of concepts and controversies. *Int J Dent.* 2010;2010:249073. doi: 10.1155/2010/249073. Epub 2010 Jun 24. PMID: 20652078; PMCID: PMC2905714.

22 Blum IR. Contemporary views on dry socket (alveolar osteitis): a clinical appraisal of standardization, aetiopathogenesis and management: a critical review. *Int J Oral Maxillofac Surg.* 2002;31(3):309–17.

23 Al-Hamed FS, Tawfik MA-M, Abdelfadil E. Clinical effects of platelet-rich fibrin (PRF) following surgical extraction of lower third molar. *Saudi J Dent Res.* 2017;8(1–2):19–25.

24 Larsen PE. The effect of a chlorhexidine rinse on the incidence of alveolar osteitis following the surgical removal of impacted mandibular third molars. *J Oral Maxillofac Surg.* 1991;49(9):932–7.

25 Shepherd J. Pre-operative chlorhexidine mouth rinses reduce the incidence of dry socket. *Evid Based Dent.* 2007;8(2):43.

26 Renton T, Al-Haboubi M, Pau A, Shepherd J, Gallagher JE. What has been the United Kingdom's experience with retention of third molars? *J Oral Maxillofac Surg*. 2012;70(Suppl 1):48–57.

27 Dodson TB. The management of the asymptomatic, disease-free wisdom tooth: removal versus retention. (review). *Atlas Oral Maxillofac Surg Clin North Am*. 2012 Sept;20(2):169–76.

28 Rango JR, Szkutnik AJ. Evaluation of 0.12% chlorhexidine rinse on the prevention of alveolar osteitis. *Oral Surg Oral Med Oral Pathol Oral Radiol Endod*. 1991;72:524–6.

29 Worrall SF, Riden K, Haskell R, Corrigan AM. UK National Third Molar project: the initial report. *Br J Oral Maxillofac Surg*. 1998 Feb;36(1):14–18.

30 Miloro M, editor. *Peterson's principles of oral and maxillofacial surgery*, 2nd edition. Hamilton: B.C. Decker, Inc., 2004, 1500 pp. Odontogenic Infections, Chapter 69.

31 Meurman JH, Rajasuo A, Murtomaa H, Savolainen S. Respiratory tract infections and concomitant pericoronitis of the wisdom teeth. *BMJ*. 1995 Apr 1;310(6983):834–6.

32 Sandor GKB, Low DE, Judd PL, Davidson RJ. Antimicrobial treatment options in the management of odontogenic infections. *J Can Dent Assoc*. 1998;64(7):508–14.

33 Odell W. *Clinical problem solving in dentistry*, 3rd edition. Edinburgh: Churchill Livingstone, 2010, 151–153, 229–233.

34 Singh S. PG student at PDM Dental College & Research Institute. Published on 2014 Feb 19.

35 Palmersheim LA, Hamilton MK. Fatal cavernous sinus thrombosis secondary to third molar removal. *J Oral Maxillofac Surg*. 1982 Jun;40(6):371–6.

36 Dhali I. Spread of oral infections. Published in: Education, 2011 Feb 19.

37 Hupp JR, Ellis E, Tucker MR. *Contemporary oral and maxillofacial surgery*, 5th edition. St. Louis, MO: Mosby Elsevier, 2008, 317–33.

38 Murray AD, et al. Deep neck infections. Medscape, 2014 Mar 28.

39 Smith JK, Armao DM, Specter BB, Castillo M. Danger space infection: infection of the neck leading to descending necrotizing mediastinitis. *Emerg Radiol*. 1999;6:129–32.

40 Potoski M, Amenabar JM. Dental management of patients receiving anticoagulation or antiploatelet treeatment. *J Oral Sci*. 2007;49(4):253–8.

41 Susarla SM, et al. Third molar surgery and associated complications. *Oral Maxillofacial Surg Clin N Am*. 2003;15:177–86.

42 Ramström G, Sindet-Pedersen S, Hall G, Blombäck M, Alander U. Prevention of postsurgical bleeding in oral surgery using tranexamic acid without dose modification of oral anticoagulants. *J Oral Maxillofac Surg*. 1993 Nov;51(11):1211–16.

43 Bandrowsky T, Vorono A, Borris T, Marcantoni H. Amoxicillin-related postextraction bleeding in an anticoagulated patient with tranexamic acid rinses. *Oral Surg Oral Med Oral Pathol Oral Radiol Endod*. 1996;82(6):610–2.

44 de Boer MP, Raghoebar GM, Stegenga B, et al. Complications after mandibular third molar extraction. *Quintessence Int*. 1995;26:779–84.

45 Baab D, Ammons W, Selipsky H. Blood loss during periodontal flap surgery. *J Periodontol*. 1977;48(11):693–8.

46 Moghadam HG, Caminiti MF. Life-threatening hemorrhage after extraction of third molars: case report and management protocol. *J Can Dent Assoc*. 2002;68(11):670–4.

47 Libersa P, Roze D, Cachart T, et al. Immediate and late mandibular fractures after third molar removal. *J Oral Maxillofac Surg*. 2002;60:163–5.

48 Krimmel M, Reinert S. Mandibular fracture after third molar removal. *J Oral Maxillofac Surg*. 2000;58:1110–12.

49 Hudson JW. Osteomyelitis and osteoradionecrosis. In Fonseca RJ, editor. *Oral and maxillofacial surgery*, Vol. 5. Philadelphia: W.B.Saunders, 2000.

50 Marx RE. Chronic osteomyelitis of the jaws. *Oral Maxillofac Surg Clin North Am*. 1991;24(2):367–81.

51 Schlieve T, et al. *Management of complications in oral and maxillofacial surgery*, 1st edition. 2012, 31–2.

52 Samman N, Cheung LK, Tideman H. The buccal fat pad in oral reconstruction. *Int J Oral Maxillofac Surg*. 1993;22(1):2–6. doi:10.1016/S0901-5027(05)80346-7.

53 Khandelwal P, Hajira N. Management of oro-antral communication and fistula: various surgical options. *World J Plast Surg*. 2017 Jan;6(1):3-8. PMID: 28289607; PMCID: PMC5339603.

54 Oberman M, Horowitz I, Ramon Y. Accidental displacement of impacted maxillary third molars. *Int J Oral Maxillofac Surg*. 1986;15:756–8.

55 Tumuluri V, Punnia-Moorthy A. Displacement of a mandibular third molar root fragment into the pterygomandibular space. *Aust Dent J*. 2002;47(1):68–71.3.

56 Nusrath MA, Banks RJ. Unrecognised displacement of mandibular molar root into the submandibular space. *Br Dent J*. 2010 Sept 25;209(6):279–80.

57 Yadav RK, et al. Accidental aspiration/ingestion of foreign bodies in dentistry: a clinical and legal perspective. *Natl J Maxillofac Surg*. 2015 Jul-Dec;6(2):144-51. doi: 10.4103/0975-5950.183855. PMID: 27390487; PMCID: PMC4922223.

4

Workspace

Equipment, Instruments, and Materials

The workspace of the general dentist and oral surgeon is similar, but with important differences. General dentists often sit in a relatively static position for long periods of time; oral surgeons usually work standing and are frequently moving to improve access, visualization, and the application of force. The oral surgeon's workspace is usually larger than the general dentists. General dentists place instruments on a small, moveable instrument tray; oral surgeons place instruments on a large surgical table positioned directly over a fully reclined patient. Visualization is critical for both dentists and surgeons, but good visualization is somewhat more important for the surgeon who frequently works near vital structures. Finally, the equipment, instruments, and materials used by the oral surgeon are often different from those used by the general dentist.

In the ADA's Health Screening Program of 2012, 56.4% of participating dentists had musculoskeletal symptoms. Thirty-seven percent were working 15 to 30 years. Thirty percent had symptoms over 10 years. Seventy-nine percent had symptoms that were worsening or unchanging. Forty-four percent believed that their pain was due to repetitive actions during work. Sixty-one percent of the currently practicing dental professionals reported regularly experiencing pain, tingling, or numbness. The most commonly reported symptoms were located in the back (51.0% reported) and neck (51.1%).[1] A good, ergonomically designed operatory with equipment that is supportive to the practitioner while allowing easy access to the oral cavity can help to avoid these injuries.[2]

According to the International Standards Organization, the following actions can improve workspace ergonomics and reduce musculoskeletal disorders:[3]

Adapt workspace and equipment to account for operator and work being performed with preferred body postures.

1) Provide sufficient space for body movements.
2) Provide variety in tasks and movements to avoid static muscle tension caused by postural constraints.
3) Design work to allow machinery to do and assist highly repetitive tasks.
4) Avoid extreme posture when exerting high force.

Compliance with these recommendations is possible when a dentist performs exodontia from the standing position. In a seated posture the pressure in the lumbar discs increases by 50% as compared to standing.[4]

Impacted Third Molars, Second Edition. Edited by John Wayland.
© 2024 John Wiley & Sons, Inc. Published 2024 by John Wiley & Sons, Inc.

$1200

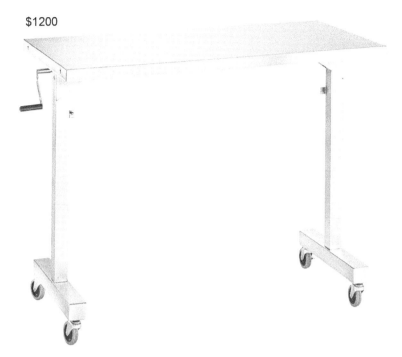

Figure 4.1   Rolling Table Adjusts From 31" to 46" Tall. (Reproduced with permission of Salvin Dental Specialties Inc.).

Workspace ergonomics can be significant for the general dentist whose practice has a heavy emphasis on exodontia and the removal of impacted third molars. The ergonomic demands of exodontia require a large operatory with room to move. Flat surfaces are needed for surgical motors, irrigation pumps, instruments, and materials. Surgical tables and chairs, loupe magnification, and loupe lighting improve efficiency, quality of treatment, and ergonomics.

Equipment

Surgical Tables and Chairs, Magnification, and Lighting

Surgical tables can significantly improve workspace ergonomics, efficiency, and productivity. Although most routine exodontia can be completed with a handful of instruments, some extractions require the use of specialized instruments. The seasoned surgical assistant can anticipate the surgical instrument and effortlessly pass it to the dentist. There is no need to leave the room in search of a unique instrument. A large surgical table (24″ × 39″), positioned above the reclined patient's chest, allows the placement of many instruments within easy reach. (See Figure 4.1.)

Surgical chairs are used by most oral surgeons for two reasons; patient access and chair height. (See Figure 4.2.) Both of these considerations are closely related to ergonomics. Oral surgery chairs are designed to allow the best possible access to the patient's oral cavity when seated or standing. Reaching and leaning are reduced compared to a traditional dental chair designed for work from the 11 o'clock or 1 o'clock position. Optimum ergonomic chair height should provide a 90-degree angle between the upper arm and lower arm. This is often difficult or impossible to achieve when working in a standing position with a traditional dental chair.

Busy exodontia practices should consider equipping one large operatory with a surgical table and chair. This investment will result in increased efficiency and production and a reduction in musculoskeletal disorders.

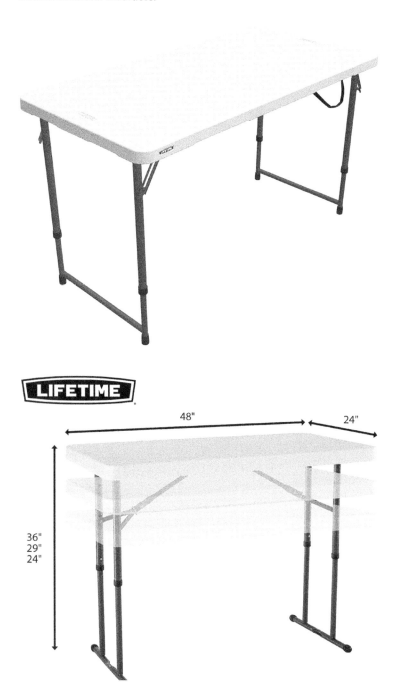

About this Item

- All purpose table constructed of powder-coated steel and high-density polyethylene plastic
- 48-inch × 24-inch molded table
- Folds in half for easy storage and transport
- Adjustable Height Settings (22-Inch, 24-Inch, 29-Inch and 36-Inch)
- Convenient carry handle; Table weight: 19 lbs. Table Top Thickness: 1. 4 inch. Frame tubing diameter: 25 mm
- Tested to hold 200 lbs. evenly distributed

The routine use of magnification in dentistry is a relatively new innovation. The author was in dental school from 1977 to 1981. The only dentists using magnification at that time were a handful of instructors. They were thought to be "nerds" or "geeks." Today most dental schools recommend or require the use of magnification.[5] Loupes make it possible to comfortably reach and see the third molar region. Loupes help to prevent nerve injury and other complications when removing bone and sectioning third molars. Magnification also improves a dentist's ability to distinguish between tooth structure and alveolar bone.[6]

Schoeffl et. el. were able to prove that microsurgical success is directly related to optical magnification. Sixteen participants of microsurgical training courses had to complete artery and nerve surgery. Each surgery had to be performed with an unaided eye, surgical loupes, and a regular operating microscope. This study showed a direct relationship of error frequency and lower optical magnification. The highest number of microsurgical errors occurred with the unaided eye.[7]

There are many variables to consider when choosing loupes. Prices range from a few hundred dollars to thousands of dollars. Optical resolution is very important when considering loupes. The image viewed through the oculars should be crisp and uniformly clear from edge to edge. Quality loupes are made with glass optics. High-quality optics improve the image and lessens the potential for eye fatigue. Plastic optics, found in less expensive loupes, do not offer the highest level of visual acuity.[8] Another decision point is the choice between through the lens (TTL) and flip up (FU) loupes.

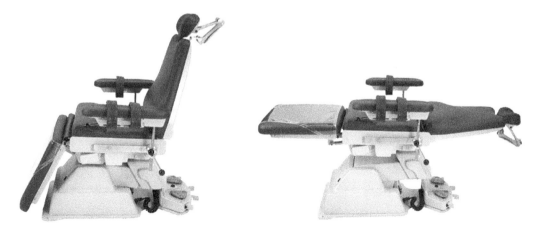

Figure 4.2   Oral surgery Chair. (Reproduced with permission of BOYD Industries, Inc.)

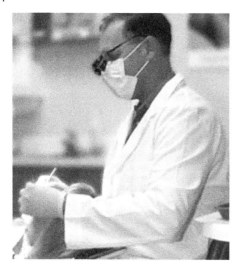

Figure 4.3   Loupe magnification can improve posture.

The choice of through the lens or flip up loupes is up to personal preference. TTL loupes never need adjustment because the lens is mounted directly on the loupe glass. They are customized to the exact pupillary distance of each dentist. FU loupes can be adjusted and shared with other users. Working distance and angle of the loupes can affect posture. Properly fitted and adjusted loupes will decrease neck and back stress, an important aspect when considering our field. (See Figure 4.3.)

Another ergonomic decision involves lighting. Adequate lighting is essential for surgery and other dental procedures. Loupe lights are mounted between the loupe lenses, directly on the loupe frame. This position provides bright, shadow-free light for the dentist/surgeon. Traditional operatory lighting cannot provide the shadow free, bright light of loupe lights. (See Figure 4.4.)

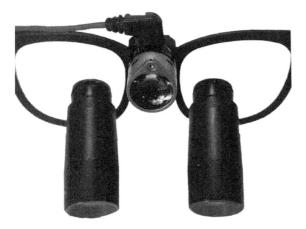

Figure 4.4   Loupe lighting can improve posture.

Surgical Drills and Motors

Surgical drills used for the removal of impacted third molars are powered by compressed gas or electricity. The cost of surgical drill systems ranges from a few hundred dollars to more than $20,000. Surgical drills can be classified as high-speed compressed air, low-speed pneumatic or, low-speed electric. The most economical surgical drills are high-speed handpieces (similar to operative dental handpieces) that run on compressed air.

High-Speed Compressed Air

High-speed restorative handpieces should not be used for oral surgery. Compressed air from these handpieces can enter the surgical site resulting in surgical emphysema, also known as subcutaneous emphysema. Subcutaneous emphysema occurs when air is forced into soft tissue through a reflected flap. The air invades adjacent tissues, leading to pain, infection, swelling, crepitus on palpation, and occasionally spreading through fascial planes.[9] This can be a life-threatening complication.

Affordable, high-speed surgical drills have been developed to address this problem. (See Figures 4.5a and 4.5b.) The cost of a high-speed surgical drill is about the same as a standard restorative handpiece. These surgical handpieces have a 45-degree angled head to improve access and visibility and a rear exhaust to prevent subcutaneous emphysema. Examples are the Impact Air 45 and the Sabra OMS45. These surgical drills run at 400,000 to 500,000 RPM and deliver slightly more torque than a standard dental handpiece. They are capable of removing bone and sectioning teeth, but don't have the high torque of traditional, straight surgical drills. The high-speed surgical drill chuck does not hold a surgical bur securely like a straight surgical handpiece. The high-speed surgical bur is short and does not turn concentrically which leads to chatter and bur breakage.

Low-Speed Nitrogen

In 1963, Dr. Robert Hall introduced the Surgairtome (also known as the "Hall") surgical drill. An example of this type of surgical drill is shown in Figures 4.6a and 4.6b. This was one of the first

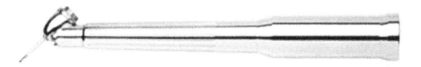

Figure 4.5a   Impact Air 45. (Reproduced with permission of Palisades Dental, LLC.).

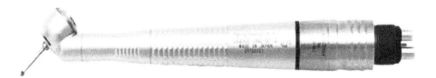

Figure 4.5b   Sabra OMS45. (Reproduced with permission of Sabra Dental).

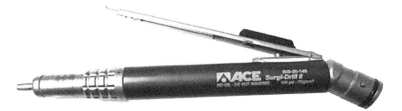

Figure 4.6a   Hall type surgical drill.

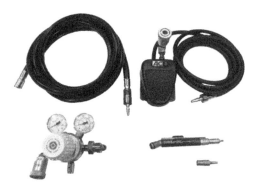

Figure 4.6b   Hall type drill and accessories.

high-torque pneumatic drills used in oral surgery. The Hall runs on compressed nitrogen at 100 psi and 90,000 rpm. It is available in straight configurations. The torque of this drill is many times greater than that of an air driven surgical drill.

The Hall type surgical drill is ideal for efficiently removing bone and sectioning teeth. The Hall uses a long bur, 44.5 mm to 70 mm in length. Most of the bur is within the handpiece chuck. This allows the bur to turn concentrically and improves torque and cutting efficiency.

It is completely sealed, does not require lubrication, and is extremely durable. Nitrogen is used to power the Hall drill to prevent oxidation of the sealed contents. Additionally, nitrogen does not support combustion.

The nitrogen driven surgical drill requires a quick disconnect hose, bur guard, compressed nitrogen, and a regulator. (See Figure 4.6b.) The straight drill design, heavy hose, and lever actuator may be challenging for first time users. An optional foot pedal actuator is available. This drill is very loud.

Low-Speed Electric
Electric surgical drills are not as durable as pneumatic surgical drills, but have many advantages. These drills are powered by a portable electric motor that is placed on a counter, cart, or Mayo stand near the dentist or surgeon. The Osteomed system features an electric surgical drill. (See Figures 4.7a, 4.7b, and 4.7c.)

Electric surgical motors are very versatile and can be used for many dental procedures including oral surgery and implantology. The typical surgical system includes an electric motor, micromotor, cable, surgical handpiece (attachment), peristaltic pump for irrigation, and foot pedal. The micromotor is

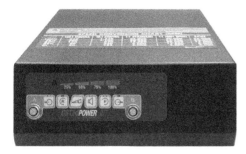

Figure 4.7a   Motor.

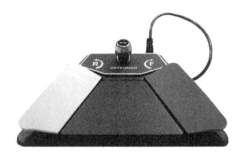

Figure 4.7b   Foot pedal. (Reproduced with permission of Osteomed, Inc.)

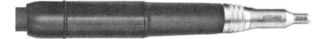

Figure 4.7c   Drill.

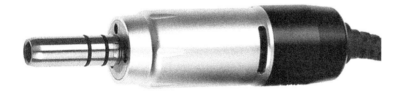

Figure 4.8   E-type micromotor with flat connecting surface.

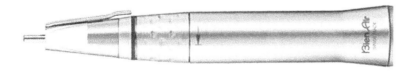

Figure 4.9   Author's surgical drill compatible with E-Type micromotor. (Reproduced with permission of Bien Air, USA.).

considered an "E-type" motor if it has a flat surface for coupling with the handpiece. (See Figure 4.8 and 4.9.) E-type micromotors are interchangeable with attachments from many manufacturers.

Surgical handpiece attachments used with E-type connections are available in straight or angled configurations. They are quiet when compared to the pneumatic surgical drill. Electric surgical micro motors used for the removal of impacted third molars usually run between 40,000 and 100,000 rpm. The drill speed can be doubled with 1:2 increasing gears in the handpiece. However, the high torque of these systems is more important than rpm when removing bone and sectioning third molars. Electric systems tend to be expensive with frequent maintenance when compared with gas driven drills. The "X Cube" is an example of an affordable electric surgical system. (See Figure 4.10.)

There are advantages and disadvantages to each system. (See Table 4.1.) The high-speed 45-degree surgical handpiece is affordably priced, but does not have the cutting power (torque)

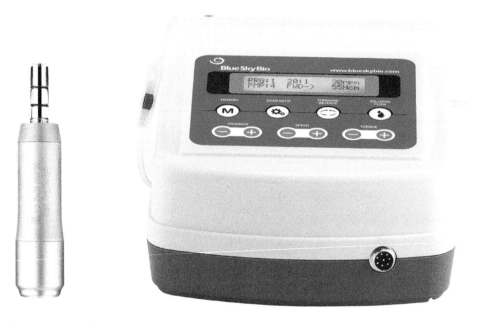

Figure 4.10   "X Cube" motor and "E" type micromotor. (Reproduced with permission of Blue Sky Bio).

Table 4.1   Characteristics of surgical drill systems.

Surgical Drill System	Cost	RPM	Torque	Cutting Efficiency	Durability	Multiple Attachments (E-Type)	Bur Type
High-speed air	Low	400,000–500,000	Low	Low	Moderate	No	High-Speed Friction Grip
Low-speed nitrogen	Moderate	90,000–100,00	High	High	High	No	44.5–70 mm
Low-speed electric	Moderate–High	0–100,000	High	High	Low–Moderate	Yes	44.5–70 mm

of a straight surgical drill. The nitrogen driven surgical drill system is moderately priced and very durable. It has high torque and cuts smoothly and efficiently. Electricity is not required. The straight drill chuck holds a long bur securely which eliminates chatter. Unfortunately, it is very loud and requires a tank of nitrogen and a long high-pressure hose to operate. Electric surgical drill systems are relatively quiet. E-type micromotors can fit various attachments including a straight or angled (20 degrees) surgical handpiece. Like nitrogen driven surgical drills, electric surgical drill system's chuck holds a long bur securely to cut smoothly and eliminate chatter. Most electrical systems have a wide range of torque and rpm. The main disadvantage of these systems is cost.

The choice of systems usually depends on frequency of use. The high-speed surgical handpiece may be the right choice for a dentist removing impactions once a month. An expensive electrical system may be the right choice for someone removing impactions every day.

Instruments

Instrument Manufacturing and Care

There are literally thousands of instruments used in oral surgery. Surgical instruments are manufactured by many different companies throughout the world. The quality and characteristics of surgical instruments can vary depending on the manufacturer's design and the quality of steel. High-quality surgical instruments are handmade which can lead to some minor variations in the dimensions of instruments, particularly between manufacturing sets. A 301 elevator manufactured by Miltex may feel and function differently than the same numbered elevator made by Hu-Friedy. Many surgeons prefer one instrument brand over another and may have an assortment of their favorite instruments from different manufacturers.

Most surgical instruments are stainless steel. Steel is made stainless by adding nickel and chromium in measured quantities. There are over 150 grades of stainless steel. Medical grade stainless steel is an alloy containing nickel and chromium in very specific quantities. Most medical grade stainless steel is Type 304, sometimes called T304. Carbon can be added to the steel to make the metal harder when a sharp instrument edge is desired, but the addition of carbon makes surgical instruments more likely to corrode. This problem can be solved for hinged instruments by the addition of tungsten carbide inserts. Tungsten carbide is among the hardest materials known and is very resistant to wear and corrosion. Tungsten carbide inserts are used in surgical instruments to enhance their performance and longevity. Needle holders and forceps made with tungsten carbide grasp more securely and are more durable than their stainless-steel counterparts. Tungsten carbide scissors cut better and need much less sharpening than stainless steel. A gold handle on scissors, forceps, or needle holders indicates they have tungsten carbide inserts on the working surfaces. They are approximately twice as expensive as standard instruments, but can last five times longer. This can be very cost effective in the long run.

New instruments are more likely to corrode than old instruments because they have a thin layer of chromium oxide on their surface. This layer thickens with age and increases the resistance of the instruments to corrosion. New instruments are particularly vulnerable to detergents, inadequate lubrication, and the corrosive environment of an autoclave. New instruments often show markings while old instruments are unmarked. Maximizing the chromium oxide layer is the basis of sound instrument care.

The chromium oxide layer can be maintained and thickened through proper cleaning and maintenance. Surgical instruments should be scrubbed with a soft brush to remove blood and debris, run in an ultrasonic cleaner for 10–15 minutes, immediately rinsed, and steam autoclaved until the full drying cycle is complete. Any moisture left on instruments or in overlapping joints will result in staining, pitting, and corrosion. The use of a surgical "milk" lubricant for hinged instruments prior to sterilizing will prevent corrosion and spotting from mineral deposits left behind by water. Silicone grease can be used in the joint of hinged instruments to improve performance. Lubrication is the most important action one can take to extend the life of hinged instruments.

Impacted Third Molar Instruments

A basic instrument setup for the surgical removal of impacted third molars consists of a limited number of instruments. A fundamental goal in any efficient surgical procedure requires that individual instruments are used as seldom as possible. Accomplished surgeons routinely complete difficult procedures with a handful of their favorite instruments. A good analogy would be the beginning golfer, with a bag full of clubs, who cannot break 100 on the golf course. Any professional golfer could easily break 100 with 3 clubs. However, there are times when every surgeon needs an instrument that is not in their basic setup. For the purpose of this chapter these instruments will be termed "specialty instruments." A specialty instrument for one operator may be a member of the basic setup for another operator. Specialty instruments are used when instruments in the basic setup are inadequate. The author's basic instruments can be seen in Table 4.2 and Figure 4.11.

Forceps are conspicuously missing from the surgical setup. By definition, impacted third molars cannot be removed with forceps. Universal forceps or a rongeur may be useful to grasp a luxated third molar or root.

Table 4.2 Author's basic surgical instrument setup.

Straight elevator – serrated 46R	Aspirating syringe (2)	Surgical drill	Scalpel handle (2)
Periosteal elevator – #9 molt	Bite block – child	1703L surgical bur	#12 scalpel blade
Curette – 2/4 double ended molt	Needle holder – carbide tungsten	Tissue forceps	#15 scalpel blade
Minnesota retractor	Scissors – carbide tungsten	412 Monoject syringe (2)	3.0 PGA suture
Weider retractor – medium	Curved hemostat – KLS Marin tooth grabber	4×4 and 2 × 2 filled 8 ply gauze	Sterile bowl
Root tip pick	Magnification	Loupe light	Mask
Small and large (2) surgical suction	Lidocaine 2% epinephrine 1:100,000	Marcaine .5% epinephrine 1:200,000	Gloves

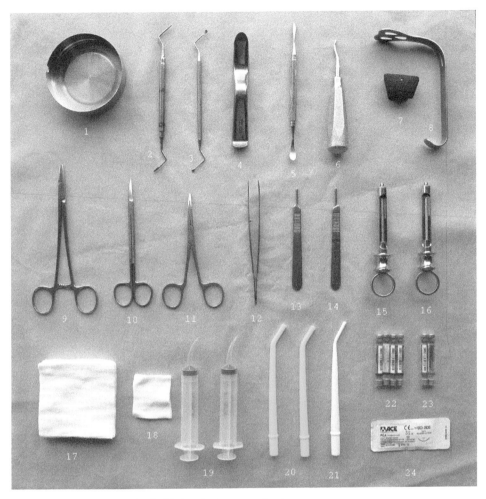

Figure 4.11   Photo of Author's third molar instrument setup.

Basic Impacted Third Molar Instrument Setup

1) Sterile bowl for irrigation
2) Root tip pick
3) Surgical curette
4) Minnesota retractor
5) #9 periosteal elevator
6) 46R elevator
7) Child mouth prop
8) Weider retractor.
9) Needle holder with carbide inserts
10) Surgical scissors with carbide tips
11) Curved hemostat
12) Cotton plier
13) #12 scalpel
14) #15 scalpel

15) 30 gauge long anesthetic syringe
16) 27 gauge long anesthetic syringe
17) 4×4, 8 ply, filled gauze
18) 2×2, 8 ply, filled gauze
19) Irrigation syringes
20) 1/4″ large surgical suction (2)
21) 1/16″ small surgical suction
22) Lidocaine 2% with epinephrine 1:100,000 (4)
23) Marcaine .5% with epinephrine 1:200,000 (2)
24) 3.0 polyglycolic acid absorbable suture (pga)

The Weider retractor is used in most oral surgery offices. (See Figures 4.12a and 4.12b.) It is rarely used in general dentistry practices. The instrument isolates the surgical site and protects the patient's tongue. It also prevents aspiration of fluids and solid objects when used with a gauze pharyngeal screen. This combination is especially useful when patients are sedated.

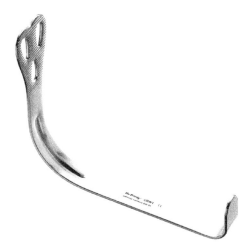

Figure 4.12a   Weider retractor. (Reproduced with permission of Hu-Friedy Dental).

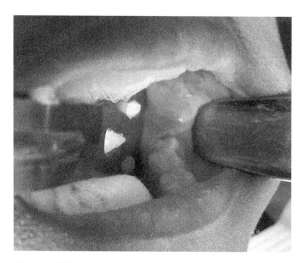

Figure 4.12b   Weider retractor in position.

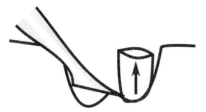

Figure 4.13   Wheel and axle.

The heart shaped paddle is inserted between the tongue and lingual surface of the mandible. The L-shaped handle can be used to retract the tongue, but usually functions as ballast allowing the assistant to use both hands for suctioning, irrigation, and other functions. The Weider retractor is available in small, medium, and large sizes.

Elevators

Elevators used in oral surgery are examples of two simple machines, the wheel and axle and inclined plane. The wheel and axle and incline plane change the direction or magnitude of force to gain mechanical advantage. Elevators can be found in many shapes and sizes for different situations when removing teeth and fractured roots.

Wheel and axle elevators usually have sharp tips that are offset from the instrument shank. (See Figure 4.13.)

They are always found as a left and right pair. They are often referred to as pennant or flag instruments due to their characteristic triangular shaped tip resembling a flag. These elevators develop significant torque when bone is used as a fulcrum. They are usually used to remove roots when there is an empty adjacent socket. The sharp point is used to engage the remaining fractured root tip. A #30 or #31 Cryer elevator can be used to remove a mesial third molar root after the distal root has been removed. (See Figures 4.14a and 4.14b.) The sharp instrument tip can push through interseptal bone to engage the mesial root cementum. Cryer elevators and other similar flag instruments come in many different sizes and shapes.

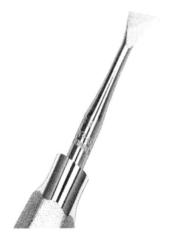

Figure 4.14a   #30 Cryer elevator. (Reproduced with permission of Hu-Friedy Dental).

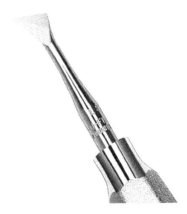

Figure 4.14b   #31 Cryer elevator. (Reproduced with permission of Hu-Friedy Dental).

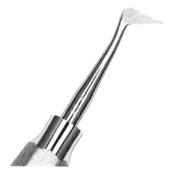

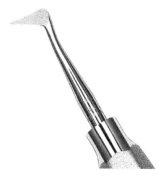

Figure 4.15a Seldin elevator #1 L. (Reproduced with permission of Hu-Friedy Dental).

Figure 4.15b Seldin elevator #1 R. (Reproduced with permission of Hu-Friedy Dental).

Another flag elevator that resembles the Cryer elevator is the Seldin #1L and #1R. (See Figures 4.15a and 4.15b.) The Cryer and Seldin elevators are mainly used in the mandible. These elevators should be sharpened regularly.

The Crane Pick and Cogswell B elevators are two more examples of wheel and axle elevators. (See Figures 4.16 and 4.17.) These elevators can be used to remove teeth and roots in the maxilla and mandible. The Crane Pick and Cogswell B are very similar in appearance and are often

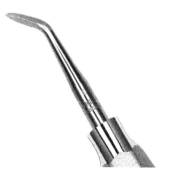

Figure 4.16 Crane Pick. (Reproduced with permission of Hu-Friedy Dental).

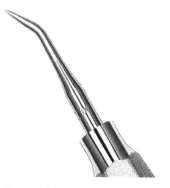

Figure 4.17 Cogswell B. (Reproduced with permission of Hu-Friedy Dental).

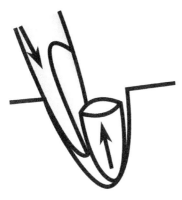

Figure 4.18   Incline plane displaces the root or tooth.

confused with each other. The handle, shank, and offset tip are nearly identical. However, the Crane Pick tip has a sharp pointed tip that is triangular in shape. The tip of the Cogswell B is smooth and rounded. Both instruments work well when a purchase point is drilled in a tooth or root. The instrument tip is placed in the purchase point and a bony fulcrum used to remove the tooth or root.

The inclined plane principle is illustrated in Figure 4.18. These elevators work on the principle that two objects cannot occupy the same space at the same time. Straight elevators are wedged into the periodontal ligament space between bone and tooth structure to luxate teeth and roots. The shank of a straight elevator should parallel the long axis of the tooth or root when used properly. Once the periodontal ligament is severed, the instrument can be rotated clockwise and counter clockwise to further luxate the tooth or root.

Inclined plane elevators are normally called straight elevators. They have a straight or slightly curved shank and a tapering, concave tip. Common straight elevators are the 301 and 34. (See Figures 4.19 and 4.20.) The main difference between the 301 and 34 is the size of the tip and the amount of force that can be applied. Straight elevators can be used to elevate all teeth in addition to third molars. There are many versions of these versatile elevators.

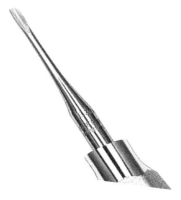

Figure 4.19   301 Elevator. (Reproduced with permission of Hu-Friedy Dental).

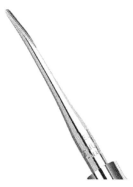

Figure 4.20   34 elevator. (Reproduced with permission of Hu-Friedy Dental).

The author's favorite elevator for the removal of third molars is the 46R. This instrument is very similar to the 77R. The main feature of the instrument is a gradual curve in the instrument shaft. This curve provides easier access to third molars. Serrations at the working end of the instrument increase the grip on the tooth. (See Figure 4.21.)

Another elevator used by the author to remove impacted third molars is the Hu-Friedy EL3CSM. (See Figure 4.22.) The number 3 indicates that the working tip is 3 mm wide. The EL CSM

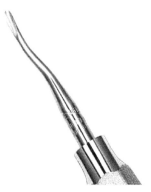

Figure 4.21   46R elevator. (Reproduced with permission of Hu-Friedy Dental).

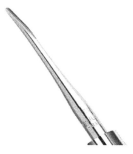

Figure 4.22   Hu-Friedy El3CSM. (Reproduced with permission of Hu-Friedy Dental).

elevators are available from Hu-Friedy with tips ranging from 2 mm to 5 mm. This elevator is very similar to the generic 301 elevator with some important differences. The shaft has a gradual curve that improves access when used as an incline plane. The tip is slightly concave and is very strong. This elevator is especially useful when removing vertical and distoangular impactions. The tip is placed in the periodontal ligament space on the buccal surface with the shaft parallel to the long axis of the tooth. Force is applied and the tooth is elevated in an occlusal direction.

The inclined plane straight elevators previously described are among the most popular elevators used in the United States for the removal of impacted third molars. However, many wheel and axle elevators are also used, especially when removing maxillary third molars and space is limited. The 19/20, 190/191, and Potts elevators are other examples of wheel and axle elevators. (See Figures 4.23a and 4.23b, Figures 4.24a and 4.24b, Figures 4.25a and 4.25b.)

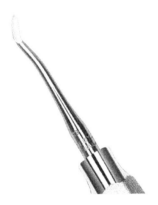

Figure 4.23a   #19 Warwick-James. (Reproduced with permission of Hu-Friedy Dental).

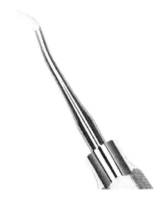

Figure 4.23b   #20 Warwick-James. (Reproduced with permission of Hu-Friedy Dental).

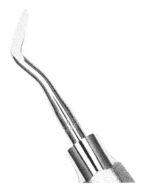

Figure 4.24a   #190 Modified Woodward. (Reproduced with permission of Hu-Friedy Dental).

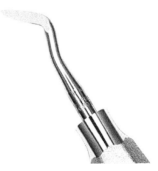

Figure 4.24b   #191 Modified Woodward. (Reproduced with permission of Hu-Friedy Dental).

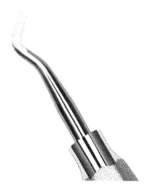

Figure 4.25a #6 Potts. (Reproduced with permission of Hu-Friedy Dental).

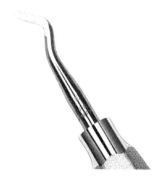

Figure 4.25b #7 Potts. (Reproduced with permission of Hu-Friedy Dental).

Periotomes, Proximators, and Luxators (PPL)

PPL instruments, like straight elevators, are wedged between tooth roots and bone to sever the periodontal ligament and displace a tooth or fractured root. The tip of PPL instruments is very sharp, and relatively flat when compared to a straight elevator. A periotome is smaller than a proximator, a proximator is usually smaller than a luxator, and a luxator is usually smaller than a straight elevator. (See Figure 4.26, 4.27, and 4.28.) The previously mentioned EL3CSM is sometimes called a "luxating elevator" because it combines the characteristics of a luxator and an elevator. PPL instruments are often used when the dentist's goal is an atraumatic extraction.

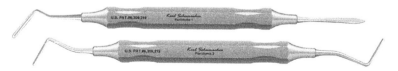

Figure 4.26 Periotome. (Reproduced with permission of Schumacher Dental.)

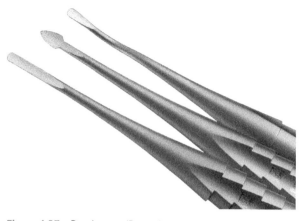

Figure 4.27 Proximator. (Reproduced with permission of Schumacher Dental).

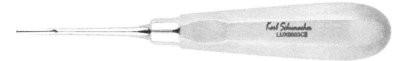

Figure 4.28   Luxator (luxating elevator) (Reproduced with permission of Schumacher Dental).

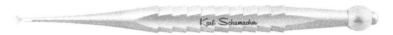

Figure 4.29   Spade Proximator. (Reproduced with permission of Schumacher Dental).

Periotomes, proximators, and luxators are used in the periodontal ligament space prior to the application of a straight elevator. The progressive application of larger instruments expands the bony socket. The use of a traditional elevator may not be necessary since the tooth or fractured root is often avulsed without a prying motion.

All PPL instruments work on the principle of the inclined plane. They are inserted along the long axis of the tooth into the PDL space to sever the periodontal ligament and expand the socket. Periotomes, proximators, and luxators can be used in succession to enlarge the PDL space and socket. Unlike straight elevators, these instruments are not rotated clockwise and counter clockwise once they are wedged in place. PPL instruments are used with finesse to avoid chipping of the sharp tip. They are wedged in several places around the tooth/root and gradually displace the tooth/root from the socket. PPL instruments are manufactured in many different sizes.

The spade proximator deserves further discussion. (See Figure 4.29.) The author has had success using this instrument to remove impacted third molar root tips. The spade proximator is unique because it has a thin, strong, and sharp tip that can be rotated clockwise and counterclockwise, or used with a prying motion, without breaking. The spade-shaped instrument tip can be wedged between the retained root and the wall of the socket.

The number of instruments designed to remove teeth can be overwhelming. One manufacturer's website (Hu-Friedy) displays 123 elevators over 14 pages! Furthermore, there are hundreds of manufacturers worldwide with a wide range of quality and design for the same instrument.

Oral surgeons have favorite instruments for different situations. It is recommended that the reader try different instruments and manufacturers to discover their "favorite" instruments. It's not possible to know what instrument feels right and works best for you unless you try it. For example, a 190/191 elevator from one manufacturer may feel, and function, very differently from a 190/191 from another manufacturer.

Materials

Materials used in oral surgery for the removal of impacted third molars are many and varied. For the purpose of this discussion, materials are grouped into two categories.

1) Personal protective equipment
2) Disposable materials

Personal Protective Equipment (PPE)

PPE is designed to protect the skin and the mucous membranes of the eyes, nose, and mouth from exposure to blood or other potentially infectious material.[10] Use of rotary surgical instruments and air-water syringes creates a visible spray that contains primarily large-particle droplets of water, saliva, blood, microorganisms, and other debris. This spatter travels only a short distance and settles out quickly, landing on the floor, nearby operatory surfaces, dental health care providers, or the patient. The spray also might contain certain aerosols (i.e., particles smaller than 10 μm that can be inspired). Aerosols can remain airborne for extended periods. However, they should not be confused with the large-particle spatter that makes up the bulk of the spray from handpieces. Appropriate work practices, including the use of a throat pack and high-velocity evacuation, should minimize the spread of droplets, spatter, and aerosols.[11]

The use of personal protective equipment (PPE) and universal precautions in healthcare is closely related to the AIDS outbreak in the 1980s. Kimberly Bergalis developed AIDS after visiting HIV positive Dr. David Acer in 1987 for the removal of a molar. This incident is the first known case of clinical transmission of HIV.[12] Initially, the CDC and media believed HIV was transmitted to Ms. Bergalis via unclean dental instruments. It was later learned that Dr. Acer intentionally infected the patient. This incident led to the implementation of Universal Precautions.

Universal precautions in healthcare refer to the practice of treating every patient as if they are infected.[13] Universal precautions include good hygiene habits (hand washing), correct handling of needles and scalpels, aseptic techniques, and the use of barriers such as gloves, face masks, eye protection, and barrier gowns or lab coats.

Gloves

Gloves reduce the spread of germs to patients and protect the hands of the surgeon. Surgical latex gloves come with or without powdered cornstarch to make them easier to put on the hands. In the late 1980s latex glove use in dentistry exploded after the Aids outbreak and implementation of Universal Precautions. According to projections from a report published by Global Industry Analysts (GIA), the market for disposable medical gloves will be worth $4 billion in 2017.[14] Gloves used in dentistry are primarily made of natural latex rubber or synthetic nitrile rubber. (See Figures 4.30a and 4.30b.)

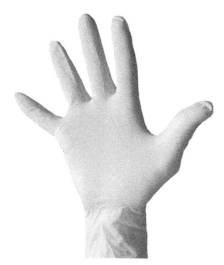

Figure 4.30a   Latex glove.

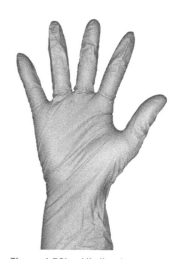

Figure 4.30b   Nitrile glove.

Most surgeons prefer latex gloves due to superior fit and the ability to stretch which improves tactile feel. However, the incidence of latex allergy has prompted an increase in the use of synthetic gloves such as nitrile gloves. It is estimated that 8–12% of health care workers are latex sensitive with reactions ranging from irritant contact dermatitis and allergic contact sensitivity to anaphylaxis.[15] Regarding powdered gloves, one should consider that the cornstarch powder in latex gloves may cause wound healing issues, postoperative complications, and facilitate latex allergy exposure.[16]

Wearing gloves does not eliminate the need for hand washing. Hand washing should be performed immediately before putting on gloves. Gloves can have small defects or can be torn during use increasing the risk of wound contamination and exposure to microorganisms from patients. Bacteria can multiply rapidly in the moist environments underneath gloves. Therefore, hands should be completely dry before donning gloves and washed again immediately after glove removal.[17]

Masks

Surgical masks prevent the transmission of body fluids to patients and protect the surgical team from being splashed in the mouth with body fluids. (See Figure 4.31.) They can also reduce the spread of infectious liquid droplets that are created when the wearer coughs or sneezes. They are a constant reminder for the surgical team to not touch their mouth or nose which could transfer viruses and bacteria. Evidence supports the effectiveness of a mask with >95% bacterial filtration efficiency in reducing the risk of infection.[18]

All procedures performed with the use of surgical handpieces cause the formation of aerosol and splatter which are commonly contaminated with bacteria, viruses, fungi, and blood.[19]

Eyewear

Eye protection includes face shields and goggles. (See Figure 4.32.) Protective eyewear with solid side shields or a face shield should be worn during procedures likely to generate splashes or sprays of blood or body fluids. Goggles and face shields protect mucous membranes in the surgical team

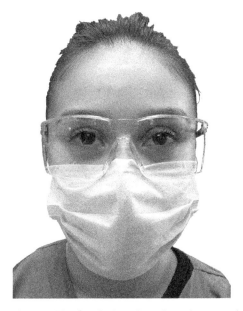

Figure 4.31   Surgical masks reduce the transmission of infectious disease.

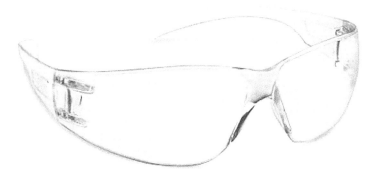

Figure 4.32 Goggles and face shields protect against transmission of disease.

eyes from blood and other bodily fluids. Protective eyewear for patients shields their eyes from splatter or debris generated during surgical procedures.

Gowns

The Occupational Safety and Health Administration (OSHA) Bloodborne Pathogens Standard requires that personal protective clothing (e.g., gowns, lab coat) have sleeves long enough to protect the forearms, have a high neck, and be knee length. (See Figure 4.33.) Street clothes or scrubs are usually not intended to be personal protective equipment and are worn under a lab coat or gown.

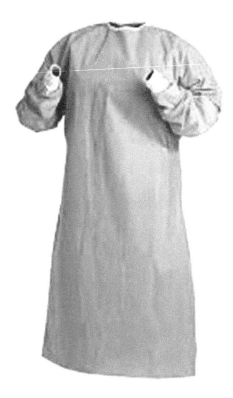

Figure 4.33 Surgical gowns and lab coats protect against transmission of disease.

Disposable Materials

The removal of impacted third molars requires the use of many disposable materials. Most of these materials are essential, but may vary by manufacturer and the surgeon's preference. A list of disposable materials used by the author when removing impacted third molars is shown in Table 4.3.

The use of some materials shown in Table 4.3 is anecdotal, but has worked well for the author for more than 30 years. The author's reason for using these materials is presented in the following section. The scientific basis for the material use is included when available.

Lidocaine and Marcaine

The author uses lidocaine 2% in all four quadrants. Bupivacaine (Marcaine) .5% is used in addition to lidocaine in lower quadrants. Marcaine appears to be more effective than lidocaine in reducing postoperative pain following the removal of impacted mandibular third molars.

Brajkovi et al. studied the effects of lidocaine vs bupivacaine in reducing postoperative pain following the surgical removal of mandibular third molars. They concluded that bupivacaine .5% (Marcaine) controlled postoperative pain more efficiently after lower third molar surgery than lidocaine 2% with epinephrine 1:80,000.[20]

Another study by Naichuan et al. found bupivacaine better than the lidocaine in dental operations that take a relatively long time, especially in endodontic treatments or where there is a need for postoperative pain management. Specifically, 0.5% levobupivacaine had higher success rates and was better in postoperative pain control than 2% lidocaine.[21]

Suction

Disposable surgical suction is available in three lumen sizes: 1/16″, 1/8″, and ¼″. The plastic surgical suction is sterilized prior to use. Two disposable surgical suctions are part of the author's surgical setup, green ¼″ and white 1/8″. (See Figure 4.34.) The green suction is used for most of the surgery. The ¼″ large lumen minimizes clogging and the suction power is almost the same as

Table 4.3 Disposable materials used by the author when removing impacted third molars.

Lidocaine 2%, epi 1:100,000 Marcaine .5%, epi 1:200,000		PGA 3.0 suture	4 × 4 Gauze 2 × 2 Gauze
Surgical suction		12 and 15 scalpel	Irrigation syringes

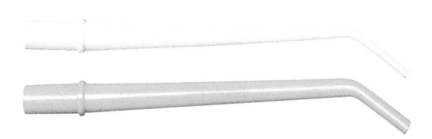

Figure 4.34 Disposable surgical suction is sterilized prior to use.

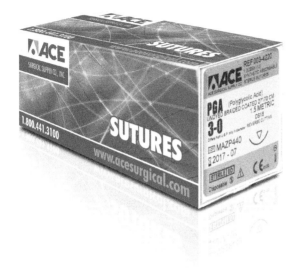

Figure 4.35   Polyglycolic acid absorbable suture handles like silk and absorbs like gut.

HVE. The strong suction is useful if debris or fluid find its way behind the pharyngeal screen. The small white 1/8″ suction is used inside flaps or when visualization is paramount; for example, when removing root tips.

Suture

The use of needle and thread to close wounds is several thousand years old dating back to ancient Egypt. Classical period literature (800–200 BC) contains many descriptions of surgery involving sutures. Two physicians from that period, Hippocrates and Galen, described sutures and suturing technique.[22]

Various types of suture materials were used for thousands of years. Needles and thread were made from bone or metal such as gold, silver, copper, and bronze. Suture thread was made of metal wire, plant, or animal material. Silk eventually became the number one non-absorbable material. Catgut (bovine, sheep, goat intestine) became the standard absorbable suture material near the end of the 19th century.

The first synthetic suture was developed in the 1930s followed by polyglycolic acid suture (PGA) in the 1960s. (See Figure 4.35.) Many synthetic sutures are now available with different characteristics. The majority of sutures used today are synthetic. Silk and gut are the only remaining natural sutures from ancient times. Gut sutures have been banned in Europe and Japan owing to concerns regarding bovine spongiform encephalopathy (mad cow disease). Most sutures manufactured today are sterilized by ethylene oxide or gamma irradiation.

Suture material can be classified as absorbable or non-absorbable, natural or synthetic. Absorbable suture from natural sources, such as catgut, is absorbed enzymatically. Absorbable suture from synthetic polymer sources is hydrolyzed. Sutures are absorbed at different rates. This is important since surgery may require a strong suture of long duration or a weak suture of short duration. Suture ½ life is described as the amount of time for the suture to lose ½ of its original tensile strength. Suture rate of absorbability and ½ life can be as short as a few days or more than a month. Suture ½ life is influenced by type of material, thread diameter, type of tissue, and general condition of the patient. Non absorbable materials used in oral surgery must be removed. This suture type includes natural materials such as silk, cotton, or steel and synthetic materials such as prolene, polypropylene, polyester, or nylon.

Another important characteristic of sutures is thread structure. Sutures can be considered monofilament or multifilament (usually braided). Monofilament sutures are comprised of one strand. Catgut is a monofilament suture. Monofilament sutures pass through tissue smoothly and are resistant to infection. However, monofilament sutures bend and crimp easily which can lead to breakage and loss of tensile strength. Multifilament suture consists of several strands braided or twisted together. This structure increases tensile strength, but increases the rate of infection and drag through tissue.

Multifilament sutures are can be coated to decrease drag when passing through tissue. Monofilament sutures and coated multifilament sutures make it easier to tie a surgical knot, but the knot is more likely to come untied. Coatings can also increase the ½ life of sutures. For example, coated chromic gut will maintain its integrity and strength longer than standard gut suture.

Suture thread is sized by numbers; the smaller the number, the larger the thread. The smallest suture is 10.0 which is the thickness of a human hair. The largest suture is 00 which may be as large as a fishing line. Oral surgery procedures usually require suture between 3.0 and 5.0. 3.0 sutures are most commonly used for impacted third molar flaps. 4.0 or 5.0 suture may be used to repair mucosal tears or to close vertical incisions.

Needles are selected based on size, type, and shape. Needle size can be tiny for ophthalmic procedures or huge for abdominal procedures. Most needles used in oral surgery are moderate in size. There are two fundamental types of suture needles; tapered or cutting. Tapered needles are used where tissue is easy to penetrate such as bowel or blood vessels. These needles are round in cross section and taper to a point. Cutting needles are triangular in cross section which makes it easier to penetrate tough tissue with less trauma. Cutting needles are either conventional cutting or reverse cutting. The apex of conventional cutting needle triangle is on the inside, concave, surface of the needle. Reverse cutting needles are similar to a conventional cutting needle, but the triangle apex is on the outside, convex, surface of the needle. Reverse cutting needles, often used in oral surgery, decrease the chance of sutures tearing tissue and pulling through the incision edge. (See Figures 4.36a, 4.36b, and 4.36c.)

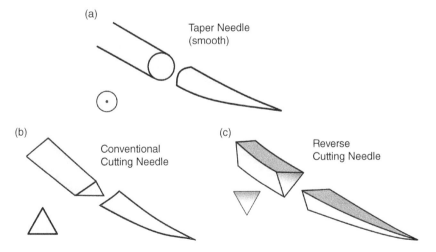

Figure 4.36 (a) Tapered needle. (b) Conventional cutting needle. (c) Reverse cutting needle. Drawings by Michael Brooks.

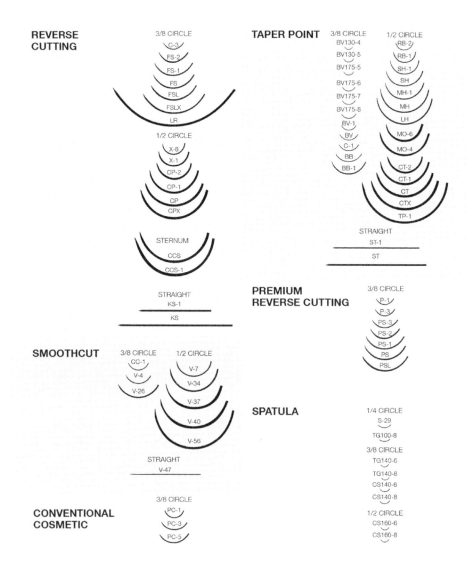

REVERSE CUTTING

3/8 CIRCLE
C-3
FS-2
FS-1
FS
FSL
FSLX
LR

1/2 CIRCLE
X-8
X-1
CP-2
CP-1
CP
CPX

STERNUM
CCS
CCS-1

STRAIGHT
KS-1
KS

SMOOTHCUT

3/8 CIRCLE
CC-1
V-4
V-26

1/2 CIRCLE
V-7
V-34
V-37
V-40
V-56

STRAIGHT
V-47

CONVENTIONAL COSMETIC

3/8 CIRCLE
PC-1
PC-3
PC-5

TAPER POINT

3/8 CIRCLE
BV130-4
BV130-5
BV175-5
BV175-6
BV175-7
BV175-8
BV-1
BV
C-1
BB
BB-1

1/2 CIRCLE
RB-2
RB-1
SH-1
SH
MH-1
MH
LH
MO-6
MO-4
CT-2
CT-1
CT
CTX
TP-1

STRAIGHT
ST-1
ST

PREMIUM REVERSE CUTTING

3/8 CIRCLE
P-1
P-3
PS-3
PS-2
PS-1
PS
PSL

SPATULA

1/4 CIRCLE
S-29
TG100-8

3/8 CIRCLE
TG140-6
TG140-8
CS140-6
CS140-8

1/2 CIRCLE
CS160-6
CS160-8

Figure 4.37 The 3/8 circle shape is normally used for third molar surgery.(See Figure 4.37) (Reproduced by permission of Riverpoint Medical).

Suture needles are available in many different shapes including straight and "fish hook" shape. However, most suture needles are partial circles ranging from ¼ circle to ½ circle. (See Figure 4.37.)

Although there are hundreds of suture and needle configurations, there are only a few possibilities for each surgical application. Flap design, access, and procedure dictate suture and needle choice when removing impacted third molars. Flaps created for the removal of impacted third molars are full thickness mucoperiosteal flaps with or without a releasing incision. Third molar sutures dissolve or are removed within 2 weeks. This timeline limits absorbable sutures to gut, rapid PGA, or other fast resorbing synthetic sutures. Silk is another option, but not a good choice due to patient non-compliance with appointments. Also, silk is often difficult to remove after third molar procedures due to limited access and patient sensitivity. Absorbable sutures are recommended.

Two surgical situations determine suture selection when removing impacted third molars.

1) Releasing incisions and the repair of mucosal tears determine needle and thread size. 5.0 suture is typically used to approximate edges of delicate oral mucosa. The thread diameter and friable tissue dictate a small, ½ circle, reverse cutting needle.
2) Full thickness mucoperiosteal flaps without releasing incisions or mucosal tears are typically closed with 3.0 suture thread and 19 mm, 3/8 circle, reverse cutting needle.

Experienced surgeons choose their favorite sutures based on flap design, procedure, absorbability, and handling characteristics. PGA suture is the author's favorite suture. It handles like silk and resorbs like gut.

Scalpel Blades

Scalpel blades are made of hardened and tempered steel, stainless steel, or high-carbon steel. Titanium blades are available for surgical procedures performed with MRI guidance. Scalpel blades are also made with zirconium nitride-coated edges to improve sharpness and edge retention. Other manufacture blades are polymer coated to enhance lubricity during a cut.

Scalpels consist of re-useable handles and disposable blades. Like sutures, scalpel blades come in many sizes and shapes. (See Figure 4.38.)

The choice of scalpel blade is based on the surgical procedure. There are dozens of scalpel blades designed for different surgical procedures. For example, the # 10 blade is a relatively large blade with a smooth curve used for skin incisions and abdominal surgery. The most common blades used for the removal of impacted third molars are the #12 and #15. (See Figure 4.39.)

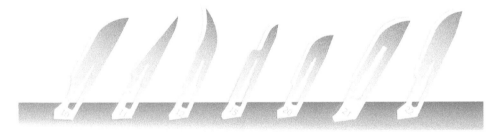

Figure 4.38   Scalpel blades are available in many sizes and shapes. (Reproduced by permission of Exel International).

Figure 4.39   #12 and #15 blades are commonly used when removing impacted third molars. (Reproduced by permission of Exel International).

The #12 blade is sometimes used for an incision distal to a maxillary second molar and tuberosity. The curved blade allows easy access to this area. The #15 blade is used for small, precise incisions and is ideal for most oral surgery procedures, including third molar removal.

Gauze

A fundamental premise in oral surgery is to prepare for complications and prevent them. The aspiration of root fragments, debris, or blood during exodontia can be prevented with gauze. Gauze used to prevent accidental aspiration or swallowing is variously known as a pharyngeal drape, screen, or throat pack.

Gauze should be placed in the pharynx, posterior to the tongue, during every exodontia procedure. 4×4, 8 ply, filled gauze, used in conjunction with a Weider retractor, protects the airway and throat. (See Figures 4.40 and 4.41.)

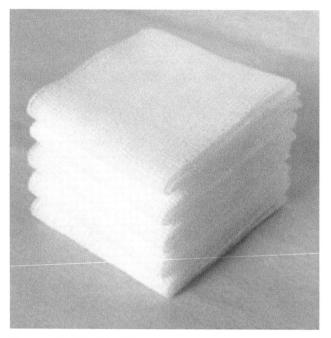

Figure 4.40 Filled 4 × 4 Gauze.

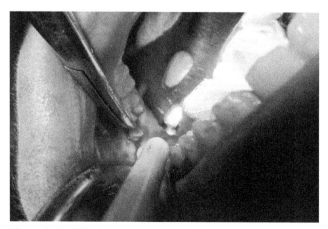

Figure 4.41 Filled gauze 4 × 4 pharyngeal screen.

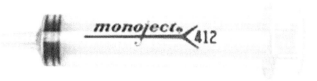

Figure 4.42   Irrigation syringes are used to irrigate the surgical site and flap.

Pharyngeal screens keep the surgical field dry and clean and increase visibility. This simple device should be part every dentist's exodontia algorithm.

Irrigation Syringe

Irrigation syringes are an essential part of any exodontia procedure. The flap should be thoroughly irrigated with sterile fluid to flush out debris. The extraction site should be suctioned and inspected following flap irrigation. The Monoject 412 syringe or similar syringe is recommended. These syringes can be sterilized without melting. (See Figure 4.42.) Irrigation is also needed to reduce heat from rotary instruments when removing bone or sectioning teeth.

Bloodborne Pathogen Standard

OSHA personal protective clothing regulations are specific and can be found in Section 1910 of the bloodborne pathogen standard.[22]

1) Provision. When there is occupational exposure, the employer shall provide, at no cost to the employee, gowns and lab coats. Personal protective equipment will be considered "appropriate" only if it does not permit blood or other potentially infectious materials to pass through to or reach the employee's work clothes, street clothes, undergarments, skin, eyes, mouth, or other mucous membranes under normal conditions of use and for the duration of time which the protective equipment will be used.

2) Use. The employer shall ensure that the employee uses appropriate personal protective equipment unless the employer shows that the employee temporarily and briefly declined to use personal protective equipment when, under rare and extraordinary circumstances, it was the employee's professional judgment that in the specific instance its use would have prevented the delivery of health care or public safety services or would have posed an increased hazard to the safety of the worker or co-worker. When the employee makes this judgment, the circumstances shall be investigated and documented in order to determine whether changes can be instituted to prevent such occurrences in the future.

3) Accessibility. The employer shall ensure that appropriate personal protective equipment in the appropriate sizes is readily accessible at the worksite or is issued to employees.

4) Cleaning, laundering, and disposal. The employer shall clean, launder, and dispose of required personal protective equipment at no cost to the employee.

5) Repair and replacement. The employer shall repair or replace personal protective equipment as needed to maintain its effectiveness, at no cost to the employee. The employer must pay for replacement PPE, except when the employee has lost or intentionally damaged the PPE.

6) Removal. If a garment(s) is penetrated by blood or other potentially infectious materials, the garment(s) shall be removed immediately or as soon as feasible. All personal protective equipment shall be removed prior to leaving the work area. When personal protective equipment is removed, it shall be placed in an appropriately designated area or container for storage, washing, decontamination, or disposal.

Personal protective equipment is especially important during surgical procedures. Removal of impacted third molars requires a mucoperiosteal flap, bone removal, and sectioning of teeth. These actions create an open wound that allows access of bacteria into a normally sterile blood stream and surgical site. The use of personal protective equipment minimizes the transfer of bacteria from the surgical team into the surgical site.

The workplace, equipment, instruments, and materials used to remove impacted third molars are an important consideration for every dentist. Workplace conditions affect the health of the patient and surgical team. Equipment, instruments, and materials affect procedure efficiency and surgical success.

References

1 HaEstrich C, Caruso T, Gruninger S, Pleva D. Musculoskeletal complaints among dental practitioners. *Occup Environ Med*. 2014;71(Suppl 1):A50.

2 ADA Professional Product Review. Ergonomics and dental practice: preventing work-related musculoskeletal problems. 2014 Nov 01.

3 Silverstein B. When to take action to reduce risk: work-related musculoskeletal disorders (lecture). Dental Ergonomics Summit 2000, ADA, Chicago.

4 Fisk JW. *Your painful neck & back*. London: Arrow, 1987.

5 Clark DJ. Operating microscopes and zero-defect dentistry, micro restorative dentistry. 2008, 37–42.

6 Mamoun J. Use of high-magnification loupes or surgical operating microscope when performing dental extractions. *N Y State Dent J*. 2013 Apr;79(3):28–33.

7 Schoeffl H, Lazzeri D, Schnelzer R, Froschauer SM, Huemer GM. Optical magnification should be mandatory for microsurgery: scientific basis and clinical data contributing to quality assurance. *Arch Plast Surg*. 2013 Mar;40(2):104–8.

8 Pencek L. Benefits of magnification in dental hygiene practice. *J Prac Hyg*. 1997;6(1):13–1.

9 Romeo U, Galanakis A, Lerario F, Daniele GM, Tenore G, Palaia G. Subcutaneous emphysema during third molar surgery: a case report. *Braz Dent J*. 2011;22(1):83–6.

10 Centers for Disease Control and Prevention. Personal protective equipment. http://www.cdc.gov/niosh/ppe. Accessed 2014 Feb 20.

11 CDC. Recommended infection-control practices for dentistry, 1993. *MMWR*. 1993;42(No.RR-8):(inclusive page numbers)

12 Johnson B. A life stolen early. People. 1990 Oct 22. Retrieved 2008 Dec 24.

13 Centers for Disease Control. Recommendations for prevention of HIV transmission in health-care settings. *MMWR*. 1987;36(suppl no. 2S):(inclusive page numbers).

14 Global Industry Analysts, Inc. Disposable medical gloves – a global strategic business report. 2014 Apr.

15 United States Department of Labor, Occupational Health and Safety Administration. Healthcare wide hazards, latex allergy, website. 2015.

16 Milt Hinsch–Technical Services Director, Regent Medical Surgical Services Management. Choosing gloves is a hands – on process. *Relias Media*. 2000 Apr;6(4):36–42.

17 Larson EL. APIC guideline for hand washing and hand antisepsis in health-care settings. *Am J Infect Control*. 1995;23:251–69.

18 MacIntyre CR, Chughtai AA. Facemasks for the prevention of infection in healthcare and community settings. *BMJ* (Clinical research ed). 2015 Apr 9;350:h694.

19 Ann SJ. Dental bioaerosol as an occupational hazard in a dentist's workplace. *Agric Environ Med.* 2007 Dec;14(2):203–7.

20 Brajkovi D, et al. Quality of analgesia after lower third molar surgery: a randomised, double-blind study of levobupivacaine, bupivacaine, and lidocaine with epinephrine. *Vojnosanit Pregl.* 2015;72(1):50–6.

21 Su N, et al. Efficacy and safety of bupivacaine versus lidocaine in dental treatments: a meta-analysis of randomised controlled trials. *Int Dent J.* 2014 Feb;64(1):34–45.

22 United States Department of Labor, Occupational Safety and Health Administration. Section 1910 of the bloodborne pathogen standar.

5

Surgical Principles and Techniques

The removal of impacted third molars can be predictable. A thorough knowledge of oral anatomy, proper case selection, and good surgical principles and techniques is necessary to avoid complications. This chapter will discuss surgical principles and techniques for the removal of impacted third molars.

Surgical Principles

Successful impacted third molar surgery follows fundamental surgical principles. Following these principles will increase success and decrease complications. The following list is a guide for surgical protocol.

1) **Preparation for surgery**
2) **Patient management**
3) **Speed and efficiency**
4) **Surgical access**
5) **Osteotomy and sectioning**
6) **Surgical site debridement**
7) **Soft tissue management**
8) **Postoperative care**

1) Preparation for surgery

Operating room sterility is required for hospital procedures. All surfaces are sterile and the surgical team is "scrubbed in" to the operating room. Even room air is exchanged periodically to reduce airborne microbes. Patients are pre-medicated and prepared for surgery well before the actual procedure. All instruments are sterile and equipment is ready for use. The anesthesiologist and surgeon have completed informed consent. The surgical team is a cohesive unit that follows established protocol. This pre-surgical routine is completed for every patient.

Preparation for the removal of impacted third molars is also important. The operatory, instruments, equipment, medication, and documentation should be ready prior to surgery. Preparation will decrease complications and increase surgical speed and efficiency.

Impacted Third Molars, Second Edition. Edited by John Wayland.
© 2024 John Wiley & Sons, Inc. Published 2024 by John Wiley & Sons, Inc.

Asepsis

There is debate regarding aseptic technique for in office oral surgery and exodontia. Several studies have shown that operating room asepsis is not necessary for minor in office oral surgery.[1] There are more than 10^{13} microbes on all surfaces of the body, yet the underlying tissues and the bloodstream are usually sterile. One study observed bacteremia in 55% of the patients after third-molar surgery.[2]

In spite of these findings, several studies have found no difference between clean and sterile conditions when used for minor in office surgery. (See Figure 5.1.)

Chui et al. completed a randomized prospective study to evaluate postoperative complication rates after mandibular third molar surgery performed with either sterile or clean gloves.

> The microbiological profiles of the tooth sockets and glove surfaces were also evaluated and compared. A total of 275 ASA I, non-smoking and non-drinking patients consented to be randomly assigned into two groups for lower wisdom tooth surgery, performed by operators wearing either sterile or clean gloves. All the patients returned for a post-operative assessment visit one week later. An additional 40 patients were recruited and randomized into the sterile glove group (n = 20) or the clean glove group (n = 20) for the microbiology study. Specimens were taken from the glove surfaces and the post-operative socket wounds during wisdom tooth surgery. This clinical trial showed no significant difference between the sterile and clean glove groups in the incidence of acute inflammation, acute infection, and dry sockets in the wounds. No single peri-operative factor had a statistically significant effect on post-operative pain intensity. Most of the bacterial isolates from the clean gloves were Gram-positive cocci or spore-forming bacilli. The total number of colony forming units and the variety of bacterial isolates from the socket wounds in the sterile and clean glove groups were similar.[3]

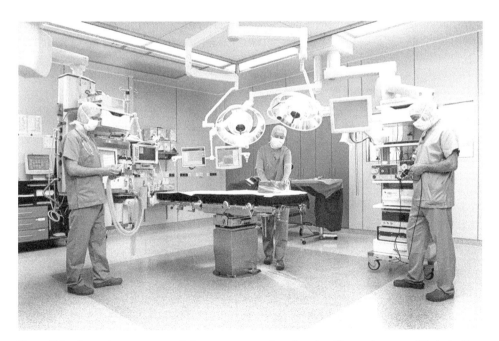

Figure 5.1 Operating room asepsis is not necessary for minor in office oral surgery. (Photo by Bureau of Labor Statistics, US Department of Labor, *Occupational Outlook Handbook, 2016–17 Edition*, Surgical Technologists).

The study concluded that there was no advantage in using sterile surgical gloves rather than clean gloves to minimize postoperative complications in third molar surgery. There was also no apparent relationship between the bacteria contaminating the clean glove surfaces and those isolated from the socket wounds.

Another study looked at success rates of osseointegration for implants placed under sterile versus clean conditions. A retrospective analysis was done comparing the success rate of osseointegration at stage 2 of implants placed under "sterile" versus "clean" conditions. "Sterile" surgery took place in an operating room setting with strict sterile protocol. "Clean" surgery took place in a clinic setting with the critical factor that nothing touched the surface of the implant until it contacted the prepared bone site. A total of 273 implants in 61 cases were placed under sterile conditions with a fixture success rate of 98.9% and a case success rate of 95.1%; 113 implants were placed under clean conditions in 31 cases with a fixture and case success rate of 98.2% and 93.5%, respectively as judged clinically at stage 2. The difference in the success rates was not statistically significant. The results of this analysis indicate that implant surgery can be performed under both "sterile" and "clean" conditions to achieve the same high rate of clinical osseointegration.[4]

A third prospective study suggested that routine exodontia can be safely performed by a surgeon wearing non-sterile, but surgically clean, gloves without increasing the risk of postoperative infection. One hundred twenty-four patients, who showed no clinical evidence of acute infection, were not taking antibiotics, and were to undergo routine removal of erupted teeth were studied. Patients were alternately assigned to surgeons who were wearing sterile or clean gloves. Surgery was performed in the usual manner and no postoperative antibiotics were prescribed. None of the patients was found to be infected postoperatively.[5]

A fourth study looked at clean vs sterile technique for pediatric dental patients in the operating room. Recommendations on the need for clean or sterile technique were made based on personal experience. This retrospective analysis of 100 children and adolescents who received dental treatment in the operating room showed no statistical difference in morbidity or postoperative complications between patients treated with clean or sterile operating room techniques.[6]

The author recommends a common sense approach to operatory asepsis when removing impacted third molars. All surfaces should be disinfected. Sterile gloves are recommended, but not required. The use of an over the patient surgical table, as mentioned in the previous chapter, is highly recommended. The work surface or table should be covered with a sterile drape. All instruments, equipment, suction, irrigation fluid, and gauze that make direct contact with the surgical site should be sterile.

A busy oral surgeon or general dentist may remove more than 100 impacted third molars per day. It is not practical or necessary to achieve hospital operating room asepsis for these procedures.[2,3,5] Wearing personal protective equipment, sterilizing all critical instruments, and following CDC disinfection guidelines is an evidence-based and logical approach to asepsis. The operatory should be in full compliance with the Centers for Disease Control (CDC) guidelines for infection control.

According to the CDC, dental instruments are classified into three categories depending on the risk of transmitting infection. The classifications of critical, semi-critical, and noncritical are based on the following criteria.

1) **Critical** instruments are those used to penetrate soft tissue or bone, or enter into or contact the bloodstream or other normally sterile tissue. They should be sterilized after each use. Sterilization is achieved by steam under pressure (autoclaving), dry heat, or heat/chemical vapor. Critical instruments include forceps, scalpels, bone chisels, scalers, and surgical burs.

2) **Semi-critical** instruments are those that do not penetrate soft tissues or bone but contact mucous membranes or non-intact skin, such as mirrors, reusable impression trays, and amalgam condensers. These devices also should be sterilized after each use. In some cases, however, sterilization

is not feasible and, therefore, high-level disinfection is appropriate. A high-level disinfectant is registered with the US Environmental Protection Agency (EPA) as a "sterilant/disinfectant" and must be labeled as such.

3) **Non-critical** instruments are those that come into contact only with intact skin such as external components of X-ray heads, blood pressure cuffs, and pulse oximeters. Such devices have a relatively low risk of transmitting infection; and, therefore, may be reprocessed between patients by intermediate-level or low-level disinfection. An intermediate-level disinfectant is EPA-registered as a "hospital disinfectant" and will be labeled for "tuberculocidal" activity (e.g., phenolics, iodophors, and chlorine-containing compounds). A low-level disinfectant is EPA-registered as a "hospital disinfectant" but is not labeled for "tuberculocidal" activity (e.g., quaternary ammonium compounds). The tuberculocidal claim is used as a benchmark to measure germicidal potency. Germicides labeled as "hospital disinfectant" without a tuberculocidal claim pass potency tests for activity against three representative microorganisms: *Pseudomonas aeruginosa*, *Staphylococcus aureus*, and *Salmonella choleraesuis*.

All critical instruments used to remove third molars must be sterile. These instruments include plastic irrigation syringes and surgical suction. The dental surgeon and surgical team should wear personal protective equipment including gowns, masks, and eye protection.

Antibiotics

Surgical preparation includes prescribing necessary antibiotics. Although the routine use of prophylactic antibiotics is controversial, a substantial number of studies have shown that the use of antibiotics decreases the incidence of alveolar osteitis; especially when bone is removed or the procedure is long or complicated.

Martin et al. reviewed the available literature regarding the use of prophylactic antibiotics for the removal of third molars. They found many studies that advocated or disapproved of the use of antibiotics in the removal of third molars. They concluded that there is no advantage in patients where bone removal is not required.[7]

A second study by Arora et al. found no statistically significant difference between the test group and the control group with regard to erythema, dehiscence, swelling, pain, trismus, and infection based on microbial load. The data were statistically significant for alveolar osteitis, with the occurrence of alveolar osteitis (14.58%) in the placebo group. They concluded that postoperative antibiotics are recommended only for patients undergoing contaminated, long-duration surgery.[8]

A third study found that antibiotics reduced the risk of AO and wound infection only when the first dose was given before surgery. They concluded that systemic antibiotics given before surgery were effective in reducing the frequencies of AO and wound infection after third molar surgery.[9]

The author routinely prescribes prophylactic antibiotics. The number of postoperative complications has been extremely low, far below published percentages. More than 35,000 impacted third molars have been removed resulting in 5 subperiosteal infections and 8 dry sockets. Most of the patients were under age 25.

Antiseptic Mouthwash

Preoperative antiseptic mouthwash (e.g., chlorhexidine) has been shown to decrease intraoral bacterial counts and alveolar osteitis. In order to show the effectiveness of preoperative antiseptic mouthwash Kosutic et al. undertook a prospective study in 120 patients who underwent elective surgery under general or local anesthesia. Patients were allocated to one of 4 groups, depending on whether the oral cavity was washed preoperatively with 1% cetrimide, chlorhexidine, povidon-iodine or sterilized normal saline solution (control group). Aerobic and anaerobic bacterial samples were taken from the inferior vestibular mucosa before surgery, 5 min after the start of the operation, and at the end of the procedure. The results show a statistically significant reduction in bacterial counts during procedures in which antiseptics were used to wash the oral cavity preoperatively; 1% cetrimide solution was the most successful in reducing intraoral bacterial counts and produced the longest-lasting antiseptic effect. Chlorhexidine is a good option for procedures longer than 1 hour, while povidon-iodine is recommended for procedures lasting up to 1 hour. Normal saline rinse reduced bacterial counts in the specimen taken 5 min after washing but this short-lasting effect was due to mechanical cleansing rather than the antiseptic effect.[10]

Another study published in the *Journal of Maxillofacial Oral Surgery* found the incidence of alveolar osteitis was 8% when patients did not use 0.2% chlorhexidine gluconate rinse perioperatively.[11] The incidence of AO was reduced significantly by using 0.2% chlorhexidine gluconate mouth rinse twice daily, 1 day before and 7 days after the surgical extraction of impacted mandibular third molars.

Pain Medication

There is evidence that nonsteroidal anti-inflammatory drugs (NSAIDS) combined with acetaminophen are more effective in controlling acute pain than narcotics. Hersh et al. found the combination of ibuprofen and acetaminophen works better than the combination of an opioid drug and acetaminophen. Furthermore, the ibuprofen and acetaminophen combination was safer than combinations that include opioids. The combination may work best when administered prior to the start of surgery.[12]

Documentation

All forms, including medical history and consent forms, should be completed prior to seating the patient. The patient's vital signs should be recorded and entered in the patient's record. Informed consent should be completed with the patient prior to administering medication.

2) **Patient management**

A successful surgical procedure requires the cooperation of the patient. Ideally, the patient will not move during the procedure. A cooperative patient improves efficiency, speed, and the quality of surgery. Select patients can have their third molars successfully removed with local anesthesia. Many factors must be considered when determining if local anesthetic without sedation is appropriate.

- Patient anxiety
- Difficult local anesthesia
- Difficult procedure
- Dentist
- proficiency

A study was completed by Aznar-Arasa et al. to determine if patient anxiety influences the difficulty of impacted lower third molar removal. A total of 102 extractions done under local anesthesia were assessed. The study found that impacted lower third molar extraction is significantly more difficult in anxious patients.[13]

Patients with high anxiety are not good candidates for local anesthetic without sedation. The removal of impacted third molars often requires significant pressure which will be unacceptable for the anxious patient. Constant management of the patient demands the dentist's attention. Surgical complications are more likely to occur.

Patients who are "difficult to numb" may need sedation or general anesthesia. The difficult to numb patient may have aberrant nerve pathways, low pain thresholds, or psychological issues such as dental phobias.

The difficulty of the procedure and dentist's proficiency are important factors when deciding if sedation is necessary. Difficult surgeries and inexperienced dentists will increase appointment length. Patients may become less cooperative during long procedures. These surgeries may require additional local anesthetic, sedation, or general anesthesia.

Sedation combined with local anesthetic is recommended for most impacted third molar patients. Local anesthetic alone should be reserved for cooperative patients and predictable surgeries.

Please see Chapter 12 for a detailed discussion of patient management.

3) **Efficiency and speed**

Efficiency and speed can increase office production and improve surgical results. Many studies have shown that long surgical procedures result in increased complications and delayed healing. Bello et al. studied 120 patients with an age range of 19–42 years. Operation time was determined by the time lapse between incision and completion of suturing. The study concluded that increasing operating time and advancing age are associated with more postoperative morbidity.[14]

Daley et al. found that the duration of an operation correlates with complications and time longer than a statewide established standard carries higher risk. To reduce risk of complications, study data supports expeditious surgical technique.[15]

The coordinated efforts of the surgical team can make an impressive difference in efficiency and speed. The steps required for the removal of impacted third molars should be completed in sequence for every patient. Instruments should be arranged in the order of use on the surgical table. The orderly sequence of events is a key factor in efficiency and predictability. Surgical assistants cannot be efficient when procedures are completed in a haphazard manner.

A real-life example will illustrate efficiency. This dental team actually exists. The office is designed for the efficient removal of third molars. Three rooms are equipped with high torque, straight surgical drills, surgical tables, and a very competent surgical assistant.

GP dentist, Dr. X, has removed more than 200,000 third molars. Dr. X is very proficient at removing impacted third molars. There is no wasted motion. Patients are sedated. Retractors are used to improve access and visibility. A surgical table is placed over the patient. Instruments are inches from the patient's mouth. All instruments are quickly and efficiently passed to Dr. X without discussion.

A nurse anesthetist prepares each patient ahead of Dr. X. The anesthetist has more than 30 years of experience. Patients are sedated in a safe and predictable manner. Local anesthetic is provided in each quadrant. We will begin this example with patients seated in all three rooms.

Dr. X has just completed the removal of four third molars in room 1 with the anesthetist. The surgical assistant provides postoperative instructions, dismisses the patient, prepares the operatory, and seats the next patient. After completing surgery in room 1, Dr. X completes informed consent in room 3 while the patient in room 2 is sedated by the nurse anesthetist.

Dr. X then removes four third molars in room 2 with the anesthetist. The surgical assistant provides postoperative instructions, dismisses the patient, prepares the operatory, and seats the next patient. After completing surgery in room 2, Dr. X completes informed consent in room 1 while the patient in room 3 is sedated by the nurse anesthetist.

Dr. X then removes four third molars in room 3 with the anesthetist. The surgical assistant provides postoperative instructions, dismisses the patient, prepares the operatory, and seats the next patient. After completing surgery in room 3, Dr. X completes informed consent in room 2 while the patient in room 1 is sedated by the nurse anesthetist.

This organized sequence of events continues throughout the day. Dr. X removes about 120 third molars per day, 4 every 15 minutes. He works two days a week. Very few oral surgeons remove 120 third molars in a day. However, the Dr. X example clearly illustrates how organization and teamwork can increase productivity and procedure speed while decreasing complications.

4) **Surgical access**

Surgical incisions should be as conservative as possible while providing unobstructed access and vision for the surgeon. This fundamental principle is especially important when removing impacted third molars. Many factors affect surgical access and vision in the oral cavity.

- Surgical site
- Mucosa
- Saliva
- Coronoid process
- Tongue

Third molars are located in the posterior portion of the mouth. Access requires a vertical releasing incision or a large envelope flap to gain access and vision. Mucosa is difficult to handle and usually requires a small needle and suture to close. Alternatively, a large envelop flap can be used to gain access. The large envelop flap is usually closed with 3.0 suture.

Saliva can be viscous or watery. Watery saliva tends to increase the flow of blood requiring constant suction to maintain good vision. A dry mouth with viscous saliva is preferable to watery saliva.

The coronoid process can be particularly troublesome when removing maxillary third molars. The coronoid process can press against the maxillary alveolus when the mouth is opened wide. This may make surgical access very difficult. In this case a large envelope flap may be needed.

Patients may have a large, active tongue combined with a small alveolus. The tongue may actually cover the mandibular posterior teeth. A Weider retractor is recommended to retract the tongue and isolate the surgical site.

5) **Osteotomy and sectioning**

The removal of bone and sectioning of third molars allows access for instruments and elevation of the third molar. Straight oral surgery drills, either compressed gas or electric, should be used to remove impacted third molars. Surgical drills have several advantages over restorative handpieces when used to remove bone and section third molars: (1) Efficient cutting (2) Decreased heat (3) Decreased vibration 4) Rear exhaust. Oral surgery drills are designed to address the limitations of the restorative handpiece. (See Table 5.1.)

Table 5.1   Surgical drill advantage compared to restorative handpiece.

Characteristic	Restorative handpiece	Compressed Gas	Electric handpiece
Efficient cutting	No	Yes	Yes
Decreased vibration	No	Yes	Yes
Decreased heat	No	Yes	Yes
Rear exhaust	No	Yes	Yes

The removal of impacted third molars requires cutting bone and sectioning teeth. Cutting efficiency is a balance between the speed and torque delivered to the bur. Air driven restorative handpieces run at 400,000 to 500,000 rpm. Pneumatic (gas driven) and electric handpieces operate between 60,000 and 100,000 rpm, but their torque is much higher than restorative handpieces. Torque is more applicable to how efficient a handpiece will be than speed. Drills designed specifically for use in oral surgery offer smooth, constant torque that does not vary as the bur meets resistance. High torque results in more cutting efficiency and less heat at the bone bur interface.

Several studies have shown that increased heat from drills can cause bone necrosis.[16] One study measured bone temperature rise during drilling of bovine cortical bone specimens. A straight surgical drill (Stryker-100) was fitted with a custom-designed speedometer for monitoring the rotational speed during the drilling, and the drill was mounted on a specially constructed drill press. The tests were conducted at variable speeds (20,000–100,000 rpm) and at different constant forces (1.5–9.0 N). The results revealed that the temperature rise and the duration of temperature elevation decreased with speed and force, suggesting that drilling at high speed and with large load is desirable. High torque (larger load) can only be accomplished with a straight surgical handpiece.

In a second study, Augustin et al. found that, during the drilling of bone, temperature could increase above 47 degrees C and cause irreversible osteonecrosis. The aim of the study was to find an optimal condition where the increase in bone temperature during bone drilling process would be minimal. The study concluded that for all combinations of parameters used, external irrigation maintained the bone temperature below 47 degrees C. External irrigation was the most important cooling factor.[17]

Most oral surgeons use straight surgical handpieces, which are either electric or driven by nitrogen gas which exhausts to the rear. Straight surgical handpieces use a long surgical bur; typically, 44 mm to 70 mm in length. The added length, with more bur shank in the straight drill chuck, creates higher torque and a more concentric bur rotation that results in less vibration and heat. The use of electric or pneumatic straight handpieces eliminates the possibility of subcutaneous air emphysema.

Although uncommon, subcutaneous air emphysema has been reported in both the medical and dental literature. This condition can be minor or life threatening. It is often the result of trauma such as stabbings, gunshot wounds, or car accidents. It has been reported in root canal treatment, dental restorations, ultrasonic scalers, standard dental air-water syringes, and extraction of maxillary and mandibular teeth. "The most common cause of subcutaneous air emphysema involves the surgical extraction of mandibular third molars. It is a result of air under pressure being driven into the subcutaneous tissues in the head and neck. It is generally associated with the use of a high-speed, air-driven, restorative handpiece which allows air to be vented toward the bur. This air under pressure can get into the subcutaneous tissues when either a flap is reflected or the gingival attachment to the alveolus is compromised. Air is forced beneath the soft tissue and subcutaneous air emphysema results."[18]

One alternative to the straight surgical handpiece is the high-speed surgical handpiece. The Impact Air 45 and Sabra OMS45 are similar to a restorative handpiece, but have higher torque and rear exhaust. They are available with fiberoptics and connect to the standard dental unit. These surgical handpieces are a good choice for the general dentist who seldom removes impacted third molars.

The use of a surgical drill is a fundamental surgical principle when removing impacted third molars. Efficient bone removal with irrigation reduces vibration, heat, and bone necrosis. Surgical drills eliminate the possibility of subcutaneous air emphysema.

6) **Surgical site debridement**

Surgical site debridement can prevent infection and improve healing,[19,20] The socket should be gently irrigated with sterile saline following the removal of the impacted third molar. A small surgical suction allows for close inspection of the surgical site and removal of small particles of bone and tooth. The socket walls should be gently curetted to remove loose bone, tooth remnants, and soft tissue.

Aggressive use of the surgical curette in a mandibular third molar socket could damage nearby structures such as the fragile lingual plate, inferior alveolar nerve, or lingual nerve. The thin bone of the maxillary sinus floor can be damaged creating an opening into the sinus. Any sharp bony edges around the socket should be smoothed using a bone file, #9 periosteal elevator, or rongeur. Soft tissue flaps accumulate debris from troughing and sectioning. All debris must be removed from flaps to prevent subperiosteal infections. Forceful irrigation between the flap and lateral border of the mandible is required to flush out debris. Irrigation is followed by close inspection and suctioning of the flap bone interface to remove all debris. (See Figure 5.2.)

Contrary to aggressive flap irrigation, studies have shown that aggressive irrigation of the extraction socket can impede healing and cause alveolar osteitis. Tolstunov evaluated the role of socket irrigation with normal saline on the development of alveolar osteitis after the removal of impacted mandibular third molars.[21] The study was conducted as a split mouth study. One side was irrigated with normal saline; the opposite side received no irrigation. The study found a "noticeable difference of dry socket syndromes (77.8% on the irrigated versus 22.2% on non-irrigated side) between the traditional extraction protocol versus the modified approach without the end-of-surgery irrigation. The study demonstrated that the post-extraction socket bleeding is very important for proper uncomplicated socket healing. If it's not washed away with irrigation solution at the end of extraction, the normal blood clot has a higher likelihood to form, and therefore, can potentially lead to an uncomplicated socket healing without development of alveolar osteitis. Socket bleeding at the extraction site creates a favorable environment for the formation of a blood clot, a protective dressing, necessary for a favorable osseous healing of the socket." Gentle irrigation of post extraction sockets is recommended.

7) **Soft tissue management**

Most dentists have experienced frustration while attempting to remove a fractured tooth after breaking off the clinical crown. The constant and prolonged effort to remove the tooth fragment is a nightmare for both the dental surgeon and patient. The use of soft tissue flaps in exodontia can facilitate the removal of teeth and decrease trauma for the patient. Many flap designs have been proposed for the removal of impacted third molars. All of the designs have certain principles in common.

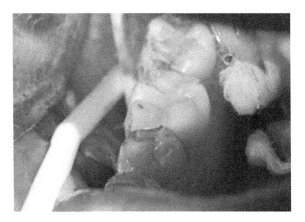

Figure 5.2 Inspection of flap following irrigation.

All flaps should have a broad base which assures a good blood supply to the flap margins. The flap should be tension free and large enough to provide access to the surgical site. A tension free flap prevents accidental tearing of delicate tissue. A large flap heals as fast as a small flap and prevents surgical errors resulting from poor access and vision. Non-tension closure of soft tissue flaps is a universally accepted surgical principle. However, primary vs secondary flap closure is controversial.

Silverstein et al. stated in the *Journal of Oral Implantology*, "Establishing non-tension primary wound closure of various soft tissue flaps is paramount for optimal postsurgical wound healing. Surgical procedures that require clinical flap manipulation, such as those used with traditional periodontal therapy, periodontal plastic cosmetic surgery, hard and soft tissue regeneration, and the excision of pathologic tissue, also require excellence in execution."[22]

Primary closure may not be the best choice in every case. Several studies have found that secondary closure improves wound healing following the removal of impacted third molars when compared to primary closure. The findings of one study suggest that the procedure of choice after removal of impacted mandibular third molars is a secondary closure and healing by secondary intention. The research concluded that secondary closure appears to minimize post extraction swelling, pain, and trismus and thus contributes to enhanced patient comfort.[23]

Jay Reznick, DDS, MD, maxillofacial surgeon, advocates one suture between the first and second molars. The incision distal to second molars is left open to drain.[24] The author has used full thickness envelope flaps with distal wedge for more than 30 years. One suture is placed distal to the second molar. The flaps heal by secondary intention. Swelling, pain, and trismus are usually minimal or gone one week following surgery. These results are consistent with many of those reported in the literature.

8) **Postoperative care**

A review of surgical principles would not be complete without discussing postoperative care. The importance of comprehensive postoperative instructions cannot be overstated. Instructions must be reviewed orally with the patient, parent, or guardian. The postsurgical review increases compliance and reduces postoperative complications. Translation may be required when English is a second language.

Patients sedated during the removal of third molars require special postoperative attention. Many drugs used in oral and IV sedation have prolonged clearance from the body. For example, diazepam has a half-life of up to 96 h in elderly patients.[25] Compliance with postoperative instructions may be negatively affected for these patients. Follow up phone calls are recommended to review instructions and assure compliance.

Surgical sites should remain undisturbed for at least 24 hours. Initial healing begins with coagulation of blood and a blood clot within the socket. Rinsing, spitting, or drinking through a straw should be avoided. Patients should be cautioned to not chew food, brush their teeth, or touch the area of surgery for 24 hours.

Patients should not be discharged until bleeding is controlled. Most patients presenting for the removal of third molars know if they have a bleeding disorder. However, postoperative complaints of excessive bleeding should be taken seriously. The author has had one patient with an undiagnosed bleeding disorder. This case clearly illustrates the need for patient follow-up and monitoring; especially, when bleeding is excessive.

A healthy 16-year-old male, with an unremarkable medical history, presented for the removal of four impacted third molars. The procedure was uneventful and postoperative bleeding appeared normal. The patient was discharged in the custody of his father.

At 8 pm the father called complaining of excessive bleeding. Instructions were given to bite on a moist tea bag, avoid unnecessary movement, and call again in 2 hours if there was no improvement. Another call was received at 10 pm reporting no improvement. The patient was advised to drink lots of fluids and report to the emergency room if he developed symptoms of hypovolemia.

The next morning the patient was seen in my office. Bleeding was still excessive. He was referred to the emergency room and subsequently admitted to the hospital where he was diagnosed with Von Willebrand's disease.

A follow-up phone call the evening of surgery can reduce the number and severity of complications. Reinforcement of proper home care increases compliance with postoperative instructions. Patients often have questions that they forgot to ask at their appointment. How much bleeding is normal? How long should the numb sensation last? When should the swelling go away? Patients should have a postoperative appointment to check for normal healing.

The surgical principles discussed in this chapter are general guidelines for success. Following these fundamental principles will streamline your procedures and help to avoid complications.

Surgical Technique

There is no universally accepted technique for the removal of impacted third molars. Schools in Great Britain advocate a lingual approach for removal while US schools tend to favor a buccal approach. Toughing bone and sectioning teeth can be accomplished with a round bur, fissure bur, or Lindemann bone cutting bur. (See Figures 5.3a, 5.3b, and 5.3c.)

Third molars are usually sectioned with a surgical drill, but some operators still prefer mallet and chisel. The management of soft tissue is extremely variable. Many flap designs exist that use various incisions. Wound closure can be primary with several sutures or secondary with no sutures.

The remainder of this chapter reviews various surgical techniques used for the removal of impacted third molars. A technique is recommended based on a review of the literature and the authors 35 years of experience.

Mandibular Third Molars

The removal of mandibular impacted third molars can be separated into 7 steps.

1) **Flap**
2) **Trough**
3) **Section**

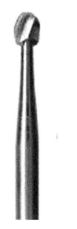
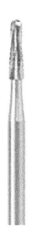
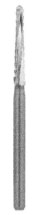

Figure 5.3a   Round.   Figure 5.3b   Fissure.   Figure 5.3c   Lindemann.

4) **Split**
5) **Delivery**
6) **Debridement**
7) **Closure**

1) FLAP

All third molar flaps are designed to separate periosteum from the underlying bone to gain surgical site access. Many flap designs and incisions have been used to remove mandibular impacted third molars. (See Figures 5.4a, 5.4b, 5.4c, and 5.4d) Regardless of design, all third molar flaps should be full thickness with a broad base.

Many studies have been completed to determine the best flap design for the removal of impacted mandibular third molars. The majority of these studies found no difference in postoperative healing among different designs.

Sulieman evaluated four flap designs for postoperative pain, swelling, and trismus. Sixty patients were divided into four groups based on flap design; envelope flap, triangular, modified triangular, and S-flap. Pain and swelling were evaluated subjectively while trismus was evaluated by measuring the maximum mouth opening ability (in mm) between the right upper and right lower central incisors. No significant difference was found on the postoperative sequela among the four groups.[26]

A second study compared the two most commonly used flap designs, envelope and triangular, to evaluate periodontal healing and postoperative complications. Twenty-four mandibular third molars were extracted from 12 patients with an average age of 16 years. Patients were included in the study when radiographs at the time of surgery showed that only the crown of the germ was formed. Each patient underwent 2 extractions, using a triangular flap on one side and an envelope flap on the other. Periodontal probing was recorded at the preoperative visit, and 7 days, 3 months, and 6 months after extraction. Postoperative complications were recorded using a questionnaire completed by the patient for the week after the extraction.

The examination performed 7 days after extractions demonstrated a deeper probing depth in all teeth examined. This increase was statistically greater for the first and second molars when an envelope flap was used. However, after 3 months, the probing depths returned to preoperative values. No significant differences were seen between the 2 flap designs when postoperative complications were considered.[27]

The author prefers large envelope flaps. (See Figure 5.5) Owing to the broad base, blood supply is excellent and the design facilitates easy closure and repositioning. Envelope flaps, completed efficiently with one incision and suture, decrease surgical time and swelling. Large envelope flaps improve access and visibility and heal as fast as small flaps. Small, "conservative," flaps that require multiple incisions and/or sutures may actually increase swelling due to increased surgical time.[14,15]

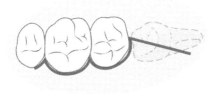

Figure 5.4a   Envelope.

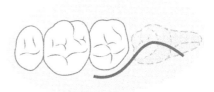

Figure 5.4b   S Shape.

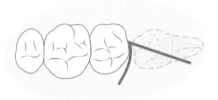

Figure 5.4c   Triangle.

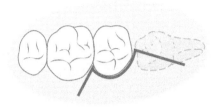

Figure 5.4d   Modified Triangle.

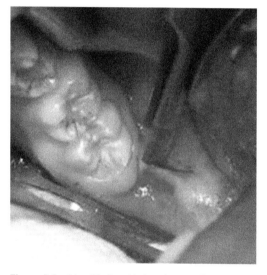

Figure 5.5   Mandibular third molar envelope flap incision.

The S flap is useful when orthodontic patients have arch wires and brackets. This flap is completed with an incision below the mucogingival junction for mandibular third molars. The mucosa is then elevated away from bone. Papillae are not elevated as is done with the envelope flap. This flap design avoids arch wires and brackets. A triangular flap is recommended for ortho patient's maxillary third molars.

The initial incision for a mandibular envelope starts 1–1.5 cm distal to the second molar and ends near the central groove of the second molar. The incision starts on the buccal near the external oblique ridge and can be extended as needed for access. DO NOT place incisions directly distal to the second molar. Never place incisions or use instruments on the lingual of the surgical site. You may cause lingual nerve paresthesia. (See Figures 5.7a and 5.7b.) Maxillary envelope flap incisions start in the hamular notch distal to the tuberosity and end between the central groove and distal buccal cusp of the second molar. Mandibular and maxillary envelope flaps should end distal to the second premolar. The papilla between first molar and second premolar is included in the flap.

The scalpel blade stays on bone throughout the incision. The incision should be completed in one smooth stroke to create a flap with clean edges. A #9 periosteal elevator is used to open the flap. (See Figure 5.6.)

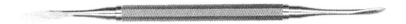

Figure 5.6   # 9 Periosteal elevator.

The small end of the elevator is used to elevate the papilla between second premolar and first molar, followed by elevating the papilla between the first molar, second molar, and the tissue distal to the second molar. The small end of the elevator is also used to elevate the flap beginning at the anterior portion of the flap and moving posterior. The large end of the elevator improves efficiency after the flap is started with the small end. The flap will open easily once dissected past the mucogingival junction. The flap should be passive, mobile, and allow the placement of a Minnesota retractor in the "pocket" created between the lateral surface of the mandible and the flap periosteum.

One significant advantage of the large envelope flap is the ability to place a Minnesota retractor in the "pocket" created between the lateral surface of the mandible and the flap. This technique, when combined with a Weider retractor on the lingual, isolates the surgical site and improves access and visibility. (See Figure 5.7.)

Another unique characteristic of the envelope flap is the ability to extend and enlarge the flap as needed. This is not possible when releasing incisions are used.

2) TROUGH

Full bony impactions and germectomies require removal of bone covering the impaction prior to creating a trough. This can be accomplished using a surgical drill and bur. The tooth location is determined after assessing a panoramic X-ray and patient arch form.

A buccal trough next to the impacted mandibular third molar creates space for elevators. (See 5.8 and 5.9.)

The trough is completed using a surgical drill and bur. The author recommends a 1703L bur. (See Figure 5.10.) The working end of the bur is 7.8 mm in length and 2.1 mm in diameter at the tip. The tip is rounded to facilitate smoothing bone.

The depth of the trough can be estimated using the 7.8 mm working end of the 1703L bur. When the junction of bur shank and working end is even with the crown CEJ, the bur tip is approximately 8 mm past the CEJ. The trough should be as deep possible without injuring the IAN. The IAN is almost invariably located laterally with respect to the roots of the third molar.[28] It's important to

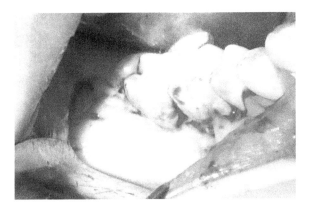

Figure 5.7   Minnesota retractor in flap "pocket".

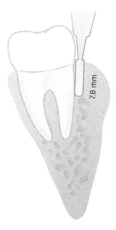

Figure 5.8 Troughing coronal view.

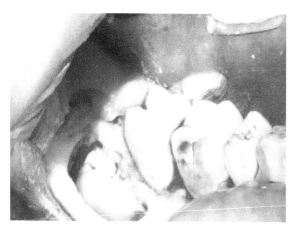

Figure 5.9 Trough complete.

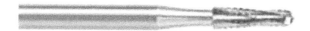

Figure 5.10 1703L surgical bur working end is 7.8 mm.

visualize the local anatomy in three dimensions. The depth and path of the trough will vary based on individual anatomy. This can be assessed with a quality digital panoramic film.

The trough allows for the placement of elevators and mobilization of the tooth. It should continue in a mesial direction to a point adjacent to the distal buccal line angle of the second molar. Bone surrounding the second molar is not removed. The mesial extension of the trough facilitates placement of instruments mesial to the impacted third molar. The ideal trough follows the course of the IAN; it is deeper on the mesial than on the distal. (See Figure 5.11a.) The triangular area mesial to mandibular third molar roots can be considered an IAN "safe zone." (See Figure 5.11b.)

The bur should "hug" the crown of the impacted third molar to preserve bone. The impacted tooth enamel will feel harder than the surrounding bone. This is especially true when using a

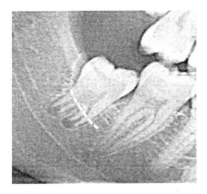
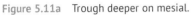
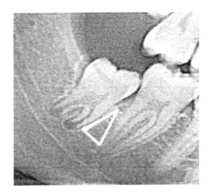

Figure 5.11a Trough deeper on mesial.   **Figure 5.11b** IAN "safe zone".

Table 5.2 Ideal trough characteristics and rationale.

Characteristic	Rationale
Deep as possible without injury to IAN	Access for instruments and tooth mobilization
Extends mesial to second molar	Allow mesial elevator access
Deeper on mesial than on distal	IAN is more apical on mesial
Close to tooth surface	Preserves bone
Extends past height of contour	Removes undercuts

straight, high torque, surgical drill. The trough should always extend apically past the impacted third molar height of contour to prevent undercuts. Ideally, the trough should have the characteristics shown in Table 5.2.

3) SECTION

Sectioning and troughing of mandibular third molars creates space and is best accomplished with the 1703L bur. Elevation of the entire tooth prior to sectioning mobilizes the tooth and decreases the chance of root fracture. The section should attempt to divide the tooth into mesial and distal halves. (See Figure 5.12.)

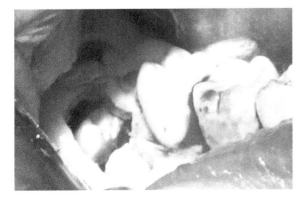

Figure 5.12 Section complete.

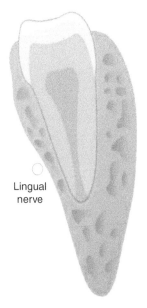

Figure 5.13 Cross section of the mandible and third molar.

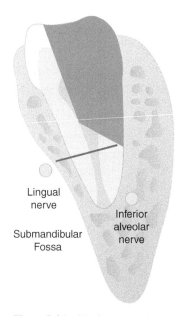

Figure 5.14 Ideal section shown in green.

A cross section of the mandible near the third molar reveals the submandibular fossa, a depression on the medial surface of the mandible, inferior to the mylohyoid muscle. (See Figure 5.13.) This concavity contains the submandibular salivary gland and may contain the lingual nerve. The lingual nerve enters the sublingual space by passing between the superior constrictor and mylohyoid muscles; at this location the nerve is immediately beneath the periosteum and at risk from trauma.

The horizontal section should cut approximately 2/3–3/4 through the tooth stopping short of the lingual plate.[28] (See Figure 5.14.) The green area in Figure 5.14 indicates a safe zone for sectioning. The red line indicates potential lingual nerve injury if the section is too deep on the lingual side of the tooth.

This is analogous to troughing deeper on the mesial than on the distal to avoid injury to the inferior alveolar nerve. It is important to visualize local anatomy in three dimensions to avoid nerve injury. Ideally, the section should have the characteristics shown in Table 5.3.

Third molar dimensions vary considerably; however, the buccolingual diameter of third molars is normally 9.5 mm–10.0 mm. Crown length is normally 6.5 mm–7.0 mm. (See Table 5.4) The 7.8 mm cutting surface of the bur can be used as a gauge to avoid vital structures when troughing and sectioning. In all cases of sectioning the cut should be kept within the tooth structure to prevent damage to the lingual tissues or the inferior alveolar canal.

4) SPLIT

An ideal section stops short of the lingual plate and inferior alveolar canal. The tooth is then "split" into separate segments. The split is usually accomplished with a straight elevator, such as an EL3CSM, or 46R. The tip of the elevator is placed deep into the section and rotated along its long axis. An audible "pop" is heard accompanied by tactile sensation when the tooth is divided into segments. (See Figure 5.15.)

5) DELIVERY

The EL3CSM and 46R elevators are commonly used for delivery. (See Figure 5.16) A Hu-Friedy EL3CSM luxating elevator is helpful when used on the straight buccal of vertical and distoangular impactions. The Cogswell B is recommended when purchase points are placed. The Cogswell B has smooth surfaces at the tip and is less likely to cause fracture than a Crane pick. The purchase point should be placed deep into substantial tooth structure to elevate the tooth segment without fracture. Excessive force can result in root fracture, unnecessary bone loss, or even fracture of the mandible. Adequate troughing and sectioning provide an unobstructed pathway for delivery. Multiple sections may be required.

Table 5.3   Ideal section characteristics and rationale.

Characteristic	Rationale
Divide tooth into mesial and distal halves	Equal halves are easier to remove
Extend to furcation	Section into individual roots
Lingual as possible without injury to LN	Avoid incomplete split
Deeper on buccal than on lingual	Avoid submandibular fossa and LN
More lingual occlusal direction (~3/4)	Avoid submandibular fossa and LN
Less lingual apical direction (~2/3)	

Table 5.4   Third molar crown length and diameter relative to 7.8 mm bur working end.

	Crown Length	Root Length	Crown MD	Diameter FL[+]	Curvature	
					M	D
Maxillary Teeth						
Central incisor	10.5	13.0	8.5	7.0	3.5	2.5
Lateral incisor	9.0	13.0	6.5	6.0	3.0	2.0
Canine	10.0	17.0	7.5	8.0	2.5	1.5
1st premolar	8.5	14.0	7.0	9.0	1.0	0.0
2nd premolar	8.5	14.0	7.0	9.0	1.0	0.0
First molar	7.5	B 12, L 13	10.0	11.0	1.0	0.0
Second molar	7.0	B 11 L 12	9.0	11.0	1.0	0.0
Third molar	6.5	11	8.5	10.0	1.0	0.0
Mandibular Teeth						
Central incisor	9.0	12.5	5.0	6.0	3.0	2.0
Lateral incisor	9.5	14.0	5.5	6.0	3.0	2.0
Canine	11.0	16.0	7.0	7.5	2.5	1.0
1st premolar	8.5	14.0	7.0	7.5	1.0	0.0
2nd premolar	8.0	14.5	7.0	8.0	1.0	0.0
First molar	7.5	14.0	11.0	10.5	1.0	0.0
Second molar	7.0	13.0	10.5	10.0	1.0	0.0
Third molar	7.0	11.0	10.5	9.5	1.0	0.0

* Average measurements in millimeters
÷ FL – faciolingual, buccolingual, labiolingual
Adapted from Ash MM, Nelson SJ: Wheeler's Dental Anatomy, Physiology. and Occlusion (8th edition). Philadelphia: WB Saunders, 2023.

6) DEBRIDEMENT

The surgical site must be thoroughly cleaned following the removal of third molars. This includes debridement of all particulate bone, tooth fragments, soft tissue, and follicle. Sharp or rough edges around the socket should be removed. This is accomplished with double ended surgical curettes,

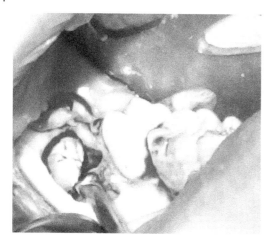

Figure 5.15   Split with 46R elevator.

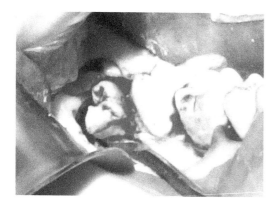

Figure 5.16   Elevator delivery with 46R.

2/4 molt curettes, bone files, burs, rongeurs, and Kelly hemostats. The socket is gently irrigated, suctioned, and inspected with magnification. (See Figures 5.17a and 5.17b.)

Debridement includes irrigation of the full thickness flap. Irrigation is completed with a Monoject 412 syringe and sterile saline. The passive flap is retracted and saline is injected with pressure between the lateral surface of the mandible and flap. The flap is suctioned and inspected with magnification and loupe light to assure that all debris has been removed. A small suction tip is necessary to reach the apical portion of the flap.

Meticulous debridement of the flap is necessary to avoid subperiosteal infections. Fifty percent of third molar postoperative infections are localized subperiosteal abscess-type infections occurring approximately 2–4 weeks after surgery.[29] This infection results from debris left in the flap following surgery. Healing is normal at one week followed by acute swelling 2–4 weeks after the procedure. Definitive treatment involves re-opening the flap, debridement, irrigation, and antibiotics.

7) CLOSURE

Primary closure of lower third molar surgical sites is controversial. Some surgeons are proponents of tight suturing to assist in hemostasis, whereas other surgeons believe that loose suturing leads to less edema and allows for drainage of the wound.[30]

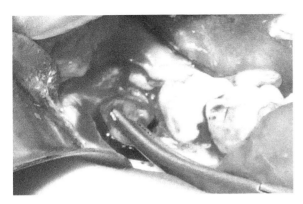

Figure 5.17a   Debridement of socket.

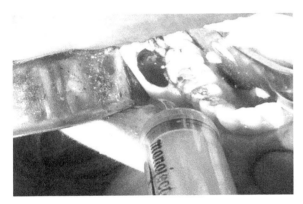

Figure 5.17b   Thorough irrigation of flap.

A study conducted in 2005 by Pasqualini et al. compared postoperative pain and swelling following removal of impacted mandibular third molars. Two hundred patients with impacted third molars were randomly divided into two groups of 100. Panoramic radiographs were taken to assess degree of eruption and angulation of third molars. Teeth were extracted, and in Group 1 the surgical site was closed by primary intention. In Group 2 a distal wedge of tissue was removed adjacent to the second molar to obtain secondary healing. Swelling and pain were evaluated for 7 days after surgery. Pain and swelling were less severe with secondary closure than with primary closure.[31]

A second study in 2012 found similar results. Chaudhary et al. studied the effects of primary vs secondary closure on pain and swelling following the removal of impacted mandibular third molars.[30] Twelve patients, under 30 years of age were divided into two groups. In Group A, closure was done by primary intention and in Group B, by secondary closure. A comparison between both groups was done with regards to postoperative pain and swelling. The study found that secondary closure is better than primary closure for removal of impacted mandibular third molar with regards to postoperative pain and swelling.

The author prefers an envelope flap with distal wedge and secondary closure using PGA suture. A simple interrupted suture can be placed just distal to the second molar. (See Figure 5.18.) Care must be taken to keep the suture needle from penetrating tissue below the level of the lingual alveolar bone. Penetrating the tissue below this level increases the risk of injury to the lingual nerve.[24]

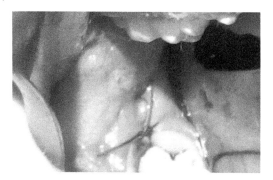

Figure 5.18   Single suture closure.

Mandibular third molar flaps can be closed with 3.0 silk or gut. Non absorbable silk sutures should not remain in place for more than a week due to increased risk of infection. Gut sutures normally resorb in three to five days, chromic gut in ten days. A third possibility is polyglycolic acid suture which handles like silk and resorbs in three to four weeks. In delicate non-keratinized mucosa, 5.0 suture with a small needle is preferred. 5.0 suture is recommended to close vertical releasing incisions or tears in the flap.

Proper flap closure requires that the suture needle is held approximately 2/3 of the way from the tip of the needle. Holding a 3.0 suture needle in this position allows the needle and suture to easily penetrate the flap's mobile buccal tissue and fixed lingual tissue in one pass. The tying technique is a double throw, followed by a locking throw in the opposite direction. Although non-absorbable silk sutures encourage patients to return for suture removal, some surgeons prefer sutures that will resorb if patients do not return. Pressure should be held on the repositioned flap for 10–15 seconds to adapt the soft tissue and papilla

Maxillary Third Molars

The removal of maxillary impacted third molars can be separated into 4 steps

1) **Flap**
2) **Delivery**
3) **Debridement**
4) **Closure**

1) FLAP

The maxillary third molar flap is similar to the mandibular third molar flap. A large envelope flap is recommended. The initial incision begins distal to the tuberosity near the hamular notch. A #12 scalpel blade improves access distal to the tuberosity. The incision ends between the second molar central groove and distobuccal cusp. The tip of the #12 scalpel blade should remain on bone during the incision. The papilla distal to the second premolar is included in the flap. (See Figures 5.19a and 5.19b.)

The flap is reflected with a # 9 periosteal elevator beyond the mucogingival junction. A Minnesota retractor is used to retract the flap. The flap will be easier to retract when incisions are made ending at the distobuccal cusp of the second molar. This is important when removing deep impactions.

Maxillary flap incisions distal to the second molar should be completed with caution. Incisions that are too far distal and buccal can expose the buccal fat pad. Exposure of the buccal fat pad results in fat extruding from the incision site and restricting vision. High volume suction should be

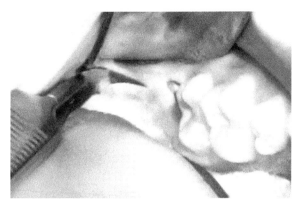

Figure 5.19a   #12 blade improves access.

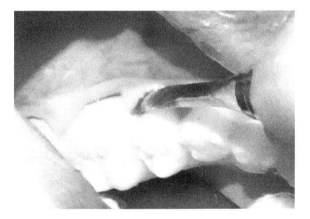

Figure 5.19b   Flap includes premolar papilla.

avoided to prevent further extrusion of the fat pad. Repositioning the buccal fat pad can be compared to replacing toothpaste into the toothpaste tube. Experienced surgeons may be able to work around the fat and complete the procedure.

Surgeons with limited experience should attempt to reposition the extruded fat as much as possible and abort the procedure. The surgical site usually heals without complications and the procedure can be attempted again when healing is complete. Sutures are usually not needed.

2) DELIVERY

Most impacted maxillary third molars can be easily removed with EL3CSM or 46R elevators. (See Figure 5.20)

Flag elevators are especially useful when access is limited. Examples include the 190/191, Woodward, Potts, or other paired elevators. A Minnesota retractor, periosteal elevator, or Laster retractor should be placed distal to the tuberosity to prevent displacement into the infratemporal fossa. (See Figures 5.21a and 5.21b.) The risk of this complication increases when the third molar is deep and palatal which is often the case with germectomies. Although rare, this is a serious complication due to the contents of the infratemporal fossa. The infratemporal fossa contains many vital structures including the pterygoid plexus, maxillary artery, and the mandibular nerve. Damage to these structures can affect function and may be fatal.

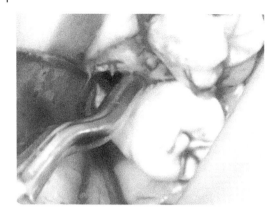

Figure 5.20   Delivery with 46R elevator.

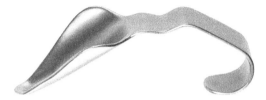

Figure 5.21a   Laster retractor.

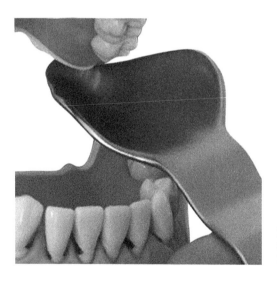

Figure 5.21b   Laster retractor in position.
(Reproduced with permission of Salvin Dental
Specialties Inc.).

The overlying bone in the maxilla is typically thin and can be removed with hand instruments such as a #9 periosteal elevator. The pointed end of the elevator is used to pry away buccal bone covering the tooth. (See Figures 5.22a and 5.22b.)

In some cases, a surgical drill may be required when maxillary third molars are in a palatal position or buccal bone is thick. The drill is used to create a shallow vertical groove in the buccal bone mesial to the third molar. The #9 periosteal elevator can be placed in the groove to remove buccal bone and gain access to the third molar. Once access is gained, an EL3CSM straight elevator, 46R elevator, 190/191 or similar instrument is used to deliver the tooth.

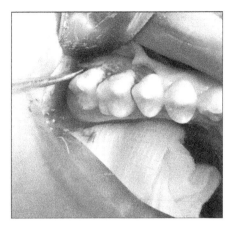

Figure 5.22a Removal of bone.

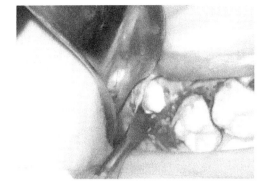

Figure 5.22b Removal of bone.

Delivery is usually easier in the maxilla than in the mandible for two reasons. First, the maxillary impaction is usually covered with thin cancellous bone when compared to the mandibular impaction. Second, the periodontal ligament space is wide because the impacted tooth has not experienced occlusal loading.[28] Due to these factors, sectioning is normally not required to remove a maxillary impaction. However, it should be noted that a difficult maxillary impaction is much more difficult than a difficult mandibular impaction due to limited access and vision.

Maxillary third molars with divergent roots or thick bone may require sectioning. This should be considered only as a last resort because small segments can be displaced into the sinus or infratemporal fossa.

3) DEBRIDEMENT

The surgical site should be thoroughly debrided with a surgical curette. All bone fragments and tissue should be removed from the socket. Sharp edges should be smoothed. The surgical site should be palpated to confirm that all sharp edges have been removed. Irrigation is not required unless a surgical drill was used. (See Figures 5.23a and 5.23b.)

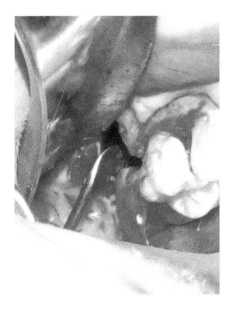

Figure 5.23a Removal of tissue with curette.

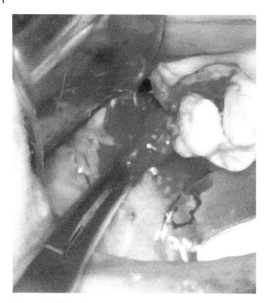

Figure 5.23b   Removal of tissue with hemostat.

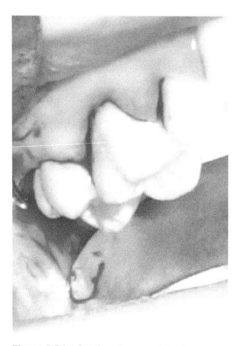

Figure 5.24   Passive closure without suture.

Horizontal

The crown of horizontal impactions is often "trapped" under the height of contour of the second molar. A straight surgical handpiece is used to section the crown. The objective is to remove the crown and create space for the subsequent removal of the roots. The sectioned crown must be

4) CLOSURE

Maxillary third molar envelope flaps usually do not require suturing because they are held in place by gravity, the coronoid process, and the surrounding soft tissues. Pressure should be held on the repositioned flap for 10–15 seconds to adapt the soft tissue and papilla. (See Figure 5.24.)

Angulations

The surgical technique used for the removal of impacted mandibular third molars is universal. However, individual angulations require minor modifications when sectioning and elevating.

Mesioangular

Mesioangular impactions usually offer good access for sectioning. A straight surgical handpiece is used to section the long axis of the tooth. The most common problem, when sectioning along the tooth's long axis, is not dividing the tooth into equal halves. This is caused by the second molar obstructing access and results in a section that is too far distal. The solution to this problem involves making the section 1–2 mm more mesial than originally planned. Sectioning more mesial is especially important when sectioning vertical and distoangular impactions.

When roots are divergent, the section should end near the furcation. The distal root is removed first after splitting the tooth through the furcation. The mesial root can be elevated distally into the available space. (See Figure 5.25.)

The removal of horizontal impactions by removing the tooth crown will be discussed in the next section. Horizontal impactions can also be removed with the mesioangular technique – by sectioning the long axis of the tooth. (See Figure 5.26.) This usually requires a second section of the mesial root before elevation.

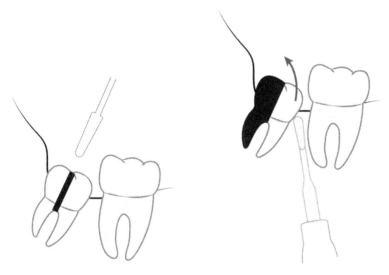

Figure 5.25 Technique for removal of mesioangular impaction.

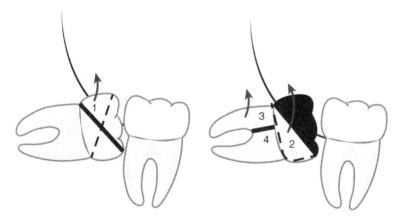

Figure 5.26 Horizontal section should be narrow apically and wide coronally (solid line).

narrower on the bottom than on the top to facilitate removal. (See Figure 5.25). Multiple crown sections are often required.

Following crown removal, remaining roots are moved mesial into the vacated space where they are easily removed. This is usually accomplished with a 190/191, Cryer elevator or similar flag elevator. A purchase point can be helpful. Divergent or hooked roots may require sectioning through the furcation. The distal root is removed followed by the mesial root.

Vertical

Deep vertical impactions always require sectioning. (See Figure 5.27.) A 50% section on the long axis of the tooth is usually not possible due to limited access. However, sectioning as close as possible to the long axis is the goal. This usually results in sectioning a distal portion of the tooth. A purchase point and Cogswell B may help to elevate the tooth until obstructions block further elevation. Repeated sections may be required as the tooth is slowly elevated from its socket. Avoid forces that move the tooth in a distal direction (See the Red Arrow Figure 5.27.)

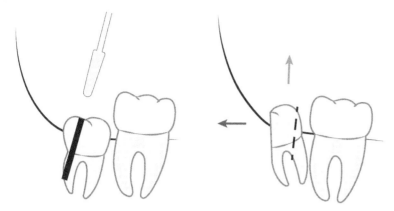

Figure 5.27 Deep vertical impactions usually require slow elevation and multiple sections.

Distoangular

Most distoangular impactions will be more difficult than expected. Sectioning always results in a less than ideal section. The steps required for removal of a distoangular impaction are very similar to the vertical impaction. (See Figure 5.27.) Removal of distal bone may be required while keeping in mind the possibility of lingual nerve injury.

Following the initial section, the tooth should be slowly elevated and sectioned repeatedly as needed. A purchase point and Cogswell B, or luxating elevator, can be used to move the tooth in a straight vertical direction (See the green arrow Figure 5.27). Removal of the crown followed by the roots may be necessary. Never remove the crown until the tooth is luxated and elevated.

Germectomy

There is little debate regarding the benefits of early third molars removal (Chapter 2). The removal of third molars prior to full root development, during the teenage years, is predictable and decreases surgical complications. Most surgeons agree that the ideal time to remove third molars is when the roots are 1/2–3/4 developed, usually in the later teenage years. Eruption follows the development of roots and can be seen as early as 13–14 years of age or as late as the third decade of life. The third molar crown is typically visible on radiographs by 14–15 years of age. (See Figure 5.28.)

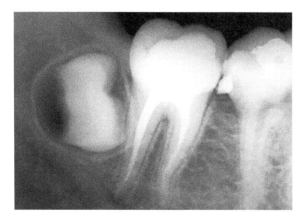

Figure 5.28 Third molar crown at 14–15 years of age.

Germectomy is defined as the removal of teeth with one third or less root development. The removal of third molars with little or no root development is controversial. Detractors argue against removal prior to root development for two reasons; the tooth has not erupted and is covered with bone and the tooth can "spin" or move in the bone crypt.

Advocates argue that removal of third molars as germectomies is predictable with fewer complications because roots have not developed. (See Table 5.5.) Dilacerated, divergent, or thin roots are no longer subject to fracture with displacement of fragments into the maxillary sinus, infratemporal fossa, or submandibular space. Modified technique for different tooth angulations is not necessary. The surgical technique is the same for all germectomies. Sinus openings are reduced and nerve injuries from third molar roots virtually eliminated. The developing tooth has a large follicular space which allows for easy placement of elevators and reduced force when elevating. The removal of third molars becomes routine and predictable.

Chiapasco et al. found no difference in the incidence of complications when removing third molars between ages 9–16 and 17–24.[32] The study included 1500 mandibular impactions for 868 patients aged 9 to 67 years. The patients were divided into three groups.

Group A, patients aged 9 to 16 including germectomies;

Group B, patients aged 17 to 24; and

Group C, patients older than 24.

The incidence of complications was 2.6% in group A, 2.8% in group B, and 7.4% in group C. All complications were temporary except in one instance of inferior alveolar nerve paresthesia that occurred in a group C patient. This study showed no significant difference in the complication rate between group A (including germectomies) and group B, but complications significantly increased in group C.

The germectomy procedure always requires a full thickness mucoperiosteal flap and bone removal. The steps to remove a mandibular third molar are nearly identical to partial or full bony impactions. The tooth germ is always sectioned and may require a second section in a mesial distal direction. The section creates a flat surface that prevents "spinning." Elevators are often unnecessary. The tooth fragments can be removed with cotton pliers or similar instruments. Maxillary germectomies can be problematic when they are in a deep Gregory Pell class C position. Maxillary germectomies in Gregory Pell A and B positions are easily removed with minimal force due to the large follicular space. One exception is the maxillary germectomy positioned near the palate. Extreme caution must be used when removing these teeth due to their proximity to the infratemporal fossa.

It is not always possible to remove impacted third molars at the ideal time when roots are 1/2–3/4 developed. Dentists proficient in the removal of impacted third molars should consider removal as germectomies when access and position is favorable.

Table 5.5 Removal of third molars at the germectomy stage of development has many advantages.

Germectomy Advantages		
Eliminates fractured roots	Eliminates divergent roots	Decreases sinus openings
Eliminates displaced roots	Eliminates tooth angulations	Increases follicular space
Eliminates dilacerated roots	Decreases nerve injury	Increases predictability

References

1 Li X, Kolltveit KM. Tronstad L, Olsen I. Systemic diseases caused by oral infection. *Clin Microbiol Rev.* 2000 Oct;13(4):547–58.

2 Heimdahl A, Hall G, Hedberg M, Sandberg H, Söder PO, Tunér K, Nord CE. Detection and quantitation by lysis-filtration of bacteremia after different oral surgical procedures. *J Clin Microbiol.* 1990 Oct;28(10):2205–9.

3 Chiu WK, et al. A comparison of post-operative complications following wisdom tooth surgery performed with sterile or clean gloves. *Int J Oral Maxillofac Surg.* 2006 Feb;35(2):174–9.

4 Scharf DR, Tarnow DP. Success rates of osseointegration for implants placed under sterile versus clean conditions. *J Periodontol.* 1993 Oct;64(10):954–6.

5 Giglio JA, Rowland RW, Laskin DM, Grenevicki L, Roland RW. The use of sterile versus nonsterile gloves during out-patient exodontia. *Quintessence Int.* 1993 Aug;24(8):543–5.

6 Helpin ML, Duncan WK. Clean vs sterile technique for pediatric dental patients in the operating room. *ASDC J Dent Child.* 1988 Nov-Dec;55(6):449–51.

7 Martin MV, Kanatas AN, Hardy P. Antibiotic prophylaxis and third molar surgery. *Br Dent J.* 2005;198:327–30.

8 Arora A, Roychoudhury A, Bhutia O, Pandey S, Singh S, Das BK. Antibiotics in third molar extraction; are they really necessary: a non-inferiority randomized controlled trial. *Natl J Maxillofac Surg.* 2014 Jul-Dec;5(2):166–71.

9 Ren Y-F, Malmstrom HS. Effectiveness of antibiotic prophylaxis in third molar surgery: a meta-analysis of randomized controlled clinical trials. *Oral Maxillofac Surg.* 2007 Oct;65(10):1909–21.

10 Kosutic D, Uglesic V, Perkovic D, Persic Z, Solman L, Lupi-Ferandin S, Knezevic P, Sokler K, Knezevic G. Preoperative antiseptics in clean/contaminated maxillofacial and oral surgery: prospective randomized study. *Int J Oral Maxillofac Surg.* 2009 Feb;38(2):160–5.

11 Sridhar V, Wali GG, Shyla HN. Evaluation of the perioperative use of 0.2% chlorhexidine gluconate for the prevention of alveolar osteitis after the extraction of impacted mandibular third molars: a clinical study. *J Maxillofac Oral Surg.* 2011 Jun;10(2):101–11.

12 Hersh EV, Moore PA. Combining ibuprofen and acetaminophen for acute pain management after third-molar extractions. *J Am Dent Assoc.* 2013 Aug 1;144:898–908.

13 Aznar-Arasa L, Figueiredo RL, Valmaseda-Castellón E, Gay-Escoda C. Patient anxiety and surgical difficulty in impacted lower third molar extractions: a prospective cohort study. *Int J Oral Maxillofac Surg.* 2014 Sept;43(9):113–16.

14 Bello SA, Adeyemo WL, Bamgbose BO, Obi EV, Adeyinka AA. Effect of age, impaction types and operative time on inflammatory tissue reactions following lower third molar surgery. *Head Face Med.* 2011;7:8.

15 Daley BJ, Cecil W, Clarke P, Cofer JB, Guillamondegui OD. How slow is too slow? Correlation of operative time to complications: an analysis from the Tennessee Surgical Quality Collaborative. *J Am Coll Surg.* 2015 Apr;220(4):550–8.

16 Symington JM. Effect of drill speed on bone temperature. *Int J Oral Maxillofac Surg.* 1996 Oct;25(5):394–9.

17 Augustin G, et al. Thermal osteonecrosis and bone drilling parameters revisited. *Arch Orthop Trauma Surg.* 2008 Jan;128(1):71–7.

18 Reznick JB. Avoiding a very preventable surgical complication. Dentaltown Magazine, 2010 Aug.

19 Robinson PD. *Tooth extraction, a practical guide.* Wright Elsevier, 2010, 77.

20 Hooley JR, Whitacre RJ. *Assesssment of and surgery for impacted third molars*, 3rd edition. Stoma Press, Inc., 1983, 62.

21 Tolstunov L. Influence of immediate post-extraction socket irrigation on development of alveolar osteitis after mandibular third molar removal: a prospective split-mouth study. *Br Dent J.* 2012;213:597–601.

22 Silverstein LH, Kurtzman GM, Shatz PC. Suturing for optimal soft-tissue management. *J Oral Implantol.* 2009;35(2):82–90.

23 Maria A, Malik M, Virang P. Comparison of primary and secondary closure of the surgical wound after removal of impacted mandibular third molars. *J Maxillofac Oral Surg.* 2012 Sept;11(3):276–28.

24 Reznick JB. Principles of flap design and closure. Dentaltown Magazine, 2016 Apr.

25 Ruscin M, Linnebur SA. Pharmacokinetics in the elderly. MSD Manual, 2014 Jun.

26 Sulieman MS. Clinical evaluation of the effect of four flap designs on the post–operative sequel (pain, swelling and trismus) following lower third molar surgery. *Al–Rafidain Dent J.* 2005;5(1):24–32.

27 Monaco G, Daprile G, Tavernese L, Corinaldesi G, Marchetti C. Mandibular third molar removal in young patients: an evaluation of 2 different flap designs. *J Oral Maxillofac Surg.* 2009 Jan;67(1):15–21.

28 Farish SE, Bouloux GF. General technique of third molar removal. *Oral Maxillofacial Surg Clin N Am.* 2007;19:23–43.

29 Figueiredo R, Valmaseda-Castellon E, Berini-Aytes L. Incidence and clinical features of delayed-onset infections afterextraction of lower third molars. *Oral Surg Oral Med Oral Pathol Oral Radiol Endod.* 2005;99:265.

30 Chaudhary M, Singh M, Singh S, Singh SP, Kaur G. Primary and secondary closure technique following removal of impacted mandibular third molars: a comparative study. *Natl J Maxillofac Surg.* 2012 Jan-Jun;3(1):10–14.

31 Pasqualini D, Cocero N, Castella A, Mela L, Bracco P. Primary and secondary closure of the surgical wound after removal of impacted mandibular third molars: a comparative study. *Int J Oral Maxillofac Surg.* 2005 Jan;34(1):52–7.

32 Chiapasco M, Crescentini M, Romanoni G. Germectomy or delayed removal of mandibular impacted third molars: the relationship between age and incidence of complications. *J Oral Maxillofac Surg.* 1995 Apr;53(4):41.

6

Pharmacology

Pharmacology is the science that deals with drugs. A myriad of drugs are available to control anxiety, pain, inflammation, and infection when removing impacted third molars. In many cases the use of particular drugs and regimens may not be appropriate. For example, the use of oral narcotics (Vicodin, Lortab, or Norco) to control pain may cause postoperative nausea and vomiting or lead to addiction. Research has shown that 600 mg ibuprofen combined with 500 mg acetaminophen is as efficacious as 10 mg of hydrocodone with minimal adverse effects and no potential for abuse.[1] A fundamental knowledge of pharmacology is necessary to provide optimal care when removing impacted third molars. The subjects of pharmacokinetics and pharmacodynamics are the foundation of pharmacology. The pharmacology of the most common drugs used by general dentists when removing impacted third molars are the focus of this chapter.

Pharmacokinetics and Pharmacodynamics

Pharmacokinetics

Pharmacokinetics describes how the body affects drugs; how drugs are absorbed, distributed, metabolized, and excreted. It refers to the movement of a drug into, through, and out of the body. Drug pharmacokinetics determines the onset, duration, and intensity of a drug's effect. (See Figure 6.1.)

The pharmacokinetic process of absorption is defined as the diffusion of a drug from the site of administration into the bloodstream. Distribution refers to the diffusion of a drug from the bloodstream into the body tissues. Metabolism refers to the process of biotransformation by which drugs are broken down so that they can be eliminated by the body. Elimination is defined as the removal of an active drug from the bloodstream.

Absorption of a drug into the bloodstream is determined by a drug's properties, formulation, and route of administration. Bioavailability is a subcategory of absorption. It is the percentage of a drug that reaches the systemic circulation. By definition, when a drug is administered intravenously, its bioavailability is 100%. The drug is then distributed in its active form to the target organ (brain, heart, kidney, liver, etc.).

The bioavailability of drugs that are administered orally is highly variable and is never 100%. Bioavailability is dependent on absorption and biotransformation. A portion of orally administered drugs is absorbed through the intestinal mucosa and enters the liver where it may be altered due to first-pass metabolism before entering the blood stream. The bioavailability of drugs administered

Impacted Third Molars, Second Edition. Edited by John Wayland.
© 2024 John Wiley & Sons, Inc. Published 2024 by John Wiley & Sons, Inc.

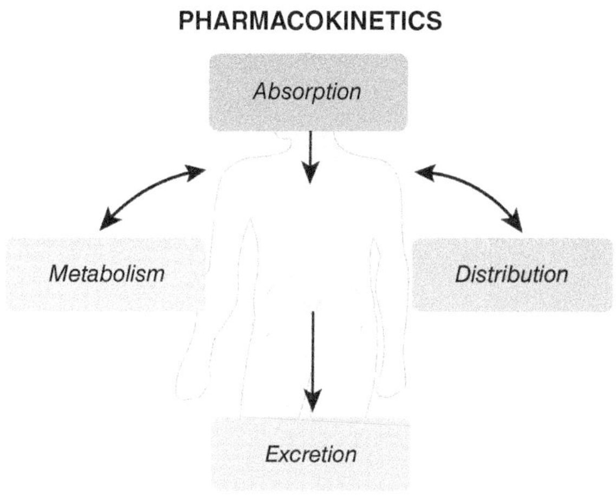

PHARMACOKINETICS

Figure 6.1   Pharmacokinetics describes how the body affects drugs.

sublingually is higher than oral, but is unpredictable because some of the drug is swallowed and is absorbed in the intestines. Therefore, the time to reach peak plasma level for sublingual drugs should be viewed as the same as oral drugs.

Absorbed drugs entering the bloodstream are either bound to plasma proteins or unbound and available for distribution. The average circulation time of blood is 1 minute. As the blood circulates, unbound drugs move from the bloodstream into the body's tissues. The amount and rate of drug distribution to body tissues is dependent on many factors including perfusion (blood flow), tissue binding, regional pH, and permeability of cell membranes.[2] Distribution is greater in highly perfused tissue such as the heart, brain, liver, and kidney. Some drugs accumulate within cells because they bind with proteins, phospholipids, or nucleic acids. Drugs that are lipid soluble are more likely to penetrate cell membranes and distribute to tissues. Tissues with permeable cell membranes receive more drug distribution than tissues with low cell membrane permeability. Drugs with a high pH (such as meperidine) have a relatively high distribution to tissues. Additionally, metabolism and excretion occur simultaneously with distribution making the process complex.

Most drugs are metabolized and transformed in the liver. Metabolism typically inactivates drugs in preparation for excretion. However, some drug metabolites are pharmacologically active. The liver's primary mechanism for metabolizing drugs is oxidation by a specific group of enzymes known as cytochrome P450 (CYP450) enzymes. The concentration of cytochrome P450 enzymes controls the rate at which many drugs are metabolized. Young children and elderly metabolize drugs more slowly than young and middle-aged adults due to altered enzymatic activity in the liver. These patients require smaller doses to achieve the same effect as young and middle-aged adults.

Elimination is accomplished through two mechanisms: (1) renal clearance by excretion into urine via the kidneys and (2) hepatic clearance by biotransformation to inactive metabolites via the liver. The term "elimination" refers to the removal of active molecules from the bloodstream, not from the body. Active drugs are transformed into inactive metabolites in the liver. This is termed hepatic clearance. Drugs that are water soluble are generally excreted in urine. This is termed renal clearance. The plasma half-life of a drug is the time required to eliminate 50% of the active drug from the bloodstream. Drugs are considered to be completely eliminated after 4 half-lives. Patients with liver or kidney dysfunction will experience longer drug elimination half-lives. For example, both renal and hepatic clearance is reduced by 50% by age 65.[3]

Pharmacodynamics

The mechanism by which a drug produces an effect is described as its action. Pharmacodynamics describes a drug's actions and how the actions affect the body. It describes observed therapeutic effects and side effects which can be positive or negative. (See Figure 6.2.)

Physiological responses are the result of the interaction of substances with molecular components of cells called receptors. Drugs that bind to receptors and initiate a response are called agonists. Drugs that bind to receptors and block a response are called antagonists. For example, the emergency drug naloxone is an antagonistic drug that blocks the effect of opioids. Naloxone has greater affinity for the CNS receptor than the opioids.

Drugs can also influence the action of enzymes. Enzyme inducers increase an enzyme's activity while enzyme inhibitors decrease an enzyme's activity. For example, non-steroidal anti-inflammatory drugs (NSAIDS) are enzyme inhibitors. NSAIDS inhibit the enzymes responsible for prostaglandin synthesis resulting in decreased pain, inflammation, and fever.

A drug's effect on the body can be evaluated in terms of potency and efficacy. Potency refers to the amount of a drug needed to produce an effect such as pain reduction or sedation. Efficacy refers to a drug's ability to produce an effect; its effectiveness.

A common misconception in dentistry is the belief that a more potent drug is more effective than a less potent drug. A drug can be less potent but more effective than another drug.[4] Drugs are considered equipotent when they produce the same effect. Fifty micrograms of fentanyl is 1000 times more potent than 50 micrograms of meperidine. However, 50 micrograms of fentanyl is no more effective than 50 milligrams of meperidine. Equipotent doses are equivalent in efficacy. Drugs belonging to the same class generally produce comparable efficacy, provided one administers appropriate doses. When choosing between drugs of comparable cost and safety, preference should be given to the one demonstrating greatest efficacy.[5]

A drug's therapeutic index is an indication of a drug's safety. It is a ratio of a clinically adequate dose and an average lethal dose. Drugs with a high index are safer than drugs with a low index and are prescribed more frequently. Drugs within the same class tend to have similar safety margins and efficacy.

The ceiling effect of a drug refers to a point where no additional effect is seen with increasing dosage. Increasing the dose further will not produce a greater response. This upper limit of dosage, above which no additional effect is seen, is called the ceiling dose. Ibuprofen has a ceiling dose of 400 mg as an analgesic. Opioids have no ceiling effect as analgesics.

The interaction of two or more drugs can have a positive or negative effect. Pharmacodynamic interactions alter the response of another drug by having an agonistic or antagonistic effect.

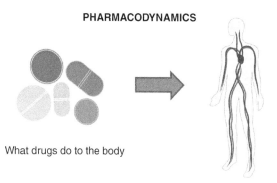

PHARMACODYNAMICS

What drugs do to the body

Figure 6.2 Pharmacodynamics describes how drugs affect the body.

Pharmacology for Third Molar Removal

Countless drugs are available to produce sedation, manage pain, reduce inflammation, and prevent or eliminate infection. Clinicians removing impacted third molars have many choices. The objective of this chapter is to reduce these overwhelming choices to a manageable number. A limited number of drugs are recommended in this book for the removal of impacted third molars.

Every drug mentioned in this chapter should be evaluated prior to use with pregnant patients. The United States Food and Drug Administration (FDA) classify drugs based on the risk they pose to the fetus. (See Box 6.1.)

Box 6.1 FDA Pregnancy Risk Categories.

FDA Pregnancy Category

A   No risk in controlled human studies: Adequate and well-controlled human studies have failed to demonstrate a risk to the fetus in the first trimester of pregnancy (and there is no evidence of risk in later trimesters).

B   No risk in other studies: Animal reproduction studies have failed to demonstrate a risk to the fetus and there are no adequate and well-controlled studies in pregnant women OR Animal studies have shown an adverse effect, but adequate and well-controlled studies in pregnant women have failed to demonstrate a risk to the fetus in any trimester.

C   Risk not ruled out: Animal reproduction studies have shown an adverse effect on the fetus and there are no adequate and well-controlled studies in humans, but potential benefits may warrant use of the drug in pregnant women despite potential risks.

D   Positive evidence of risk: There is positive evidence of human fetal risk based on adverse reaction data from investigational or marketing experience or studies in humans, but potential benefits may warrant use of the drug in pregnant women despite potential risks.

X   Contraindicated in pregnancy: Studies in animals or humans have demonstrated fetal abnormalities and/or there is positive evidence of human fetal risk based on adverse reaction data from investigational or marketing experience, and the risks involved in use of the drug in pregnant women clearly outweigh potential benefits.

Drugs in categories A and B are considered safe for use during pregnancy. Drugs in Category C can be used when the benefits to mother and fetus outweigh the risks. Drugs in category D should be avoided except in exceptional circumstances. The use of drugs in category X is strictly prohibited during pregnancy.

Sedation

Sedation is recommended for the removal of impacted third molars. Extractions and the removal of third molars are among the most feared oral surgical procedures. Patient management can be challenging when treating patients with anxiety.

Data collected by Osborne, et al, suggest that the more anxious a patient in the preoperative period, the more prone he or she is to movement during the surgical procedure.[6] Obviously, surgical complications are more likely when patients are moving. The surgical removal of impacted third molars requires a cooperative patient. Sedation can improve the patient's experience and treatment outcome.

The most common drugs used for sedation by general dentists when removing impacted third molars are triazolam, midazolam, zolpidem, and nitrous oxide. Triazolam and zolpidem are administered orally or sublingually, nitrous oxide by inhalation, and midazolam intravenously. Fentanyl, a narcotic, has both analgesic and sedative qualities. It is discussed in this chapter in the pain management section.

Triazolam (Halcion)

Triazolam belongs to a group of drugs known as benzodiazepines. Benzodiazepines possess amnesic, sedative-hypnotic, anxiolytic, and anticonvulsant qualities. More than 2000 benzodiazepines have been synthesized since 1933. Benzodiazepines affect GABA-mediated systems. The neurotransmitter GABA is an inhibitory neurotransmitter and controls the state of a chloride ion channel. Benzodiazepines increase the inhibitory action at the GABA receptor. Benzodiazepines are the most effective drugs currently available for the management of anxiety.[7] The efficacy of benzodiazepines is equivalent to or greater than any other class of sedatives and their safety profile is enviable. Death following an overdose of benzodiazepines alone is a virtually unheard of statistic.[8] Benzodiazepines are normally administered by the oral, sublingual, intramuscular, or intravenous route. Benzodiazepines are contraindicated in patients with acute narrow-angle glaucoma.

Paradoxical rage reactions due to benzodiazepines occur as a result of an altered level of consciousness, which generates automatic behaviors, anterograde amnesia and uninhibited aggression. These aggressive reactions may be caused by a disinhibiting serotonergic mechanism.[9] Paradoxical effects of benzodiazepines appear to be dose related, that is, likelier to occur with higher dose.[10]

Triazolam is usually used in dentistry for short- to moderate-length appointments. Its rapid onset, short duration of action, and lack of active metabolites makes it a near ideal antianxiety/sedation medication for the removal of impacted third molars. Onset of activity is usually within 30 minutes with peak blood levels occurring after approximately 75 minutes. The oral bioavailability for triazolam is only 44% but can be increased to 53% with sublingual administration.[11]

The usual adult dose for triazolam sedation ranges from 0.125 mg to 0.5 mg. The maximum recommended dose is .5 mg. Toxicity and overdose may develop at 4 times the maximum recommended dose. Baughman et al. compared triazolam 0.125, 0.25, and 0.5 mg with diazepam 5, 10, and 15 mg. Only the highest triazolam dose was consistently effective.[12] Triazolam has no major active metabolites. It is metabolized by oxidative reduction via the hepatic cytochrome P450 system. It can be influenced by aging, hepatic dysfunction, and drug–drug interactions. A small percentage of patients can have paradoxical reactions such as worsened agitation, aggression, or panic. Triazolam is contraindicated with medications that significantly impair the oxidative metabolism mediated by cytochrome P450 including ketoconazole, itraconazole, nefazodone, and several HIV protease inhibitors. (See Table 6.1.)

Triazolam is a United States FDA pregnancy category X drug. It is contraindicated in pregnant patients, patients with acute narrow-angle glaucoma, or known hypersensitivity to triazolam.

Midazolam (Versed)

Midazolam is another benzodiazepine commonly used during the removal of impacted third molars. Many routes of administration are possible including oral, intramuscular, nasal, and intravenous. The intravenous route is normally used for the removal of impacted third molars. Midazolam is available for parenteral administration in concentrations of 1 mg/ml and 5 mg/ml in 2 ml or 10 ml vials. Midazolam received FDA approval in December of 1985. (See Table 6.2.)

Table 6.1   Characteristics of triazolam.

Characteristic	Triazolam
Bioavailability	44–53%
Peak Plasma Level	75 min.
½ Life	1.5–5.5 hrs.
Availability	.125 –.25 mg
Metabolism	Hepatic CYP 450
Active metabolites	None major
Onset of activity	30 min.
Amnesia	Yes
Pregnancy category	X + not for use in nursing
DEA schedule	IV
Contraindications	1) Acute narrow-angle glaucoma 2) Ketoconazole, intraconazole, nefazodone, HIV protease inhibitors impair metabolism

Table 6.2   Characteristics of intravenous midazolam.

Characteristic	IV Midazolam
Bioavailability	100 %
Peak Plasma Level	< 1 min.
½ Life	1.5–3.5 hrs.
Availability	1 and 5 mg/ml
Metabolism	Hepatic CYP 450
Active metabolites	None major
Onset of activity	< 1 min.
Amnesia	Yes
Pregnancy category	D + caution in nursing
DEA schedule	IV
Contraindications	Acute narrow-angle glaucoma Ketoconazole, intraconazole, HIV protease inhibitors impair metabolism

Midazolam is soluble in water. Its water solubility is responsible for the absence of phlebitis and a lack of burning sensation on injection. Midazolam is metabolized in the liver by the cytochrome P450 system resulting in no major active metabolites. Onset is rapid when administered intravenously. Midazolam has been used as an induction agent for general anesthesia with induction times ranging from 55 to 143 seconds.[13] Anterograde amnesia is a characteristic of midazolam.

Midazolam can be used alone or in combination with other drugs. Titration should be slow and dosage should be reduced when used with other CNS depressants such as nitrous oxide or fentanyl. The 1 mg/ml intravenous concentration is recommended to increase the drug's safety margin.

Midazolam is a United States FDA pregnancy category D drug. Midazolam is contraindicated for patients with acute narrow-angle glaucoma or known hypersensitivity to midazolam.

Zolpidem (Ambien)

Zolpidem tartrate is a nonbenzodiazepine sedative hypnotic drug with pharmcodynamic characteristics (benefits, side effects, and risks) nearly identical to triazolam. However, the chemical structure of zolpidem is unrelated to triazolam. Zolpidem belongs to a class of sedative hypnotics known as imidazopyridines. This class of sedative hypnotics is sometimes referred to as "Z-compounds."

Zolpidem is a strong sedative with mild anxiolytic, muscle relaxant, and anticonvulsant properties. It has amnesic side effects similar to triazolam. More than 90% of zolpidem exists in its protein-bound form with a bioavailability of approximately 70%.[14] It is rapidly absorbed from the GI tract, having an onset of action of 45 minutes and a peak effect in 1.6 hours.[15] It is metabolized in the liver with and elimination half-life of 2.6 hours. Elimination is primarily renal.

Zolpidem has no major active metabolites. It is metabolized by oxidative reduction via the hepatic cytochrome P450 system. It can be influenced by aging, hepatic dysfunction, and drug–drug interactions. A minority of patients can have paradoxical reactions such as worsened agitation, aggression, or panic. (See Table 6.3.)

Zolpidem is a United States FDA pregnancy category C drug. Zolpidem is contraindicated in patients with known hypersensitivity to Zolpidem.[16]

Flumazenil (Romazicon)

Adverse drug reactions (ADRs) can occur after the administration of any drug. A major advantage of benzodiazepines and imidazopyridines is the ability of flumazenil to reverse their sedative effects. Flumazenil is a benzodiazepine and imidazopyridine antagonist that rapidly reverses the sedative effects of triazolam, midazolam, or zolpidem. Patients show an improved ability to comprehend and obey commands when flumazenil is administered intravenously. Flumazenil was FDA-approved in December 1991. (See Table 6.4.)

Table 6.3 Characteristics of oral zolpidem.

Characteristic	Zolpidem
Bioavailability	70 %
Peak Plasma Level	1.5–2.5 hrs.
½ Life	2.5–3.1 hrs.
Availability	5 mg + 10 mg
Metabolism	Hepatic CYP 450
Active metabolites	No
Onset of activity	45 min.
Amnesia	Yes
Pregnancy category	C + caution in nursing
DEA schedule	IV
Contraindications	Hypersensitivity

Table 6.4   Characteristics of IV flumazenil.

Characteristic	IV Flumazenil
Bioavailability	100%
Peak Plasma Level	1–3 min.
½ Life	54 min.
Availability	0.5mg/5ml vials
Metabolism	Hepatic CYP 450
Active metabolites	No
Onset of activity	1–3 min.
Amnesia	Reverses
Pregnancy category	C + caution in nursing
DEA schedule	None
Contraindications	History of seizures

Flumazenil's onset of action is 1 to 2 minutes following IV administration. Peak concentrations are dose dependent and occur 1 to 3 minutes after administration.[17] Flumazenil's duration of action is short. Additional flumazenil doses may be needed to reverse sedative effects when extremely large doses of sedative have been used. Resedation is highly unlikely following low or conventional doses of benzodiazepines, e.g., less than 10 mg midazolam IV.[18]

Flumazenil is a United States FDA pregnancy category C drug. Flumazenil injection is contraindicated in patients with a known hypersensitivity to flumazenil or a history of seizures.

Nitrous Oxide

Nitrous oxide is an inorganic inhalation agent that is colorless, odorless to sweet-smelling, and nonirritating to tissues. It is nonflammable but will support combustion. Given its long history of safety, it could be argued that nitrous oxide is the safest of all the modalities available for sedation in dentistry.[19] It is an ideal drug for patients with mild to moderate anxiety.

The potency of an anesthetic gas is described as its minimum alveolar concentration (MAC). Minimum alveolar concentration represents the percent concentration required to produce immobility in response to a surgical stimulus for 50% of patients. Nitrous oxide has very low potency with a MAC of 104. The concentration of nitrous oxide indicated on typical dental office equipment is drastically reduced when compared with the concentration that actually reaches the patient. Even though the machine may indicate up to 70% nitrous oxide, the actual concentration delivered to alveoli is unlikely to exceed 30% to 50%.[20] Breathing by mouth, system leaks, poorly fitting masks, and dead space all contribute to this discrepancy. It should be emphasized that nitrous oxide MAC is significantly reduced (more potent) when it is combined with other sedatives or narcotics. General anesthesia with depressed respiratory and cardiovascular function is possible when nitrous oxide is combined with other sedative hypnotic drugs or narcotics.

Nitrous oxide has the fastest onset and elimination of all anesthetic gases due to its low solubility in blood. The absorption, distribution, and elimination of nitrous oxide are the result of pressure gradients in the lungs, blood, and tissue. Nitrous oxide does not undergo biotransformation. The elimination half-life of nitrous oxide is approximately 5 minutes.[21] Nitrous oxide is eliminated unchanged from the body, almost entirely via the lungs. (See Table 6.5.)

Table 6.5   Characteristics of nitrous oxide.

Characteristic	Nitrous Oxide
Minimum alveolar concentration (MAC)	104
½ Life	5 min.
Availability	Gas cylinders
Metabolism	No
Active metabolites	No
Onset of activity	1–3 min.
Amnesia	No
Pregnancy category	C + caution in nursing
DEA schedule	No
Contraindications	History of seizures

Nitrous oxide produces analgesia in addition to sedation. It is estimated that a 20%:80% mixture of N_2O/O_2 produces the analgesic effectiveness of 10 to 15 mg of morphine.[22] The exact mechanism for the analgesic property of nitrous oxide is unknown. It is believed that there is an interaction with the endogenous opioid system. The strongest evidence is that nitrous oxide stimulates release of enkephalins which bind to opioid receptors that trigger descending noradrenergic pathways.[23] The analgesic effect of nitrous oxide can be reversed with the opioid antagonist naloxone.

There are no contraindications to the use of nitrous oxide in combination with an adequate percentage of oxygen.[24] Nitrous oxide is an FDA pregnancy category C drug.

Pain Management

The management of pain is an integral part of the practice of dentistry. This is especially true when impacted third molars are removed. The most common drugs used to manage intraoperative and postoperative third molar pain include local anesthetics, opioids, ibuprofen, and acetaminophen.

Local Anesthetics: Lidocaine, Articaine, and Bupivacaine

The ancient Incas may have used the leaves of the coca plant as a local anesthetic. Cocaine was isolated from the coca plant in 1860 and first used as a local anesthetic in 1884. Since then, several synthetic local anesthetic drugs have been developed including lidocaine in 1943, bupivacaine in 1957, and articaine in 1969. These local anesthetics are commonly used for the removal of impacted third molars. (See Table 6.6.)

The potency of a local anesthetic is determined by its lipid solubility. Lipid solubility improves diffusion through nerve cell membranes. Bupivacaine is the most lipid-soluble and potent local anesthetic. It is four times as potent as lidocaine and three times as potent as articaine.[25]

The majority of lidocaine and bupivacaine is metabobolized in the liver by cytochrome P450 enzyme pathways. In contrast, 90–95% of articaine is hydrolyzed in plasma rendering the molecule inactive. The result is that articaine is eliminated quickly when compared to lidocaine and bupivacaine. For this reason, articaine presents less risk for systemic toxicity than lidocaine or bupivacaine at equipotent doses.[26]

Table 6.6   Characteristics of xylocaine, articaine, and bupivacaine.

Anesthetic	Potency	Metabolism	Onset	Duration Pulp/Soft Tissue (minutes)	Elimination ½ life (minutes)
Lidocaine 2% 1:100,000	Least	70% Hepatic	Rapid	60/180–360	96
Articaine 4% 1:100,000	Intermediate	95% Plasma	Rapid	60–75/180–360	25
Bupivacaine .5% 1:200,000	Most	94% Hepatic	Slow	90–180/240–540	210

The time of onset of a local anesthetic is determined by the amount of anesthetic that is non-ionized. Local anesthetics with more molecules that are non-ionized have faster onset times. At the physiological pH of 7.4, lidocaine and articaine have more non-ionized molecules than bupivacaine. Therefore, lidocaine and articaine have faster onset times than bupivacaine in equipotent doses.[27]

Duration of action is determined by plasma protein binding. Bupivacaine is 95% bound to plasma protein and has an affinity for protein at the receptor site within the sodium channel. Protein binding accounts for the long duration of bupivacaine.[25]

The elimination ½ time of a drug is largely dependent on metabolism. Drugs metabolized in the blood have a shorter half-life compared with drugs metabolized in the liver. This process is clearly demonstrated when comparing the half-lives of articaine and lidocaine. The elimination half-life for lidocaine is 96 minutes as compared to 45 minutes for articaine. Bupivacaine has the longest elimination half-time due to the combination of liver metabolism and protein binding. The elimination half-life of bupivacaine is 210 minutes.

Epinephrine delays absorption of local anesthetic and provides hemostasis. Concentrations of epinephrine greater than 1:200,000 do not provide better onset or duration for inferior alveolar nerve blocks.[28] However, higher concentrations of epinephrine improve hemostasis. Delayed absorption due to the addition of vasoconstrictor decreases the risk of anesthetic toxicity, but does not eliminate it.

Maximum recommended doses must be respected. Toxic doses of local anesthetic can induce seizures. Local anesthetic is a CNS depressant when administered in high doses. This factor should be considered when local anesthetic is combined with other CNS depressant drugs. The absolute maximum adult dose of lidocaine is 300 mg, articaine 500 mg, and bupivacaine 90 mg. The absolute maximum recommendations for lidocaine, articaine, and bupivacaine are shown in Table 6.7.

Table 6.7   Maximum local anesthetic recommendations.

Anesthetic	Absolute Maximum (mg)	Maximum Carpules
Lidocaine 2% Epinephrine 1:100,000	300	7
Articaine 4% Epinephrine 1:100,000	500	6
Bupivacaine .5% Epinephrine 1:200,000	90	9

Table 6.8 Concentration of common local anesthetics.

Vasopressor Concentration	Micrograms per 2 ml Carpule
1:50,000	40 micrograms
1:100,000	20 micrograms
1:200,000	10 micrograms

A medical consultation is prudent for medically compromised patients receiving local anesthetics. The planned amount of local anesthetic and vasopressor should be expressed in milligrams and micrograms when consulting with a physician. Physicians are not familiar with dental carpule concentrations.

Daniel E. Becker, DDS and Ken Reed, DMD have proposed a simple and effective method to quickly convert anesthetic and epinephrine concentrations.[26] Consider all carpules to be 2.0 ml. This adjustment makes calculations easier and adds a margin of safety. To convert anesthetic concentration from percent to milligrams, move the decimal point one place to the right. 2% lidocaine is 20 mg/ml, 4% articaine is 40 mg/ml, and .5% bupivacaine is 5 mg/ml. One carpule of lidocaine contains 2 ml, therefore each carpule contains 40 mg of lidocaine. 2 ½ carpules of lidocaine contains 100 mg lidocaine.

Vasopressor concentrations can be converted to micrograms by remembering that a vasopressor concentration of 1:100,000 is equivalent to 10 micrograms/ml. Again, consider all carpules to be 2 ml. A 2 ml carpule of lidocaine 2% with epinephrine 1:100,000 will contain 20 micrograms of epinephrine. A concentration of 1:50,000 will contain 40 micrograms of epinephrine, and a concentration of 1:200,000 will contain 10 micrograms of epinephrine. (See Table 6.8.)

The recommended local anesthetic dose is only a guideline. The amount of local anesthetic administered is determined following a thorough patient assessment. Surgical difficulty, patient anxiety, and appointment length are variables that affect local anesthetic decisions. Dose adjustments may be necessary for medically compromised patients. The vital signs of these patients should be assessed at regular intervals following the administration of local anesthetic.

Articaine and bupivacaine are United States FDA pregnancy category C drugs. Contraindications include a known history of hypersensitivity to local anesthetics and sulfites. Lidocaine is a United States FDA pregnancy category B drug. Contraindications include a known history of hypersensitivity to local anesthetics and sulfites.

Opioids: Hydrocodone, Oxycodone, and Fentanyl

Opioids are among the world's oldest known drugs.[29] Opiates, originally derived from the opium poppy, have been used for thousands of years for both recreational and medicinal purposes. The earliest reference to opium growth and use is in 3400 B.C. when the opium poppy was cultivated in lower Mesopotamia (Southwest Asia).[30] The word opium originates from the Greek word *opion* which meant poppy juice. (See Figure 6.3.)

The word opiate was classically used in pharmacology to mean a drug derived from opium. The modern word opioid is now used to designate all substances, both natural and synthetic, that bind to opioid receptors in the central nervous system and other tissues.[31] Opioids bind to specific receptors in the central nervous system and other tissues. There are three principal classes of opioid receptors, μ, κ, δ (mu, kappa, and delta).

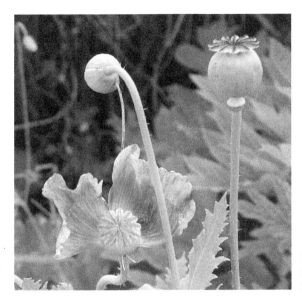

Figure 6.3 Poppy pod and flower in bloom. (Dinkum / Wikimedia Commons / Public domain / CC0 1.0.).

Opioids are strong analgesics with analgesic, sedative, and antianxiety qualities. Oral opioids are often used to control preoperative anxiety and postoperative pain when removing third molars. Intravenous opioids are usually combined with an intravenous sedative hypnotic drug during the procedure to control pain and anxiety. Opioids are CNS depressants capable of producing respiratory depression, especially when combined with other CNS depressants.

Malamed divides opioids into three categories: (1) opioid agonists, (2) opioid antagonists, and (3) opioid agonist-antagonists.[32] Opioid agonists (fentanyl) produce a physiological change. Opioid antagonists (naloxone) do not produce a physiological change. Opioid agonist-antagonists (nalbuphine) have properties of both agonists and antagonists. Agonist-antagonists are not discussed in this section since they are not commonly used for the removal of impacted third molars.

Opioid antagonists (Oas) produce analgesia, drowsiness, and euphoria. Arms and legs feel heavy, the body becomes warm, the mouth becomes dry, and itching develops around the nose and eyes. Negative side effects include nausea, vomiting, constipation and dizziness. Oas increase smooth muscle tone which can aggravate asthma in ASA III patients. However, this is unlikely to occur at therapeutic doses. Opioids are "cardioprotective" because they depress catecholamine release and obtund sympathetic reflexes to noxious stimuli such as the removal of impacted third molars. This pharmacodynamic property is especially beneficial for patients with hypertension, tachyarrhythmias, and ischemic heart disease.[19]

Common opioids used when removing impacted third molars include hydrocodone (Vicodin), oxycodone (OxyContin), and fentanyl (Sublimaze). Hydrocodone and oxycodone are administered by the oral route and fentanyl by the IV route when used for the removal of third molars.

Hydrocodone (Vicodin)

Hydrocodone was first synthesized in Germany in 1920 by Carl Mannich and Helene Löwenheim.[33] It was approved by the Food and Drug Administration in 1943 for sale in the United States. Hydrocodone is marketed in the United States under the brand names Vicodin, Lortab, and Norco. Hydrocodone is formulated with acetaminophen. It is well absorbed via the gastrointestinal tract.

Table 6.9 Characteristics of hydrocodone.

Characteristic	Oral Hydrocodone
Bioavailability	70 %
Peak Plasma Level	1 hr.
½ Life	3.3–4.4 hrs.
Availability	10 mg, 15 mg, 20 mg, 30 mg, 40 mg, and 50 mg tablets
Metabolism	Hepatic – complex metabolism
Active metabolites	Yes
Onset of activity	10–30 min.
Amnesia	No
Pregnancy category	Category C, not for use in nursing.
DEA schedule	II
Contraindications	Opioid intolerance or allergy

Oral bioavailability is 70%. Following oral administration, onset occurs after 10–30 minutes and peak plasma levels occur after about an hour. The average plasma half-life is 3.8 hours. Hydrocodone "exhibits a complex pattern of hepatic metabolism including O-demethylation, N-demethylation and 6-keto reduction to the corresponding 6-a- and 6-b-hydroxymetabolites."[34] (See Table 6.9.)

Hydrocodone is the most frequently prescribed opioid in the United States with an estimated 130 million prescriptions in 2006, up from approximately 88 million in 2000 (IMS National Prescription Audit Plus™).

Hydrocodone is contraindicated in patients with a known hypersensitivity. Hydrocodone is a United States FDA pregnancy category C drug

Oxycodone (OxyContin)

Freund and Speyer of the University of Frankfurt in Germany first synthesized oxycodone from thebaine in 1916.[35] It was first introduced to the US market in 1939. Oxycodone is available in the United States in immediate release and extended release forms. The most common brand name is OxyContin. Oxycodone is formulated with and without acetaminophen. It is well-absorbed via the gastrointestinal tract. It has an oral bioavailability of 60–87%. Following oral administration, onset occurs after 10–15 minutes and peak plasma levels occur after 30–60 minutes. The average plasma half-life is 3–4 hours. Oxycodone is metabolized in the liver by CYP3A4 to the weak analgesic noroxycodone and by CYP2D6 to the potent analgesic oxymorphone. (See Table 6.10.) It is estimated that 53 million oxycodone prescriptions are dispensed by US pharmacies annually.[36]

Oxycodone is contraindicated in patients with known hypersensitivity. Oxycodone is a United States FDA pregnancy category B drug

Fentanyl (Sublimaze)

Fentanyl was first synthesized by Paul Janssen of Janssen Pharmaceutica in 1959.[37] The FDA approved fentanyl for IV administration in February 1968. Fentanyl is the most used opioid for dental IV moderate sedation. It is approximately 100 times more potent than morphine.[38]

Table 6.10 Characteristics of oxycodone.

Characteristic	Oxycodone
Bioavailability	60–87 %
Peak Plasma Level	30–60 min.
½ Life	3–4 hrs.
Availability	Tab: 10mg, 20mg
Metabolism	Hepatic – CYP3A4 and CYP2D6
Active metabolites	Yes
Onset of activity	10–15 min.
Amnesia	No
Pregnancy category	Category B, not for use in nursing.
DEA schedule	II
Contraindications	Opioid intolerance or allergy

Fentanyl has a rapid onset and short duration of action. Following the IV administration of fentanyl, the onset of analgesia and sedation is less than one minute. Average duration of clinical action is 30 to 60 minutes, which makes fentanyl an almost ideal drug for the removal of third molars. Fentanyl does not promote histamine release. Fentanyl has an elimination half-life of 3.7 hours. Peak plasma concentration is observed after 6 minutes. It is primarily metabolized in the liver by the enzyme CYP3A4. There are no significant active metabolites. Injectable fentanyl is available in 50 mcg/ml vials. (See Table 6.11.)

Fentanyl may cause muscular rigidity, especially involving the muscles of respiration, when rapidly injected as a bolus. It should be administered slowly to avoid this potentially disastrous complication. Fentanyl is contraindicated in patients with opioid intolerance or hypersensitivity. Fentanyl is a United States FDA pregnancy category C drug.

Table 6.11 Characteristics of fentanyl.

Characteristic	IV Fentanyl
Bioavailability	100 %
Peak Plasma Time	6 min.
½ Life	3.7 hrs.
Availability	50mcg/mL vial
Metabolism	Hepatic – CYP3A4
Active metabolites	None significant
Onset of activity	< 1 min.
Amnesia	No
Pregnancy category	Category C, caution in nursing
DEA schedule	II
Contraindications	Opioid intolerance or allergy

Naloxone (Narcan)

Naloxone was patented in 1961 by Jack Fishman and Mozes J. Lewenstein. It was approved for the treatment of opioid overdose by the Food and Drug Administration in 1971.[39] Naloxone is an opioid antagonist that rapidly reverses the CNS and respiratory depressant effects of opioids. Naloxone exhibits essentially no pharmacological activity when administered in the absence of opioids.[40]

Onset of action and improvement in respiration is usually seen within 1–2 minutes following IV administration. The effect of naloxone lasts 30 to 60 minutes. In one study, the duration of action was 45 minutes following IV administration.[41] Multiple doses may be required because the duration of action of most opioids is greater than that of naloxone.[42] An IM dose of naloxone following IV administration increases the duration of clinical action. The mean serum elimination half-life has been shown to range from 30 to 81 minutes. Withdrawal symptoms are triggered when naloxone is administered to patients who are physically dependent on opioids. (See Table 6.12.)

Naloxone is contraindicated in patients with known hypersensitivity. Naloxone is a United States FDA pregnancy category C drug.

Ibuprofen (Advil)

Ibuprofen was discovered in 1961 by Stewart Adams. It was first marketed in the United States in 1974.[43] Ibuprofen is a non-steroidal anti-inflammatory drug (NSAID) used for the treatment of pain, inflammation, and fever. Its effects are due to the inhibitory actions on enzymes which reduce the synthesis of prostaglandins. Prostaglandins play an important role in the production of pain, inflammation, and fever.[44]

Preoperative use of ibuprofen has been demonstrated repeatedly to decrease the intensity of postoperative pain and swelling.[45] The concept of "pre loading" is valid if ibuprofen is administered while local anesthetic is effective. In a survey published in 2006, investigators found that ibuprofen was the most frequently recommended nonprescription peripherally acting analgesic among oral and maxillofacial surgeons for the management of postoperative pain after third-molar extractions in the United States.[46] Ibuprofen has an analgesic ceiling effect of 400 mg. Doses beyond 400 mg will not improve analgesia.

Table 6.12 Characteristics of IV naloxone.

Characteristic	IV Naloxone
Bioavailability	100 %
½ Life	30–81 min.
Availability	0.2 and 0.4 mg/ml
Metabolism	Hepatic
Active metabolites	Yes
Onset of activity	2 min.
Duration of action	30–60 min.
Pregnancy category	Category C, caution in nursing
DEA schedule	Prescription
Contraindications	Hypersensitivity to naloxone

Table 6.13   Characteristics of ibuprofen.

Characteristic	Ibuprofen
Bioavailability	95%–100 %
½ Life	1.8–2.0 hrs.
Peak plasma time	1–2 hrs.
Availability	200 mg, 400 mg, 600 mg, 800 mg
Metabolism	Hepatic, CYP450
Active metabolites	No
Onset of activity	30 min.
Duration of action	4–6 hrs.
Pregnancy category	Category C, D in third trimester, not for use in nursing
Contraindications	Hypersensitivity, blood thinners, compromised GI or renal function

There is no ibuprofen ceiling effect for inflammation. Doses of 1600 mg to 2400 mg per day may decrease inflammation following the removal of third molars. As the dose of an NSAID is increased, anti-inflammatory effects improve until maximum safe doses (2400 mg/day) preclude any further increase.[47]

Ibuprofen's bioavailability is nearly 100%. It is rapidly and widely distributed to human tissues. Onset of action is usually seen within 30 minutes with effects lasting 4–6 hours. The mean serum elimination half-life has been shown to range from 1.8 to 2.5 hours. Ibuprofen is metabolized in the liver. (See Table 6.13.)

Ibuprofen should be avoided in patients with bleeding disorders, erosive or ulcerative conditions of the GI mucosa, and those taking anticoagulants such as Coumadin. Patients with compromised renal function can experience renal failure within 24 hours of ibuprofen administration. Ibuprofen should not be prescribed for patients who have known or questionable renal function. This concern has not been found relevant with short-term use of ibuprofen (e.g., 5–7 days). Ibuprofen is a United States FDA pregnancy category B drug.

Acetaminophen (Tylenol)

Acetaminophen (paracetamol) was synthesized by Harmon Northrop Morse in 1873. This discovery was largely ignored at the time.[48] In 1948, Brodie and Axelrod linked the use of acetanilide with methemoglobinemia and determined that the analgesic effect of acetanilide was due to its active metabolite acetaminophen. They advocated the use of acetaminophen (paracetamol), since it did not have the toxic effects of acetanilide (Brodie and Axelrod 1948). The product went on sale in the United States in 1955 under the brand name "Tylenol." [49] The exact mechanism of action of acetaminophen is still poorly understood.

Oral acetaminophen is rapidly and completely absorbed from the small intestine. Its bioavailability ranges from 70% to 90% depending on dose.[50] Onset of action occurs between 30 and 60 minutes.[51] Peak plasma concentrations occur within 24 to 60 minutes. Acetaminophen has a short plasma half-life that ranges from 2 to 3 hours in healthy adults. Because acetaminophen clears rapidly from the body, it requires dosing every 4 to 6 hours in order to maintain therapeutic levels.[52]

Table 6.14   Characteristics of acetaminophen.

Characteristic	Oral Acetaminophen
Bioavailability	70%–90%
½ Life	2–3 hrs.
Peak plasma time	24–60 min.
Availability	325 mg, 500 mg
Metabolism	Hepatic
Active metabolites	Yes
Onset of activity	30–60 min.
Duration of action	4–6 hrs.
Pregnancy category	Category B, nursing safety unknown
Contraindications	Hypersensitivity to acetaminophen, hepatic impairment

Unlike ibuprofen, acetaminophen has no anti-inflammatory properties; therefore, it is not a non-steroidal anti-inflammatory drug. NSAIDS have influence on peripheral prostaglandin synthesis. Acetaminophen has no effect on peripheral prostaglandin synthesis. Instead, it is believed to inhibit prostaglandin synthesis within the CNS. This may be the reason that acetaminophen lacks anti- inflammatory qualities.

Acetaminophen has a narrow therapeutic index. This means that the common dose is close to the overdose, making it a relatively dangerous substance.[53] Hepatotoxicity is the most significant adverse effect of acetaminophen. The recommended maximum daily dose for adults is 3000 mg. Without timely treatment, acetaminophen overdoses can lead to liver failure and death within days.[49] Acetaminophen is less likely than ibuprofen to cause gastric irritation or bleeding when used in normal doses. It does not affect blood coagulation or the kidneys. When used responsibly, acetaminophen is one of the safest medications available for analgesia. (See Table 6.14.)

Acetaminophen is contraindicated in patients with severe hepatic impairment or patients with a known hypersensitivity to acetaminophen. Acetaminophen is a United States FDA pregnancy category B drug.

Ibuprofen and Acetaminophen Combination

The removal of impacted third molars is recognized as one of the more painful procedures in dentistry. Pain following the surgical removal of impacted third molars is frequently used as an analgesic model because of the intensity and consistency of postoperative pain.[54] One study found the prescription analgesics most frequently recommended by maxillofacial surgeons, for the removal of third molars, were acetaminophen-hydrocodone (Vicodin, Lortab, Norco) and acetaminophen-oxycodone (Percocet).[46] Unfortunately, the use of opioids to control postoperative pain following the removal of impacted third molars is associated with adverse events including nausea, vomiting, dizziness, and drug abuse.

The strategy of combining two analgesic agents with different sites of action has been advocated for many years. A study, published in the *Journal of the American Dental Association* in 2013, compared the efficacy of several drugs used to control postoperative pain following the removal of impacted third molars. The authors used the statistic "number needed to treat" (NNT) to rank the

Table 6.15 Efficacy of oral analgesics.

Drug (milligrams)	Number Needed to Treat (NNT)
Aspirin (600 or 650)	4.5 (4.0–5.2)
Aspirin (1,000)	4.2 (3.2–6.0)
APAP* (1,000)	3.2 (2.9–3.6)
Ibuprofen (200)	2.7 (2.5–3.0)
Celecoxib (400)	2.5 (2.2–2.9)
Ibuprofen (400)	2.3 (2.2–2.4)
Oxycodone (10) With APAP (650)	2.3 (2.0–6.4)
Codeine (60) With APAP (1,000)	2.2 (1.8–2.9)
Naproxen (500 or 550)	1.8 (1.6–2.1)
Ibuprofen (200) With APAP (500)*	**1.6 (1.4–1.8)**

*acetaminophen is N-acetyl-p-aminophenol (APAP)

efficacy of individual drugs and drug combinations. NNT has been defined as "the number of patients needed to be treated to obtain one additional patient achieving at least 50 percent maximum pain relief over four to six hours compared with placebo." The lower the NNT, the more effective the analgesic drug therapy.[55] (See Table 6.15.)

The most effective drug combination in this study was ibuprofen 200 mg combined with 500 mg acetaminophen (1.6). The combination was more effective than either drug used alone (ibuprofen 2.7 and acetaminophen 3.2) or acetaminophen combined with the opioid oxycodone (2.3). The data suggests that ibuprofen combined with acetaminophen would also be more effective than hydrocodone combined with acetaminophen, (Vicodin, Lortab, or Norco). There was little indication that adverse reactions are more frequent with the administration of the ibuprofen acetaminophen combination than with the administration of the individual components as long as maximum recommended doses of both components are not exceeded.

The analgesic ceiling effect should be considered when evaluating this study.[56] The analgesic ceilings for ibuprofen and acetaminophen are 400 mg and 1000 mg respectively.[57] It can be assumed that a combination of 400 mg ibuprofen combined with 1000 mg acetaminophen would have an NNT result lower than 1.6. To avoid adverse events, it's important that daily maximum doses of 2400 mg ibuprofen and 3000 mg acetaminophen are not exceeded.

Another effective NSAID for moderate to severe third molar pain is Ketorolac (Tramadol). Ketorolac is available as a 10 mg tablet and as a solution. The recommended oral dose is two tablets followed by one tablet every 6 hours, not to exceed 40 mg daily. Ketorolac should not be used for more than 5 days. Patients should be advised to stop the medication if they have hypersensitivity or allergic reactions. This pain medication should be used with caution when patients are allergic to ibuprofen.

Several options in addition to oral medication are available to reduce postoperative pain when removing impacted third molars. The long-acting local anesthetic bupivacaine can provide extended soft-tissue and periosteal anesthesia.[58] The corticosteroid dexamethasone is effective in limiting trismus, swelling, and pain after third-molar surgery.[59]

In summary, many medications and routes of administration are available to manage impacted third molar postoperative pain. The safest and most efficacious pharmacological choice appears to be ibuprofen combined with acetaminophen.

Inflammation

Pain, inflammation, and trismus following the removal of impacted third molars are inextricably linked. J. Ata-Ali et al. studied the effects of corticosteroids upon pain, inflammation and trismus after lower third molar surgery.[60] A total of 14 articles were included in the study. Trismus is a reduction of jaw opening caused by edema and swelling. The study found a mean reduction in opening of 24.1% the day after removal of mandibular third molars when corticosteroids were used. In 5 of the 14 articles analyzed, steroid use resulted in statistically significant reductions in pain. Seven articles found steroids reduced swelling. Eight articles found steroids reduced trismus. Few side effects were observed after short-term use of the corticosteroids.

Postoperative swelling is expected following the removal of impacted third molars. This complication can affect the social, school, and work life of patients. Pharmacological intervention has been shown to reduce postoperative swelling. Common medications used in the management of postoperative swelling include dexamethasone, methylprednisolone, and ibuprofen. Dexamethasone and methylprednisolone are glucocorticoids. Ibuprofen is a non-steroidal anti-inflammatory drug.

IV Dexamethasone

Dexamethasone was synthesized in 1957.[61] It is a potent steroid with anti-inflammatory and immunosuppressant activity. Dexamethasone phosphate is absorbed rapidly following intravenous injection. Metabolism occurs primarily in the liver by cytochrome P450 enzymes. The biological half-life of dexamethasone is about 190 minutes. Onset of action is within 1 hour. Duration of action is 36 to 54 hours. Dexamethasone phosphate can be administered IV, IM, or intraoral. (See Table 6.16.)

Many studies have shown that dexamethasone can safely reduce facial swelling using different routes of administration. For example, one study showed that the use of injectable dexamethasone phosphate, given as an intraoral injection at the time of the procedure, was effective in the prevention of postoperative swelling. In third molar surgery, pain and trismus are often directly proportional to swelling. Therefore, a patient with minimal swelling should have minimal pain and trismus.[62,63]

Table 6.16 Characteristics of injectable dexamethasone.

Characteristic	IV Dexamethasone
Bioavailability	100%
Biological ½ Life	190 min.
Peak plasma time	< 1 hr.
Availability	4.0 mg/ml and 10.0 mg/ml
Metabolism	Hepatic, CYP3A4
Active metabolites	No
Onset of activity	< 1 hr.
Duration of action	36–54 hrs.
Pregnancy category	Category C, not for use in nursing
Contraindications	Hypersensitivity to dexamethasone, systemic fungal infections

Another, more recent study, found that parenteral use of dexamethasone 4 mg, given as an intra-oral injection at the time of surgery, is effective in the prevention of postoperative edema. The study also found that increasing the dose to 8 mg provides no further benefit.[64]

Adding dexamethasone by intraoral injection may be an attractive option for dentists not certi-fied in IV sedation. Alternatively, methylprednisolone can be given orally by individual tablet.

Oral Methylprednisolone

Methylprednisolone is another potent anti-inflammatory steroid. The oral administration of meth-ylprednisolone has been shown to reduce inflammation following the removal of third molars. Acham, S., Klampfl, A., Truschnegg, A. et al. evaluated the influence of preoperative oral methyl-prednisolone on postoperative swelling, trismus, and pain.

Sixteen healthy patients were included in a prospective, randomized, placebo-controlled, dou-ble-blind study in a split-mouth design. Patients received oral methylprednisolone (40–80 mg) or a placebo 1 hour prior to surgery. The study found a significant reduction of trismus, swelling, and pain in the methylprednisolone group.[65]

Another study looked at the analgesic and anti-inflammatory efficacy when methylpredniso-lone is combined with oral ibuprofen. Methylprednisolone (32 mg) was given 12 hours before and 12 hours after removal of mandibular impacted third molars. Ibuprofen (400 mg) was given three times a day on the day of the procedure and on the two days following the procedure. Evaluation showed a 67.7% reduction in pain and a 56% reduction in swelling compared with the placebo group.[66]

Methylprednisolone is rapidly absorbed and the maximum plasma concentration is achieved around 1.1 to 2.2 hours across doses following oral administration in normal healthy adults. The absolute bioavailability of methylprednisolone in normal healthy subjects is generally high (82% to 89%) following oral administration. Methylprednisolone is widely distributed into the tissues, crosses the blood-brain barrier, the placental barrier, and is secreted in breast milk. Methylprednisolone is metabolized in the liver to inactive metabolites. Metabolism in the liver occurs primarily via the CYP3A4 enzyme. The mean elimination half-life for methylprednisolone is in the range of 1.8 to 5.2 hours. (See Table 6.17.)

Table 6.17   Characteristics of oral methylprednisolone.

Characteristic	Methylprednisalone
Bioavailability	82%–89%
Elimination ½ Life	1.8–5.2 hrs.
Peak plasma time	1.1–2.2 hrs.
Availability (Upjohn)	4 mg–100 mg
Metabolism	Hepatic, CYP3A4
Active metabolites	No
Onset of activity	1–2 hrs.
Duration of action	8–24 hrs.
Pregnancy category	Pregnancy category C, not for nursing
Contraindications	Hypersensitivity to methylprednisolone, systemic infections

Ibuprofen

Ibuprofen was previously discussed under the pain section of this chapter. Because ibuprofen has analgesic and anti-inflammatory qualities, it will be discussed again here. (See Table 6.14.)

Ibuprofen has greater potency as an analgesic and antipyretic than as an anti-inflammatory agent. Ibuprofen 400 mg is equivalent to 10 mg of oxycodone as an analgesic (NNT of 2.3). (See Table 6.16.) However, higher doses are required to achieve anti-inflammatory effects than analgesic effects. As the dose of ibuprofen is increased, anti-inflammatory effects improve until maximum safe doses preclude any further increase.[67] Doses of 1600 mg to 2400 mg per day may decrease inflammation following the removal of third molars. The maximum daily dose of ibuprofen should not exceed 2400 mg.

Inflammation is better controlled with corticosteroids than with NSAIDs.[47, 68] The anti-inflammatory and analgesic actions of corticosteroids and NSAIDs, respectively, suggest that combining dexamethasone and ibuprofen may provide beneficial inflammatory and pain relief in the absence of side effects. Jarrah et al. completed a study that confirmed the synergistic effect of corticosteroids (dexamethasone) with ibuprofen in controlling postoperative pain, trismus, and swelling as opposed to corticosteroid alone.[69]

Infection

Antibiotics play a key role in the treatment and prevention of third molar surgical site infections. The incidence of infection after the removal of third molars is very low, ranging from 1.7% to 2.7%.[70] Peterson's *Principles of Oral and Maxillofacial Surgery* states that

> infection after the removal of mandibular third molars is almost always a minor complication. In relation to third molar surgery, 50% of infections are localized subperiosteal abscess type infections occurring approximately 2–4 weeks after surgery. This type of infection is attributed to debris left under the surgically created mucoperiosteal flap and would likely not be prevented with the use of antibiotic prophylaxis. The remaining 50% of third molar surgical site infections are rarely severe enough to necessitate further surgery, antibiotics, or hospitalization. Surgical site infections within the first postoperative week after third molar surgery occurs only 0.5–1.0% of the time.[71]

Common antibiotics used in the United States for the treatment of third molar surgical site infections include amoxicillin, clindamycin, and metronidazole.

Amoxicillin (Amoxil)

The Nobel Prize in Physiology or Medicine 1945 was awarded jointly to Sir Alexander Fleming, Ernst Boris Chain, and Sir Howard Walter Florey "for the discovery of penicillin and its curative effect in various infectious diseases."[72] (See Figure 6.4.)

Amoxicillin first became available in 1972.[73] Amoxicillin is a member of a class of broad-spectrum antibiotics that contain a β-lactam ring in their molecular structure. Amoxicillin is similar to penicillin in its bactericidal action against susceptible bacteria. It acts through the inhibition of cell wall biosynthesis that leads to the death of the bacteria. Amoxicillin is active against a wide range

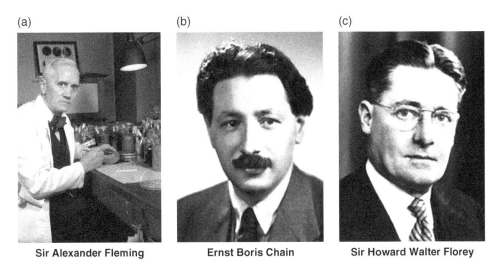

Figure 6.4 Nobel Prize winners in 1945 for the discovery of penicillin. ((a) Imperial War Museums / Wikimedia Commons / Public domain and (b and c) Nobel foundation / Wikimedia Commons / Public domain).

Table 6.18 Characteristic of amoxicillin.

Characteristic	Amoxicillin
Bioavailability	> 80%
Elimination ½ Life	61.3 min.
Peak plasma time	1.0–2.0 hrs.
Availability	250 mg–500 mg capsules
Metabolism	~ 30% Hepatic, CYP450
Active metabolites	No
Onset of activity	.5 hrs.
Duration of action	6–8 hrs.
Pregnancy category	Pregnancy: Category B, Caution in nursing.
Contraindications	Hypersensitivity to β-lactam antibiotics.

of gram-positive and a limited range of gram-negative organisms. Oral amoxicillin is the usual drug of choice within its class because it is better absorbed than other beta-lactam antibiotics.

The bioavailability and half-life of amoxicillin is superior to that of penicillin V. Amoxicillin has bioavailability greater than 80% and a half-life of 61 minutes. Amoxicillin has a peak plasma time of 1 to 2 hours. Onset of action is rapid at 0.5 hours. Duration of action is 6 to 8 hours. Approximately 30% of amoxicillin is metabolized in the liver with no active metabolites. Amoxicillin is available in many forms including 250 mg and 500 mg capsules. (See Table 6.18.)

Amoxicillin is contraindicated in patients with known hypersensitivity to Amoxicillin and or other β-lactam antibiotics. Amoxicillin is a United States FDA pregnancy category B drug.

Clindamycin (Cleocin)

Clindamycin was first made in 1966 from lincomycin.[74] Clindamycin belongs to a class of antibiotics known as lincosamides. Clindamycin is a broad-spectrum antibiotic with activity against aerobic, anaerobic, and beta-lactamase-producing pathogens. Clindamycin has a primarily bacteriostatic effect inhibiting bacterial protein synthesis by binding to the 50S bacterial ribosome subunit.[75]

A review of the literature relating to maxillofacial infections has shown this antibiotic to be highly effective in the field of dentistry.[76] Clindamycin is considered the alternative of choice in patients allergic to amoxicillin.

Clindamycin has bioavailability of 90% and a half-life of 2 ½ to 3 hours. It has a peak plasma time of 45 minutes. Onset of action is variable. Duration of action is 8 to 12 hours. Clindamycin is metabolized in the liver with active metabolites. Clindamycin is available in many forms, including 75 mg, 150 mg, and 300 mg capsules. (See Table 6.19.)

Clindamycin is contraindicated in patients with known hypersensitivity to clindamycin or lincomycin. Clindamycin is a United States FDA pregnancy category B drug.

Metronidazole (Flagyl)

Metronidazole was introduced in 1959.[77] It belongs to a class of antibiotics known as nitroimidazoles. Metronidazole is the gold standard antibiotic in the treatment of anaerobic infections because of its pharmacodynamics and pharmacokinetics, minimal adverse effects, and antimicrobial activity. Metronidazole is not recommended as single drug therapy for oral infections because it is inactive against aerobic and facultative streptococci. However, it may be combined with beta lactams (amoxicillin) when managing severe infections.[78]

The bioavailability of metronidazole is 95%. Its elimination half-life is 8 hours. Metronidazole has a peak plasma time of 1 to 2 hours. Onset of action is rapid. Duration of action is 6–8 hours. Metronidazole is metabolized in the liver and excreted primarily by the kidneys. Metronidazole is available in many forms, including 250 mg and 500 mg capsules. (See Table 6.20.)

Table 6.19   Characteristics of clindamycin.

Characteristic	Clindamycin
Bioavailability	90 %
Elimination ½ Life	2.4–3.0 hrs.
Peak plasma time	45 min.
Availability	75 mg, 150 mg, 300 mg capsules
Metabolism	Hepatic, CYP450
Active metabolites	Yes
Onset of action	Variable
Duration of action	8–12 hrs.
Pregnancy category	Pregnancy: Category B, not for use in nursing.
Contraindications	Hypersensitivity to clindamycin or lincomycin

Table 6.20   Characteristics of metronidazole.

Characteristic	Metronidazole
Bioavailability	95 %
Elimination ½ Life	8 hrs.
Peak plasma time	1–2 hrs.
Availability	250 mg–500 mg capsules
Metabolism	Hepatic, CYP450
Active metabolites	Yes
Onset of activity	Rapid
Duration of action	6–8 hrs.
Pregnancy category	Pregnancy: Category B, Caution in nursing.
Contraindications	Hypersensitivity to metronidazole

Metronidazole is contraindicated in patients with known hypersensitivity to metronidazole. Metronidazole is a United States FDA pregnancy category B drug.

Prophylactic Antibiotics

The universal use of prophylactic antibiotics to prevent third molar postoperative infection is controversial. Antibiotic resistance is now a serious problem, which was not the case 50 years ago.[79] Peterson's criterion for antibiotic use is that the surgical procedure should have a significant risk of infection.[80] Antibiotic prophylaxis may also be recommended for patients when traumatic surgical procedures have been performed.[81,82]

The risk of developing a surgical site infection, associated with the removal of impacted third molars, increases with degree of impaction, need for bone removal or sectioning, the presence of gingivitis, periodontal disease and/or pericoronitis, surgeon experience, increasing age, and antibiotic use.[83] The decision to use prophylactic antibiotics should be based on these factors and assessment of each individual patient.

Treatment of Existing Infection

Signs of surgical site infection include localized swelling, purulence, erythema, fluctuance, trismus, fever, and dehydration. Definitive treatment of surgical site infection involves incision and drainage plus the administration of antibiotics. Amoxicillin, a broad-spectrum antibiotic, is often prescribed since most oral infections are caused by a mixed flora of anaerobic and gram-positive streptococci microorganisms. Metronidazole is primarily used to treat infections caused by anaerobic microorganisms. Metronidazole can be combined with amoxicillin to treat severe infections. This combination is very effective in the treatment of subperiosteal infections. Clindamycin is a good choice of antibiotic for patients allergic to amoxicillin. Most impacted third molar surgical site infections are localized subperiosteal abscesses. Rarely, cellulitis develops or the infection spreads along fascial planes in the head and neck. In this situation, immediate referral to an oral and maxillofacial surgeon for definitive management is recommended.[84,85]

Author's Medication Regimen

Most of the authors impacted third molar patients are ASA I or II patients requiring surgical flaps, bone removal, and sectioning. The majority of these patients receive prophylactic antibiotics due to the traumatic nature of the procedure. The following regimen is used for full and partial bony impactions.

Patients arrive at the office one hour prior to the procedure and are given triazolam. (See Box 6.2.) At the appointment time the patient is seated in the operatory. The IV is started and fentanyl and midazolam are slowly titrated to the desired effect. Patients who are moderately sedated from the sublingual sedative do not receive IV midazolam. Most patients receive 50 micrograms of fentanyl (maximum of 100 micrograms) and 3 milligrams of midazolam. Sedations are more effective when fentanyl is administered before midazolam.

Box 6.2 Author's medication regimen for the removal of partial and full bony impactions.

Amoxicillin 500 mg, Disp: 15
Take one tablet one hour before appointment and continue three times a day until gone.
Ibuprofen 800 mg, Disp: 15
Take one tablet one hour before appointment and continue three times a day until gone.
Triazolam .25 mg, Disp: 2
Bring to appointment (.5 mg administered in office for ASA I and II)
*0.25 mg for elderly or medically compromised

This regimen works well for the vast majority of patients. When necessary, the patient is instructed to take Tylenol 500 mg 6 times a day in addition to prescribed ibuprofen. Hydrocodone 10 mg is added in rare cases.

References

1 Harrison L. Painful dental work: acetaminophen with ibuprofen best. *Medscape*, 2013 Aug 14.
2 Le J. Drug distribution to tissues. Merck Manuals, 2016 Apr.
3 Montamat SC, Cusack BJ, Vestal RE. Management of drug therapy in the elderly. *N Engl J Med.* 1989;321:303–9.
4 Oates JA. The science of drug therapy. In: Brunton LL, Lazo JS, Parker KL, editors. *Goodman and Gilman's the pharmacological basis of therapeutics*, 11th edition. New York, NY: McGraw-Hill, 2006, 117–36.
5 Becker DE. Drug therapy in dental practice: general principles Part 2—pharmacodynamic considerations. *Anesth Prog.* 2007;54:19–24.
6 Osborn TM, Sandler NA. The effects of preoperative anxiety on intravenous sedation. *Anesth Prog.* 2004;51(2):46–51.
7 Saïas T, Gallarda T. Paradoxical aggressive reactions to benzodiazepine use: a review. *L'Encéphale* (in French). 2008;34(4):330–6.
8 Donaldson M, Gizzarelli G, Chanpong B. Oral sedation: a primer on anxiolysis for the adult patient. *Anesth Prog.* 2007 Fall;54(3):118–29.

9 Senninger JL, Laxenaire M. [Violent paradoxal reactions secondary to the use of benzodiazepines] [Violent paradoxical reactions secondary to the use of benzodiazepines]. *Annales médico-psychologiques* (in French). 1995 Apr;153(4):278–81, discussion 281–2.

10 Mancuso CE, Tanzi MG, Gabay M. Paradoxical reactions to benzodiazepines: literature review and treatment options. *Pharmacotherapy*. 2004 Sept;24(9):1177–85. doi:10.1592/phco.24.13.1177.38089.

11 Malamed SF. *Sedation a guide to patient management*, 5th edition. St Louis Missouri 63146: Mosby Elsevier, 2010. Ch 7, 101.

12 Baughman VL, Becker GL, Ryan CM, Glaser M, Abenstein JP. Effectiveness of triazolam, diazepam, and placebos as preanesthetic medications. *Anesthesiology*. 1989;71:196–200.

13 Ouellette RG. Midazolam: an induction agent for general anesthesia. *Nurse Anest*. 1991;2:131.

14 Drover DR. Comparative pharmacokinetics and pharmacodynamics of short-acting hypnosedatives: zaleplon, zolpidem and zopiclone. *Clin Pharmacokinet*. 2004;43(4):227–38.

15 Patat A, Naef MM, van Gessel E, Forster A, Dubruc C, Rosenzweig P. Flumazenil antagonizes the central effects of zolpidem, an imidazopyridine hypnotic. *Clin Pharmacol Ther*. 1994 Oct;56(4):430–6.

16 Malamed SF. *Sedation a guide to patient management*, 5th edition. St Louis Missouri 63146: Mosby Elsevier, 2010. Ch 7, 109.

17 Malamed SF. *Sedation a guide to patient management*, 5th edition. St Louis Missouri 63146: Mosby Elsevier, 2010. Ch 25, 347.

18 Greenblatt DJ, Ehrenberg BL, Gunderman J, et al. Kinetic and dynamic study of intravenous lorazepam: comparison with intravenous diazepam. *J Pharmacol Exp Ther*. 1989;250:134–40.

19 Becker DE. Pharmacodynamic considerations for moderate and deep sedation. *Anesth Prog*. 2012 Spring;59(1):28–42.

20 Sher AM, Braude BM, Cleaton-Jones PE, Moyes DG, Mallett J. Nitrous oxide sedation in dentistry: a comparison between Rotameter settings, pharyngeal concentrations and blood levels of nitrous oxide. *Anaesthesia*. 1984;39:236–9.

21 Browne DR, Rochford J, O'Connell U, Jones JG. The incidence of postoperative atelectasis in the dependent lung following thoracotomy: the value of added nitrogen. *Br J Anaesth*. 1970 Apr;42(4):340–6.

22 Yacoub O, Doell D, Kryger MH, et al. Depression of hypoxic ventilator response by nitrous oxide. *Anesthesiology*. 1976;45:385m.

23 Zhang C, Davies MF, Guo TZ, Maze M. The analgesic action of nitrous oxide is dependent on the release of norepinephrine in the dorsal horn of the spinal cord. *Anesthesiology*. 1999;91:1401–7.

24 Wylie WD. *Churchill-Davidson HC: a practice of anesthesia*, 4th edition. Philadelphia: WB Saunders, 1978.

25 Becker DE, Reed KL. Essentials of local anesthetic pharmacology. *Anesth Prog*. 2006 Fall;53(3):98-108; quiz 109-10. doi: 10.2344/0003-3006(2006)53[98:EOLAP]2.0.CO;2. PMID: 17175824; PMCID: PMC1693664.

26 Becker DE, Reed KL. Essentials of local anesthetic pharmacology. *Anesth Prog*. 2006 Fall;53(3):98–109.

27 Chong CA. Local anaesthetic and additive drugs. Anesthesia UK, 2005 Aug.

28 Tofoli GR, Ramacciato JC, de Oliveira PC, et al. Comparison of effectiveness of 4% articaine associated with 1:100,000 or 1:200,000 epinephrine in inferior alveolar nerve block. *Anesth Prog*. 2003;50:164–8.

29 Kritikos PG, Papadaki SP. The history of the poppy and of opium and their expansion in antiquity in the eastern Mediterranean area. Bulletin on Narcotics, 1967, United Nations Office on Drug Control (3-003), 1967, 17–38.

30 Drug Enforcement Administration. Museum and Visitors Center, 2021, Pentagon City, Arlington, VA.

31 Hemmings HC, Egan TD. *Pharmacology and physiology for anesthesia: foundations and clinical application*. Elsevier Health Sciences, 2013, 253.

32 Malamed SF. *Sedation a guide to patient management*, 5th edition. St Louis Missouri 63146: Mosby Elsevier, 2010. Ch 25, 330.

33 Mannich C, Löwenheim H. Ueber zwei neue Reduktionsprodukte des Kodeins. *Archiv der Pharmazie*. 1920;258(2–4):295–316.

34 Hydrocodone bitartrate and acetaminophen: clinical pharmacology. RxList. Accessed 2009 Feb 19.

35 Sneader W. *Drug discovery: a history*. Hoboken, NJ: Wiley, 2005, 119.

36 IMS Health. National, years prescription audit1997–2013. Data Extracted 2014.

37 Lopez-Munoz, F, et al. The consolidation of neuroleptic therapy: Janssen, the discovery of haloperidol and its introduction into clinical practice. *Brain Res Bull*. 2009; 79(2):130–41.

38 Malamed SF. *Sedation a guide to patient management*, 5th edition. Mosby, 2010, Ch 25, 333.

39 Yardley W. Jack Fishman dies at 83; saved many from overdose. New York Times, 2013 Dec.

40 Malamed SF. *Sedation a guide to patient management*, 5th edition. St Louis Missouri 63146: Mosby Elsevier, 2010. Ch 25, 346.

41 McEvoy GK, editor. *Drug information 2012*. Bethesda, MD: American Society of Health-System Pharmacists, 2012, 2236–9.

42 Bosack R. *Anesthesia complications in the dental office*. John Wiley & Sons, 2015, 191.

43 Halford GM, Lordkipanidzé M, Watson SP. 50th anniversary of the discovery of ibuprofen: an interview with Dr Stewart Adams. *Platelets*. 2012;23(6):415–22.

44 Wahbi AA, Hassan E, Hamdy D, Khamis E, Barary M. Spectrophotometric methods for the determination of Ibuprofen in tablets. *Pak J Pharm Sci*. 2005 Oct;18(4):1–6.

45 Dionne RA, Campbell RA, Cooper SA, Hall DL, Buckingham B. Suppression of postoperative pain by preoperative administration of ibuprofen in comparison to placebo, acetaminophen, and acetaminophen plus codeine. *J Clin Pharmacol*. 1983;23:37–43.

46 Moore PA, Nahouraii HS, Zovko JG, Wisniewski SR. Dental therapeutic practice patterns in the U.S, II: analgesics, corticosteroids, and antibiotics. *Gen Dent*. 2006;54(3):201–7.

47 Becker DE. Pain management: Part 1: managing acute and postoperative dental pain. *Anesth Prog*. 2010 Summer;57(2):67–79.

48 Melgarejo BCM, Miller MG, with consultant, Kimberly A. *Pharmacology application in athletic training*. Philadelphia, PA: F.A. Davis, 2005, 39.

49 Acetaminophen. New World Encyclopedia, 2016 Feb 11, 16:26 UTC. 12 Sep 2016, 03:49.

50 Forrest JA, Clements JA, Prescott LF. Clinical pharmacokinetics of paracetamol. *Clin Pharmacokinet*. 1982 Mar-Apr;7(2):93–107.

51 Sattar N, Preiss D, Murray H, et al. Statins and risk of incident diabetes: a collaborative meta-analysis of randomised statin trials. *Lancet*, 2010;375:735–42.

52 McNeil. Nonprescription drugs advisory committee meeting, background package on acetaminophen. 2002 Sept 19.

53 Piletta P, Porchet HC, Dayer P. Central analgesic effect of acetaminophen but not aspirin. *Clin Pharmacol Ther*. 1991;49:350–4.

54 Hersh EV, Moore PA, Ross GL. Over the counter analgesics and antipyretics: a critical assessment. *Clin Ther*. 2000;22(5):500–48.

55 Moore RA, Derry S, McQuay HJ, Wiffen PJ. Single dose oral analgesics for acute postoperative pain in adults. *Cochrane Database Syst Rev*. 2011 Sep 7;(9):CD008659. doi: 10.1002/14651858.CD008659.pub2. Update in: Cochrane Database Syst Rev. 2015;9:CD008659. PMID: 21901726; PMCID: PMC4160790.

56 Moore PA, Hersh EV. Combining ibuprofen and acetaminophen for acute pain management after third molar extractions: translating clinical research to dental practice. *JADA*. 2013;144(8):898–908.

57 Laska EM, Sunshine A, Marrero I, et al. The correlation between blood levels of ibuprofen and clinical analgesic response. *Clin Pharmacol Ther*. 1986;40:1–7.

58 Moore PA. Bupivacaine: a long-lasting local anesthetic for dentistry. *Oral Surg Oral Med Oral Pathol*. 1984;58(4):369–74.

59 Truollos ES, Hargreaves KM, Butler DP, et al. Comparison of nonsteroidal anti-inflammatory drugs, ibuprofen and flurbiprofen, methylprednisolone and placebo for acute pain, swelling, and trismus. *J Oral Maxillofac Surg*. 1990;48(9):945–52.

60 Ata-Ali J, Ata-Ali F, Peñarrocha-Oltra D, Peñarrocha M. Corticosteroids use in controlling pain, swelling and trismus after lower third molar surgery. *J Clin Exp Dent*. 2011;3(5):e469–75.

61 Moore PA, Brar P, Smiga ER, Costello BJ. Preemptive rofecoxib and dexamethasone for prevention of pain and trismus following third molar surgery. *Oral Surg Oral Med Oral Pathol Oral Radiol Endod*. 2005;99(2):E1–7.

62 Rankovic Z, Hargreaves R, Bingham M. *Drug discovery and medicinal chemistry for psychiatric disorders*. Cambridge: Royal Society of Chemistry, 2012, 286.

63 Tiwana PS, Foy SP, Shugars DA. The impact of intravenous corticosteroids with third molar surgery in patients at high risk for delayed health-related quality of life and clinical recovery. *J Oral Maxillofac Surg*. 2005 Jan;63:55–62.

64 Messer EJ, Keller JJ. The use of intraoral dexamethasone after extraction of mandibular third molars. *Oral Surg Oral Med Oral Pathol*. 1975 Nov;40(5):594–8.

65 Acham S, Klampfl A, Truschnegg A, et al. Beneficial effect of methylprednisolone after mandibular third molar surgery: a randomized, double-blind, placebo-controlled split-mouth trial. *Clin Oral Invest*. 2013;17:1693.

66 Grossi GB, Maiorana C, Garramone RA, Borgonovo A, Beretta M, Farronato D, Santoro F. Effect of submucosal injection of dexamethasone on postoperative discomfort after third molar surgery: a prospective study. *J Oral Maxillofac Surg*. 2007 Nov;65(11):2218–26.

67 Schultze-Mosgau S, Schmelzeisen R, Frölich JC, Schmele H. Use of ibuprofen and methylprednisolone for the prevention of pain and swelling after removal of impacted third molars. *J Oral Maxillofac. Surg*. 1995 Jan;53(1):2–7.

68 Baxendale BR, Vater M, Lavery KM. Dexamethasone reduces pain and swelling following extraction of third molar teeth. *Anesthesia*. 1993;48:961–4.

69 Markiewicz MR, Brady MF, Ding EL, Dodson TB. Corticosteroids reduce postoperative morbidity after third molar surgery: a systematic review and meta-analysis. *J Oral Maxillofac Surg*. 2008;66:1881–94.

70 Jarrah MH, Al-Rabadi HF, Imrayan M, Al-share' AA. Single dose of dexamethasone with or without ibuprofen effects on post-operative sequelae of lower third molar surgical extraction. *J R Med Serv*. 2015;22(1):41–5.

71 Miloro M, Ghali GE, Larsen PE. *Peterson's principles of oral and maxillofacial surgery*, 3rd edition. Impacted Teeth, 2011, Chapter 5, 114.

72 The nobel prize in physiology or medicine 1945. Nobelprize.org. Nobel Media AB 2014. Web. 2016 Sept 19.

73 Roy J. *An introduction to pharmaceutical sciences production, chemistry, techniques and technology*. Cambridge: Woodhead Publishing, 2012, 239.

74 Ainsworth SB. *Neonatal formulary: drug use in pregnancy and the first year of life*, 7th edition. John Wiley & Sons, 2014, 162.

75 Schlecht H, Bruno C. Lincosamides, oxazolidinones, and streptogramins. In: *Merck manual of diagnosis and therapy*. Merck & Co, 2005 Nov.

76 Brook I, et al. Clindamycin in dentistry: more than just effective prophylaxis for endocarditis? *Oral Surg Oral Med Oral Pathol Oral Radiol Endod.* 2005;100:550–8.

77 Bowman WC, Rand MJ. *Treatment of trichomonas urogenitalis, textbook of pharmacology*, 2nd edition. Hoboken, New Jersey: Blackwell Scientific Publications, 36.16, 1980.

78 Becker DE. Antimicrobial drugs. *Anesth Prog.* 2013 Fall;60(3):111–23.

79 Siddiqi A, Morkel JA, Zafar S. Antibiotic prophylaxis in third molar surgery: a randomized double-blind placebo-controlled clinical trial using split-mouth technique. *Int J Oral Maxillofac Surg.* 2010;39:107–14.

80 Peterson's criterion for antibiotic use is that the surgical procedure should have a significant risk of infection4. Peterson LJ. Antibiotic prophylaxis against wound infections in oral and maxillofacial surgery. *J Oral Maxillofac Surg.* 1990;48:617–20.

81 Salmerón-Escobar JI, Del Amo-Fernández de Velasco A. Antibiotic prophylaxis in oral and maxillofacial surgery. *Med Oral Patol Oral Cir Bucal.* 2006;11:E 292–6.

82 Lawler B, Sambrook PJ, Goss AN. Antibiotic prophylaxis for dentoalveolar surgery: is it indicated? *Aust Dent J.* 2005;50:S54–9.

83 Miloro M, Kolokythas A. *Management of complications in oral and maxillofacial surgery*. Hoboken, New Jersey: Blackwell Scientific Publications, 2012, Ch 2, 27.

84 Figueiredo R, Valmaseda-Castellon E, Berini-Aytes L. Incidence and clinical features of delayed-onset infections after extraction of lower third molars. *Oral Surg Oral Med Oral Pathol Oral Radiol Endod.* 2005;99:265.

85 Goldberg MH, Nemarich AN, Marco WP. Complications after mandibular third molar surgery: a statistical analysis of 500 consecutive procedures in private practice. *J Am Dent Assoc.* 1985;111:277–9.

7

Sedation Techniques

This chapter is not intended to be a comprehensive review of sedation and anesthesia. Rather, it is a review of the three most common techniques used by general dentists when sedating adults. These three techniques – nitrous oxide, oral sedation, and IV sedation – are invaluable when removing impacted third molars. The reader is referred to Stanley Malamed's excellent book *Sedation: A Guide to Patient Management* for a comprehensive review of sedation.

It is estimated that as many as 75% of US adults experience some degree of dental fear, from mild to severe.[1–3] Approximately 5–10% of US adults are considered to experience dental phobia; that is, they are so fearful of receiving dental treatment that they avoid dental care at all costs.[4] People who are very fearful of dental care often experience a "cycle of avoidance," in which they avoid dental care due to fear until they experience a dental emergency requiring invasive treatment, which can reinforce their fear of dentistry.[5] A survey of 1000 adult Americans found "going to the dentist" to be the second most common fear, only surpassed by public speaking.[6]

Gale ranked 25 dental situations from the most fearful to the least fearful. Removal of a tooth was the most feared situation.[7] Another study conducted in 2012 evaluated the level of fear and anxiety in patients undergoing different minor oral surgery procedures. The removal of a third molar was the most feared surgical procedure in the study.[8] Fortunately, thanks to the discovery of anesthesia, dentistry and the removal of impacted third molars can now be completed with minimal discomfort and with little or no memory of the procedure.

Prior to the discovery of modern anesthesia, patients facing surgery were confronted with impossible choices; namely, suffer a prolonged, painful death from their affliction or experience excruciating surgery without effective pain control. Faced with these options, many people committed suicide.

The discovery of modern anesthesia is often credited to two dentists, Dr. Horace Wells and Dr. William T. G. Morton.[9] Dr. Wells, a New England dentist, used nitrous oxide for the extraction of one of his teeth on December 12, 1844. (See Figure 7.1.) Wells had seen nitrous oxide displayed the night before by the traveling chemist and showman, Gardner Quincy Colton, a "purveyor of laughing gas." Wells had noted that those under the influence of nitrous oxide seemed insensible to injury. Dr. Wells used nitrous oxide on a number of his patients with success.

Dr. William T. G. Morton, another New England dentist, was a former student and business partner of Wells. (See Figure 7.2.) Morton arranged for Wells to demonstrate his technique for dental extraction under nitrous oxide anesthesia at Massachusetts General Hospital. This demonstration took place on January 20, 1845 and was deemed a failure because the patient moaned during the procedure. Believing that a more potent anesthetic gas was necessary, Dr. Morton began to search for a better agent than nitrous oxide. In October 1846, he demonstrated the use of diethyl

Impacted Third Molars, Second Edition. Edited by John Wayland.
© 2024 John Wiley & Sons, Inc. Published 2024 by John Wiley & Sons, Inc.

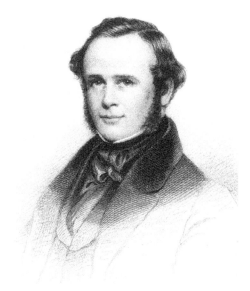

Figure 7.1   Dr. Horace Wells. (Henry Bryan Hall / Wikimedia Commons / Public domain).

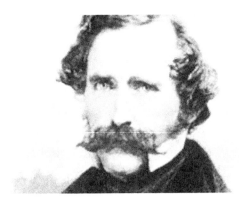

Figure 7.2   Dr. William T. G. Morton. (Unknown author / Wikimedia Commons / Public domain).

ether as a general anesthetic at Massachusetts General Hospital, in what is known today as the Ether Dome. This time, the operation was deemed a success.

Research in the control of pain and anxiety continued following the discoveries of Wells and Morton. One hundred years later, Dr. Niels Bjorn Jorgensen (another dentist), developed the Jorgenson or "Loma Linda" technique for intravenous administration of drugs to induce sedation by titration.[10] Dr. Jorgenson is considered by many to be the father of intravenous sedation in dentistry. (See Figure 7.3.)

Today, virtually all dental procedures can be completed without discomfort when topical and local anesthetics are used properly. However, difficult to numb patients, patients with long appointments or invasive procedures, and patients with high anxiety may require sedation. The goal of sedation is the elimination of anxiety and pain. Sedation is commonly used before and during impacted third molar surgery.

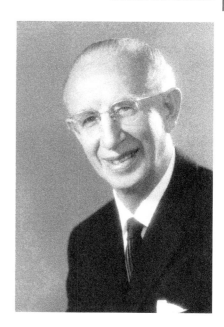

Figure 7.3 Dr. Niels Jorgenson. (Reproduced with permission of Loma Linda University Health).

Sedation as a Continuum

The concept of sedation as a continuum is the foundation of patient safety. In 2004, the American Society of Anesthesiologists made the following statement: "Because sedation and general anesthesia are a continuum, it is not always possible to predict how an individual patient will respond. Hence, practitioners intending to produce a given level of sedation should be able to diagnose and manage the physiologic consequences (rescue) for patients whose level of sedation becomes deeper than initially intended."[11] Dentists providing sedation must have the training, skills, drugs, and equipment necessary to manage patients that are more deeply sedated than intended until EMS arrives or the patient returns to the intended level of sedation.

Sedation is a continuum of levels of sedation from fully consciousness to unconsciousness (general anesthesia). (See Figure 7.4.)

The American Dental Association, Council on Dental Education, published guidelines for the use of sedation and general anesthesia by dentists in 2007. A sedation and general anesthesia policy statement was adopted by the ADA House of Delegates in 2012. The 2012 ADA policy statement contains the following definitions and clinical guidelines.[12]

Sedation is a continuum of anesthesia from fully conscious to unconscious (general anesthesia)

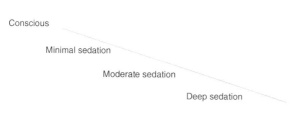

Conscious

Minimal sedation

Moderate sedation

Deep sedation

General anesthesia

Figure 7.4 Sedation continuum.

ADA Definitions

Minimal sedation (previously anxiolysis) – "a minimally depressed level of consciousness, produced by a pharmacological method, that retains the patient's ability to independently and continuously maintain an airway and respond normally to tactile stimulation and verbal command. Although cognitive function and coordination may be modestly impaired, ventilatory and cardiovascular functions are unaffected."

"Note: In accord with this particular definition, the drug(s) and/or techniques used should carry a margin of safety wide enough to never render unintended loss of consciousness. Further, patients whose only response is reflex withdrawal from repeated painful stimuli would not be considered to be in a state of minimal sedation."

"When the intent is minimal sedation for adults, the appropriate initial dosing of a single enteral drug is no more than the maximum recommended dose (MRD) of a drug that can be prescribed for unmonitored home use."

Moderate sedation (previously conscious sedation) – "A drug-induced depression of consciousness during which patients respond purposefully to verbal commands, either alone or accompanied by light tactile stimulation. No interventions are required to maintain a patent airway, and spontaneous ventilation is adequate. Cardiovascular function is usually maintained."

"Note: In accord with this particular definition, the drugs and/or techniques used should carry a margin of safety wide enough to render unintended loss of consciousness unlikely. Repeated dosing of an agent before the effects of previous dosing can be fully appreciated may result in a greater alteration of the state of consciousness than is the intent of the dentist. Further, a patient whose only response is reflex withdrawal from a painful stimulus is not considered to be in a state of moderate sedation."

Deep sedation – "A drug-induced depression of consciousness during which patients cannot be easily aroused but respond purposefully following repeated or painful stimulation. The ability to independently maintain ventilatory function may be impaired. Patients may require assistance in maintaining a patent airway, and spontaneous ventilation may be inadequate. Cardiovascular function is usually maintained."

General anesthesia – "A drug-induced loss of consciousness during which patients are not arousable, even by painful stimulation. The ability to independently maintain ventilator function is often impaired. Patients often require assistance in maintaining a patent airway, and positive pressure ventilation may be required because of depressed spontaneous ventilation or drug-induced depression of neuromuscular function. Cardiovascular function may be impaired."

The following definitions from the ADA guidelines apply to administration of minimal sedation:

Maximum recommended dose (MRD) – maximum FDA-recommended dose of a drug, as printed in FDA-approved labeling for unmonitored home use.

Incremental dosing – administration of multiple doses of a drug until a desired effect is reached, but not to exceed the maximum recommended dose (MRD).

Supplemental dosing – during minimal sedation, supplemental dosing is a single additional dose of the initial dose of the initial drug that may be necessary for prolonged procedures. The supplemental dose should not exceed one-half of the initial dose and should not be administered until the dentist has determined the clinical half-life of the initial dosing has passed. The total aggregate dose must not exceed 1.5x the MRD on the day of treatment.

The following definition from the ADA guidelines applies to moderate or greater sedation:

Titration – administration of incremental doses of a drug until a desired effect is reached. Knowledge of each drug's time of onset, peak response, and duration of action is essential to avoid over sedation.

Although the concept of titration of a drug to effect is critical for patient safety, when the intent is moderate sedation one must know whether the previous dose has taken full effect before administering an additional drug increment.

ADA Clinical Guidelines

Minimal Sedation

1) Patient Evaluation

Patients considered for minimal sedation must be suitably evaluated prior to the start of any sedative procedure. In healthy or medically stable individuals (ASA I, II) this may consist of a review of their current medical history and medication use. However, patients with significant medical considerations (ASA III, IV) may require consultation with their primary care physician or consulting medical specialist.

2) Preparation

The patient, parent, guardian, or caregiver must be advised regarding the procedure associated with the delivery of any sedative agents and informed consent for the proposed sedation must be obtained. Determination of adequate oxygen supply and equipment necessary to deliver oxygen under positive pressure must be completed. Baseline vital signs must be obtained unless the patient's behavior prohibits such determination. A focused physical evaluation must be performed as deemed appropriate. Preoperative dietary restrictions must be considered based on the sedative technique prescribed. Preoperative verbal and written instructions must be given to the patient, parent, escort, guardian, or caregiver.

3) Personnel and Equipment

At least one additional person trained in Basic Life Support for Healthcare Providers must be present in addition to the dentist. A positive-pressure oxygen delivery system suitable for the patient being treated must be immediately available. When inhalation equipment is used, it must have a fail-safe system that is appropriately checked and calibrated. The equipment must also have either (1) a functioning device that prohibits the delivery of less than 30% oxygen or (2) an appropriately calibrated and functioning in-line oxygen analyzer with audible alarm. An appropriate scavenging system must be available if gases other than oxygen or air are used.

4) Monitoring and Documentation

A dentist, or at the dentist's direction, an appropriately trained individual, must remain in the operatory during active dental treatment to monitor the patient continuously until the patient meets the criteria for discharge to the recovery area. The appropriately trained individual must be familiar with monitoring techniques and equipment. Monitoring must include oxygenation, ventilation, and circulation.

- Oxygenation
The color of mucosa, skin, or blood must be evaluated continually, and oxygen saturation by pulse oximetry should be considered.
- Ventilation
The dentist and/or appropriately trained individual must observe chest excursions and verify respirations continually.

- Circulation

Blood pressure and heart rate should be evaluated preoperatively, postoperatively, and intraoperatively as necessary (unless the patient is unable to tolerate such monitoring).

An appropriate sedative record must be maintained, including the names of all drugs administered, including local anesthetics, dosages, and monitored physiological parameters.

5) Recovery and Discharge

Oxygen and suction equipment must be immediately available if a separate recovery area is utilized. The qualified dentist or appropriately trained clinical staff must monitor the patient during recovery until the patient is ready for discharge by the dentist. The qualified dentist must determine and document that the levels of consciousness, oxygenation, ventilation, and circulation are satisfactory prior to discharge. Postoperative verbal and written instructions must be given to the patient, parent, escort, guardian, or caregiver.

6) Emergency Management

If a patient enters a deeper level of sedation than the dentist is qualified to provide, the dentist must stop the dental procedure until the patient returns to the intended level of sedation. The qualified dentist is responsible for the sedative management, adequacy of the facility and staff, diagnosis and treatment of emergencies related to the administration of minimal sedation and providing the equipment and protocols for patient rescue.

7) Management of Children

For children 12 years of age and under, the American Dental Association supports the use of the American Academy of Pediatrics/American Academy of Pediatric Dentists Guidelines for Monitoring and Management of Pediatric Patients During and After Sedation for Diagnostic and Therapeutic Procedures.

Moderate Sedation

1) Patient Evaluation

Patients considered for moderate sedation must be suitably evaluated prior to the start of any sedative procedure. In healthy or medically stable individuals (ASA I, II) this should consist of at least a review of their current medical history and medication use. However, patients with significant medical considerations (e.g., ASA III, IV) may require consultation with their primary care physician or consulting medical specialist.

2) Preparation

The patient, parent, guardian, or caregiver must be advised regarding the procedure associated with the delivery of any sedative agents and informed consent for the propose sedation must be obtained. Determination of adequate oxygen supply and equipment necessary to deliver oxygen under positive pressure must be completed. Baseline vital signs must be obtained unless the patient's behavior prohibits such determination. A focused physical evaluation must be performed as deemed appropriate. Preoperative dietary restrictions must be considered based on the sedative technique prescribed. Preoperative verbal or written instructions must be given to the patient, parent, escort, guardian, or caregiver.

3) Personnel and Equipment

At least one additional person trained in Basic Life Support for Healthcare Providers must be present in addition to the dentist. A positive-pressure oxygen delivery system suitable for the patient being treated must be immediately available. When inhalation equipment is used, it must have a fail-safe system that is appropriately checked and calibrated. The equipment must also have either (1) a functioning device that prohibits the delivery of less than 30% oxygen or (2) an appropriately calibrated and functioning in-line oxygen analyzer with audible alarm. An appropriate scavenging system must be available if gases other than oxygen or air are used. The equipment necessary to establish intravenous access must be available.

4) Monitoring and Documentation

A qualified dentist administering moderate sedation must remain in the operatory room to monitor the patient continuously until the patient meets the criteria for recovery. When active treatment concludes and the patient recovers to a minimally sedated level a qualified auxiliary may be directed by the dentist to remain with the patient and continue to monitor them as explained in the guidelines until they are discharged from the facility. The dentist must not leave the facility until the patient meets the criteria for discharge and is discharged from the facility.

Monitoring must include consciousness, oxygenation, ventilation, and circulation.
● Consciousness
The level of consciousness (e.g., responsiveness to verbal command) must be continually assessed.
● Oxygenation
The color of mucosa, skin, and blood must be continually evaluated. Oxygen saturation must be evaluated continuously by pulse oximetry.
● Ventilation
The dentist must monitor ventilation. This can be accomplished by auscultation of breath sounds, monitoring end-tidal CO_2 or by verbal communication with the patient. The dentist must observe chest excursions continually.
● Circulation
The dentist must continually evaluate blood pressure and heart rate (unless the patient is unable to tolerate and this is noted in the time-oriented anesthesia record). Continuous ECG monitoring of patients with significant cardiovascular disease should be considered.

Appropriate time-oriented anesthetic record must be maintained, including the names of all drugs administered, including local anesthetics, dosages and monitored physiological parameters. Pulse oximetry, heart rate, respiratory rate, and blood pressure must be recorded continually.

5) Recovery and Discharge

Oxygen and suction equipment must be immediately available if a separate recovery area is utilized. The qualified dentist or appropriately trained clinical staff must continually monitor the patient's blood pressure, heart rate, oxygenation, and level of consciousness. The qualified dentist must determine and document that level of consciousness; oxygenation, ventilation, and circulation are satisfactory for discharge. Postoperative verbal and written instructions must be given to the patient, parent, escort, guardian, or caregiver. If a reversal agent is administered before discharge criteria have been met, the patient must be monitored until recovery is assured.

6) Emergency Management

If a patient enters a deeper level of sedation than the dentist is qualified to provide, the dentist must stop the dental procedure until the patient returns to the intended level of sedation. The qualified dentist is responsible for the sedative management, adequacy of the facility and staff, diagnosis and treatment of emergencies related to the administration of moderate sedation and providing the equipment, drugs, and protocol for patient rescue.

7) Management of Children

For children 12 years of age and under, the American Dental Association supports the use of the American Academy of Pediatrics/American Academy of Pediatric Dentists Guidelines for Monitoring and Management of Pediatric Patients During and After Sedation for Diagnostic and Therapeutic Procedures.

Deep Sedation or General Anesthesia

1) Patient Evaluation

Patients considered for deep sedation or general anesthesia must be suitably evaluated prior to the start of any sedative procedure. In healthy or medically stable individuals (ASA I, II) this must consist of at least a review of their current medical history and medication use and NPO status. However, patients with significant medical considerations (e.g., ASA III, IV) may require consultation with their primary care physician or consulting medical specialist.

2) Preparation

The patient, parent, guardian, or caregiver must be advised regarding the procedure associated with the delivery of any sedative or anesthetic agents and informed consent for the proposed sedation/anesthesia must be obtained. Determination of adequate oxygen supply and equipment necessary to deliver oxygen under positive pressure must be completed. Baseline vital signs must be obtained unless the patient's behavior prohibits such determination. A focused physical evaluation must be performed as deemed appropriate. Preoperative dietary restrictions must be considered based on the sedative/anesthetic technique prescribed. Preoperative verbal and written instructions must be given to the patient, parent, escort, guardian, or caregiver. An intravenous line, which is secured throughout the procedure, must be established except in special circumstances (see "Pediatric and Special Needs Patients").

3) Personnel and Equipment

A minimum of three (3) individuals must be present. A dentist qualified in accordance with these Guidelines to administer the deep sedation or general anesthesia and two additional individuals who have current certification of successfully completing a Basic Life Support (BLS) Course for the Healthcare Provider are required. When the same individual administering the deep sedation or general anesthesia is performing the dental procedure, one of the additional appropriately trained team members must be designated for patient monitoring.

A positive-pressure oxygen delivery system suitable for the patient being treated must immediately available. When inhalation equipment is used, it must have a fail-safe system that is appropriately checked and calibrated. The equipment must also have either (1) a functioning device that prohibits the delivery of less than 30% oxygen or (2) an appropriately calibrated and functioning in-line oxygen analyzer with audible alarm. An appropriate scavenging system must be available if gases other than oxygen or air are used. The equipment necessary to establish intravenous access must be available. Equipment and drugs necessary to provide advanced airway management, and advanced cardiac life support must be immediately available. If volatile anesthetic agents are utilized, an inspired agent analysis monitor and capnograph should be considered. Resuscitation medications and an appropriate defibrillator must be immediately available.

4) Monitoring and Documentation

A qualified dentist administering deep sedation or general anesthesia must remain in the operatory room to monitor the patient continuously until the patient meets the criteria for recovery. The dentist must not leave the facility until the patient meets the criteria for discharge and is discharged from the facility. Monitoring must include oxygenation, ventilation, circulation, and temperature.

● Oxygenation

Mucosa, skin, or blood color must be continually evaluated. Oxygen saturation must be evaluated continuously by pulse oximetry.

● Ventilation

Respiration rate must be continually monitored and evaluated. End-tidal CO_2 must be continuously monitored and evaluated when treating intubated patients. Breath sounds via auscultation and/or end-tidal CO_2 must be continually monitored and evaluated when treating non-intubated patients.

● Circulation

The dentist must continuously evaluate blood pressure, heart rate, and rhythm via ECG throughout the procedure, as well as pulse rate via pulse oximetry.

● Temperature

A device capable of measuring body temperature must be readily available during the administration of deep sedation or general anesthesia and must be used whenever triggering agents associated with malignant hyperthermia are administered.

Appropriate time-oriented anesthetic record must be maintained, including the names of all drugs administered, including local anesthetics, doses and monitored physiological parameters. Pulse oximetry and end-tidal CO_2 measurements (if taken), heart rate, respiratory rate and blood pressure must be recorded at appropriate intervals.

5) Recovery and Discharge

Oxygen and suction equipment must be immediately available if a separate recovery area is utilized. The dentist or clinical staff must continually monitor the patient's blood pressure, heart rate, oxygenation, and level of consciousness. The dentist must determine and document that levels of consciousness, oxygenation, ventilation, and circulation are satisfactory for discharge. Postoperative verbal and written instructions must be given to the patient, parent, escort, guardian, or caregiver.

6) Pediatric and Special Needs Patients

Because many dental patients undergoing deep sedation or general anesthesia are mentally and/or physically challenged, it is not always possible to have a comprehensive physical examination or appropriate laboratory tests prior to administering care. When these situations occur, the dentist responsible for administering the deep sedation or general anesthesia should document the reasons preventing the recommended preoperative management. In selected circumstances, deep sedation or general anesthesia may be utilized without establishing an indwelling intravenous line. These selected circumstances may include very brief procedures or periods of time, which, for example, may occur in some pediatric patients; or the establishment of intravenous access after deep sedation or general anesthesia has been induced because of poor patient cooperation.

7) Emergency Management

The qualified dentist is responsible for sedative/anesthetic management, adequacy of the facility and staff, diagnosis and treatment of emergencies related to the administration of deep sedation or general anesthesia and providing the equipment, drugs, and protocols for patient rescue.

Medical Evaluation

A thorough medical evaluation is mandatory prior to administering sedative drugs (see Chapter 2). The purpose of the medical evaluation is to prevent medical emergencies while patients are sedated. Most sedation emergencies result from compromised airways and respiratory problems. Cardiovascular events are less common and typically follow a compromised airway.

The risk for complications while providing moderate and deep sedation is greatest when caring for medically compromised patients.[13] In the author's opinion, patients presenting with complicated medical histories, severe systemic disease, inability to cooperate, or unfavorable physical features should be sedated by an anesthesiologist or maxillofacial surgeon. (See Table 7.1.)

The use of sedation is contraindicated during pregnancy. The administration of sedative drugs during pregnancy, especially the first trimester, increases the chance of spontaneous abortion and fetal malformation. Antibiotics are commonly prescribed during pregnancy. Pericoronitis and other minor infections can be safely treated with antibiotics and third molar removal postponed. Amoxicillin and clindamycin are generally considered safe during pregnancy.[14] In the rare case that surgery cannot be postponed, a consultation with the patient's obstetrician-gynecologist is recommended. Local anesthetic and nitrous oxide sedation during the second trimester is the safest technique.

The American Society of Anesthesiology defines the ASA III patient as a patient with severe systemic disease. The author recommends limiting in office sedation to ASA I and II patients unless the sedation is administered by an anesthesiologist. Monitoring of ASA III patients requires the full attention of the person administering drugs.

Table 7.1   Conditions warranting referral to anesthesiologist or maxillofacial surgeon.

Medical History	Cooperation	Severe Disease	Physical Exam
Snoring and apnea	Unable to communicate	Heart	Morbidly obese
Multiple medications	Unable to understand	Lungs	Difficult airway
Prior hospitalization	Dementia	Brain	Frail
Prior adverse reaction	Psychiatric disorders	Kidney and liver	Elderly

Routes of Administration

There are ten possible routes of administration for sedative drugs used in dentistry.[15]

1) Topical
2) Intranasal
3) Transdermal
4) Subcutaneous
5) Rectal
6) Intramuscular
7) Inhalation / Nitrous oxide
8) Sublingual
9) Oral
10) Intravenous

Topical

The topical administration of medication in dentistry is limited to oral mucosa. Nusstein and Beck studied the effectiveness of 20% benzocaine as a topical anesthetic for intraoral injections.[16] The study found no difference in pain between patients with or without topical used prior to inferior alveolar nerve blocks and posterior maxillary infiltration injections.

EMLA, lidocaine-prilocaine, is a potent topical cream used when skin grafts are harvested from intact skin.[17] This potent topical anesthetic and similar compounded gels can make intraoral injections painless, but are not FDA approved for this purpose. For this reason, the author cannot recommend their use at this time.

Intranasal

The intranasal (IN) route is used primarily for pediatric and disabled patients who are uncooperative. This route is more readily accepted by these patients. The absorption and bioavailability of drugs administered by this route is similar to drugs administered intravenously.

Transdermal

A transdermal patch is a medicated adhesive patch that is placed on the skin to deliver a specific dose of medication through the skin and into the bloodstream. An advantage of a transdermal drug delivery route over other types of medication delivery is that transdermal administration provides controlled release of the medication into the patient. The first commercially available prescription patch was approved by the US Food and Drug Administration in December 1979 for the prevention of motion sickness.

The highest selling transdermal patch in the United States is the nicotine patch, which releases nicotine in controlled doses to help with cessation of tobacco smoking. Nitroglycerin patches are sometimes prescribed for the treatment of angina in instead of sublingual pills. Narcotic drugs are administered by this route to provide round-the-clock relief for severe chronic pain.

Subcutaneous (SC)

A subcutaneous injection is administered with a small gauge needle directly under dermis and epidermis. Subcutaneous tissue has few blood vessels which results in slow, sustained absorption of injected drugs. Subcutaneous injections are a common route of administration for insulin and allergy immunotherapy. Subcutaneous injections are not used in dentistry due to the slow rate of absorption.

Rectal

The administration of drugs rectally has obvious limitations. This route of administration is normally limited to children who cannot or will not take medication orally. The rectal route is also useful as a suppository for adults who vomit when taking a drug orally. Medication taken orally or rectally is absorbed by the digestive system and enters the liver where it's metabolized. Only a portion of the active drug enters the circulatory system. This process, known as "first pass" (through the liver before circulation), greatly reduces the bioavailability of the drug.

Intramuscular (IM)

The intramuscular technique is the least commonly used route in dentistry.[18] Intramuscular injections are the administrative route of choice in two situations.

1) Very young, pediatric patients in preparation for intubation or venipuncture. The very young pediatric patient is usually restrained while Ketamine is injected IM.
2) Emergencies requiring the injection of epinephrine. The fastest route to administer epinephrine in the management of anaphylaxis and bronchospasm is IM.

The main disadvantages to this route of administration are the inability to titrate or rapidly reverse drug effects in the event of an adverse drug reaction.

Inhalation – Nitrous Oxide (N_2O)

Many gases are used in dentistry to produce sedation or general anesthesia. However, nitrous oxide is the only gas routinely used in dental offices. Inhalation of nitrous oxide is the safest route of administration for patient sedation. The gas enters the circulatory system from the lungs and is effective for most patients within seconds. The ratio of nitrous oxide and oxygen can be adjusted to titrate to the desired level of sedation. Another major advantage is the ability to rapidly reverse sedation when the patient inhales 100% oxygen. Patients can leave the office unaccompanied, return to work, and even drive an automobile.

Sublingual (SL)

The sublingual route is often used in dentistry to administer sedative drugs. The main advantage of the sublingual route is that the majority of the drug is not transformed in the liver before reaching the brain. Most of the drug bypasses the GI tract and liver and enters the circulatory system directly. Onset is faster than the oral route and more drug reaches target tissue. However, some of the drug is swallowed and enters the liver. Therefore, the time to peak effect may be the same as the oral route.

The main disadvantage of this route is the inability to titrate. Another disadvantage is a bitter taste. This can be alleviated somewhat by crushing a mint lifesaver with the drug.

Oral

Oral sedation is the most common method of sedation used in dentistry. A sedative pill is easily administered, cost effective, and well received by patients. The major disadvantages are the slow absorption (first pass in the liver) and inability to titrate to desired effect. A group of patients taking the same dosage of the same drug will experience different levels of sedation. Some patients may be lightly sedated while others may be over sedated. It is recommended that patients take the oral sedative in the dental office. This guarantees patient compliance and monitoring by office staff.

Intravenous (IV)

Malamed states that "The IV route of drug administration represents the most effective method of ensuring predictable and adequate sedation for virtually all patients."[19] This route is especially effective when removing impacted third molars. Patients anticipating the removal of their wisdom teeth have increased levels of fear and anxiety when compared to less invasive dental procedures.[8] Rapid onset of action and the ability to titrate are important features of this route. Titration allows drug dosage to be customized to the desired effect for each patient. The ability to control the level of sedation increases safety when using the intravenous route.

Of the ten routes of drug administration used in dentistry, the most common routes are inhalation, oral, and intravenous. Inhalation, oral, and intravenous sedation are all capable of producing minimal, moderate, and deep sedation or general anesthesia. These three techniques can be used to control pain and anxiety when removing impacted third molars.

Inhalation (N₂O)

Nitrous oxide/oxygen inhalation sedation has maintained an excellent safety record as a single drug technique. However, when nitrous oxide/oxygen is used in combination with other CNS depressant drugs, potentially serious side effects can occur.

Health risks to patients and staff are possible if proper use of the inhaled and exhaled nitrous oxide is not monitored. Dental offices can safely use nitrous oxide to control patient pain and anxiety by adopting some general work practices.

The following are American Dental Association guidelines for using nitrous oxide.[20]

- Every nitrous oxide delivery system should be equipped with a scavenging system. A flow meter (or equivalent measuring device) should be easy to see and well maintained to ensure accuracy. The system also should have a vacuum pump with the capacity for up to 45 liters of air per minute per workstation. The system also should come with masks in various sizes to ensure a proper fit for individual patients.
- Vent the vacuum and ventilation exhaust fumes outside (for example, through a vacuum system). Do not place exhaust system in the vicinity of the fresh-air intake vents. Ensure that the general ventilation provides good room-air mixing. Chronic occupational exposure – several hours a week – to nitrous oxide has been associated with adverse health effects.[21]
- Test the pressure connections for leaks every time the nitrous system is first turned on and each time a gas cylinder is changed. High-pressure line connections can be tested for leaks quarterly. You can use a soap solution applied to the lines and connections to test for leaks. Alternatively, you can purchase a portable infrared spectrophotometer to test these connections.

- Before the initial use of the system for the day, inspect all of the system components – reservoir bag, tubing, masks, connectors – for wear, cracks, holes, or tears. Replace any damaged pieces.
- Once all of the components have passed inspection, you can connect the mask to the tubing and turn on the vacuum pump. Ensure that the flow rate is correct – up to 45 L/minute or according to the manufacturer's recommendation.
- The mask should be properly fitted to each patient. Check that the reservoir bag does not over- or underinflate while the patient is breathing oxygen, before the nitrous is administered.
- Ask the patient to limit talking during administration of the nitrous and to try to breathe through his or her nose – avoid breathing through the mouth if possible.
- During administration, watch for changes in the tidal volume of the reservoir bag, also keep an eye on the vacuum pump flow rate.
- After the procedure, deliver 100% oxygen to the patient for 5 minutes before removing the mask. This will purge the system, and the patient, of any residual nitrous oxide.
- Periodically, personnel – particularly those who work with the nitrous oxide delivery – can be assessed for exposure. This can be done by asking the staff members to wear personal dosimetry badges or by placing an infrared spectrophotometer in the room.

Patient Selection

Many experts consider nitrous oxide an inert, benign gas that has little if any influence on vital physiologic functions.[22] The inhalation of N_2O/O_2 is suitable for ASA I, II, and some medically compromised ASA III patients. Nitrous oxide does not irritate the respiratory mucosa and can be used safely for patients with respiratory disease. Asthmatic patients who are prone to bronchospasm are good candidates for sedation with N_2O/O_2 since stress is reduced. COPD patients can be safely sedated with N_2O/O_2.[19] Hypoxia is decreased with the use of N_2O/O_2 due to the increased flow of oxygen. This is particularly beneficial when treating patients with cardiovascular disease, cerebrovascular disease, and epilepsy. Patients with hepatic disorders are good candidates since the inhalation route bypasses the liver and is not biotransformed. Nitrous oxide is also effective in treating patients with severe gag reflex. All elective dental treatment should be avoided during pregnancy, especially during the first trimester. Nitrous oxide is the recommended sedation technique for pregnant women when treatment is unavoidable. Nitrous oxide does not cross the placenta and the fetus is unaffected. Consultation with the patient's OB/GYN is recommended.

Nitrous oxide can provide minimal or moderate sedation when used as a single drug technique. This technique is ideal for patients with mild anxiety. For example, patients with a fear of needles can be titrated to a comfortable level of sedation before injecting local anesthetic and returned to a lower level after injecting. Nitrous oxide has analgesic properties and can raise a patient's pain threshold for "difficult to numb" patients. In general, the nitrous oxide route is advantageous for short procedures.

Advantages and Disadvantages

There are many advantages to nitrous oxide sedation.

1) Nitrous oxide sedation is safe with very few side effects.
2) Only nitrous oxide and intravenous sedation can be titrated due to their very short latent periods. Nitrous oxide has the fastest onset among inhalation agents due its low solubility in blood and adipose tissue. Nitrous oxide can be added incrementally until the desired level of sedation is reached. Once this point is determined, patients can be rapidly sedated at this predetermined level at future office visits.

3) The patient can be rapidly "rescued" and returned to the desired level of sedation should they become over sedated or experience adverse effects.
4) Nitrous oxide is the only modality discussed in this chapter that is not metabolized by the body. Patients recover quickly after breathing 100% O_2 for 5 minutes. Most patients can leave the office unescorted. However, it is the responsibility of the treating dentist to determine if the patient can be dismissed without an escort.
5) Nitrous oxide has no adverse effects on cardiovascular, respiratory, brain, liver, or kidney.
6) The onset of action is very rapid. Patients with anxiety find relief within minutes and begin to relax.
7) Nitrous oxide has analgesic properties. In the event of a missed block or partially effective block, the analgesic properties of nitrous oxide can raise the patient's pain threshold. Patients with fear of needles can be titrated to moderate sedation prior to intraoral injections and returned to minimal sedation following injections.

Although nitrous oxide and oxygen inhalation sedation is very safe, it does have disadvantages.

1) Nitrous oxide and oxygen delivery systems can be portable or permanently installed in the office. Both systems represent a significant initial investment of several thousand dollars.
2) Regular system monitoring and maintenance is required to prevent deleterious exposure to nitrous oxide. System monitoring and maintenance increases cost to the dental office. Nitrous oxide exposure to dental staff should be minimized to prevent short-term behavioral and long-term reproductive health effects. The National Institute for Occupational Safety and Health (NIOSH) recommends no more than 25 ppm exposure to nitrous oxide during administration. Uncontrolled exposures to N_2O have exceeded 1000 ppm.
3) Patients may object to the nasal mask and hoses needed to deliver the gases.
4) The delivery of nitrous oxide in the dental office requires additional training. The American Dental Association guidelines recommend not less than 14 hours of training.

Equipment

Continuous flow delivery systems are replacing demand-flow systems in the United States. The systems consist of two cylinders of compressed gas, nitrous oxide and oxygen, and an inhalation sedation unit with flow meter. The gas cylinders can be mobile or permanently stored at a central location.

Mobile systems are normally found in offices that use inhalation sedation infrequently. (See Figure 7.5.) Color-coded gas cylinders, called "E"-type cylinders, are connected to the inhalation unit via the yoke. The yoke holds the cylinders in tight contact with the inhalation unit. Each gas cylinder has a pin configuration to fit its respective gas yoke. The pin positions are unique and correspond with the correct positions for nitrous oxide or oxygen. The cylinder will only connect to the correct equipment. The pin index system ensures the correct gas is filled into the correct cylinder.

Central storage systems connect the cylinder gases to multiple inhalation units. Each operatory contains an inhalation unit at a fixed location. The central storage

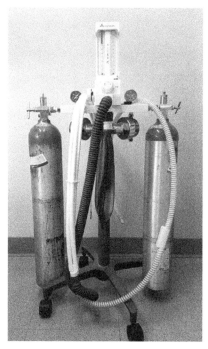

Figure 7.5 Mobile delivery system and color-coded gas cylinders.

systems are expensive to install, but relatively inexpensive to operate because the gas cylinders are large "H" cylinders. These cylinders are cost effective when compared with the smaller "E" cylinders.

All continuous flow nitrous oxide delivery systems have flow meters that permit the user to visualize the flow of gases and adjust the precise amount of each gas administered to the patient. The flow meter measures the quantity of gas flowing into a tube. Increasing the flow of gas into the tube raises a ball float in the tube. Calibrations on the tube represent liters per minute flow. State-of-the-art systems use digital flow meters that measure gas flow in 0.1 L/min increments. The total flow and percentage of O_2 are displayed digitally. (See Figures 7.6a and 7.6b.)

Other system components include regulators, manifolds, reservoir bags, and nasal hoods. Regulators reduce the cylinder compressed gas pressure to a safe and constant level at the flow meter. The manifold replaces the yoke in central storage systems and joins multiple "H" cylinders together. The reservoir bag functions as a gas reserve when the gas flow from the cylinders is insufficient; for example, when the patient takes a deep breath. Importantly, adequate respiration can be monitored by observing the reservoir bag.

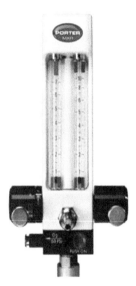

Figure 7.6a   Nitrous oxide ball float.

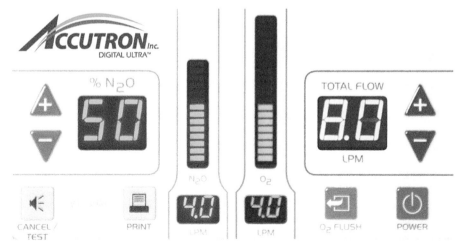

Figure 7.6b   Digital flow meter.

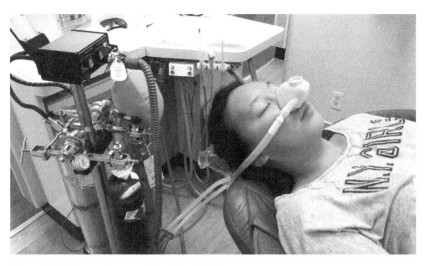

Figure 7.7 Scavenging nasal hood and tubing.

A nasal hood is connected to the reservoir bag by rubber tubing. The nasal hood adapts to the patient's nose. (See Figure 7.7.) Scavenging nasal hoods are used to minimize nitrous oxide contamination in the dental office. These devices consist of a small inner nosepiece covered by a larger outer nosepiece. Four tubes are connected to the nosepiece. Two rubber tubes provide cylinder gas to the inner hood and two separate tubes suction exhaled gas from the outer hood. Other scavenging systems use different mask designs, but the principle is the same. Unwanted nitrous oxide is removed from room air.

Many safety features in addition to scavenging nasal hoods are mandatory for inhalation units sold in the United States. The pin index system and reservoir bags have already been discussed. Additional safety features include color coding, minimum oxygen percentage, oxygen fail safe and alarm, emergency air inlet, and positive pressure connections.

System components and gas cylinders that handle oxygen are color-coded green. Nitrous oxide components and gas cylinders are colored-coded blue. Nitrous oxide and oxygen sedation systems have a minimum oxygen percentage safety feature. This feature maintains oxygen percentage at a minimum of 30%. Another safety feature, known as oxygen fail safe, terminates the flow of nitrous oxide, and sounds an alarm if oxygen pressure falls below 50 psi. Oxygen fail safe prevents the delivery of 100% nitrous oxide. The emergency air inlet safety feature is activated when the flow of gas ceases. A valve opens allowing the patient to breath room ambient air. Finally, all nitrous oxide and oxygen delivery systems are required to have quick-connect positive pressure connections.

Administration

Nitrous oxide should be titrated to effect using either constant liter flow or constant oxygen flow technique. The constant liter flow technique gradually increases nitrous flow while decreasing oxygen flow by an equal amount. For example, once oxygen flow rate is established, nitrous flow can be increased by 1 liter per minute while oxygen flow is simultaneously decreased by 1 liter per minute. Titration of nitrous oxide continues until the desired sedation is achieved. The constant oxygen technique maintains oxygen flow rate at a predetermined level while nitrous oxide flow is gradually increased. For example, oxygen flow rate is set at 4 liters per minute and nitrous oxide flow rate is gradually increased in 1 liter/minute increments until the desired sedation level is achieved.

Table 7.2   N$_2$O required for ideal sedation.

Percent of Population	Nitrous Percentage
70	30–40
12	< 30
18	> 40

Unfortunately, many dentists using nitrous oxide do not titrate when using nitrous oxide. Patients vary in their response to drugs.[23] In any given population of patients, 70% of patients will achieve ideal sedation with a nitrous oxide percentage between 30% and 40%, 12% require less than 30%, and 18% require more than 40%. (See Table 7.2.) Titrating every 60 to 90 seconds will achieve ideal sedation for most patients within 3–6 minutes.

Although nitrous oxide inhalation is very safe as a single drug technique, over sedation is possible when titration is not used. Patients may complain of nausea or dizziness, laugh uncontrollably, have disturbing dreams, respond to questions slowly, or attempt to remove the nasal hood. All of these signs and symptoms are indications that the patient is over sedated and the nitrous oxide percentage should be reduced. Over sedation can also occur during periods when the patient is not being stimulated.

No drug administration route is 100% safe. Although nitrous oxide is considered very safe, complications are more likely when it is combined with other drugs. Sedation regulations of most US states consider the single drug administration of nitrous oxide to be minimal sedation. Combining nitrous oxide with other drugs can result in deeper states of sedation or general anesthesia.

Oral Sedation

The use of modern oral sedatives began in the 19th century with the use of bromides and chloral hydrate. Bromide salts were used in medicine as mild tranquilizers and sedatives. Bromides are no longer used as sedatives due to several negative side effects including frequent urination, sweating, visual disturbances, and electrolyte disturbances. Chloral hydrate was synthesized in 1832 by the German chemist, Justus von Liebig. Chloral hydrate is a generalized CNS depressant that acts rapidly, and if given alone, is capable of inducing deep sleep in approximately 30 minutes. Although chloral hydrate was first introduced over a century ago, it remains a popular option for sedation in the pediatric practice.

Most oral sedatives in the early 20th century were barbiturates. A Prussian chemist, Adolf von Baeyer, is credited with inventing and naming barbituric acid in the early 1860s. Many pharmaceutical companies developed new barbiturates in the 1920s and 1930s. Unfortunately, barbituates produce significant cardiovascular and respiratory depressant effects. Due to their narrow margin of safety, the use of barbiturates for sedation is no longer recommended in most clinical situations. They have been replaced by safer oral sedatives (e.g., benzodiazepines).

Dr. Anthony Feck and Dr. Michael Silverman established the Dental Organization for Conscious Sedation (DOCS) in 1999. DOCS promoted oral sedation using the benzodiazepine triazolam for dental patients with fear and anxiety. The use of oral sedation in dentistry dramatically increased in the United States following the founding of DOCS.

The oral route of sedation is the oldest and most commonly used route of drug administration in dentistry. Oral drugs are easy to administer and affordable. Most patients will readily accept swallowing a pill to reduce their anxiety prior to the removal of impacted third molars.

Patient Selection

ASA I and II patients with mild anxiety are good candidates for oral sedation. Claustrophobic patients who cannot tolerate the N_2O/O_2 nasal hood may do well with the oral route. Oral sedation is also an option for patients refusing intravenous sedation.

The intended level of oral sedation should be minimal. A single maximum recommended dose (MRD), administered in the office, assures patient compliance and safety. The inability to titrate oral drugs is a severe limitation of this route. Incremental and supplemental oral dosages are discouraged because peak plasma levels are unpredictable. Oral sedation drugs are CNS depressants that can cause oversedation or general anesthesia.

Maximum drug activity of most orally administered drugs is reached approximately 60 minutes after ingestion. If deeper levels of sedation are required, moderate sedation can be achieved safely by titrating N_2O/O_2 or intravenous drugs. Titration is started after a maximum recommended oral dose has reached peak plasma level.

Oral sedation should be used with caution for children and elderly patients due to age-dependent pharmacodynamic alterations. Lower dosages and shorter acting medications are typically required in order to avoid oversedation.[24]

Advantages and Disadvantages

Oral sedation has several advantages over other routes of administration

1) Oral sedation is effective for mild to moderate anxiety.
2) Oral sedation cost is similar to inhalation (N_2O) sedation, but less than IV sedation.
3) One of the main advantages of oral sedation is the route of administration. It is the easiest way to administer drugs of all possible routes. Swallowing a small pill before the appointment is all that is required. There is no need to breathe through a mask like in nitrous oxide sedation. Patients with needle phobias do not need to have a needle in a vein as in IV sedation.
4) There are no needles, syringes, or equipment required.

Although the oral route of administration has many advantages, it also has many significant disadvantages.

1) The level of sedation is not easily reversed as it is with nitrous oxide or IV sedation. The oral route requires more monitoring than nitrous oxide sedation to insure patient safety.
2) Titration of drugs is difficult when using the oral route due to the long latent period. It can be 30–60 minutes following drug administration before a clinical effect is observed.
3) Patients may not comply with prescribed oral medication directions. When patient compliance is questionable, it's recommended that patients take their oral sedative in the office under the supervision of office staff.
4) Absorption of drugs from the GI tract is erratic and incomplete. Many variables affect the absorption of oral sedatives. Consistent clinical results are difficult to achieve.
5) The level of sedation cannot be easily increased or decreased as with nitrous oxide or IV sedation.

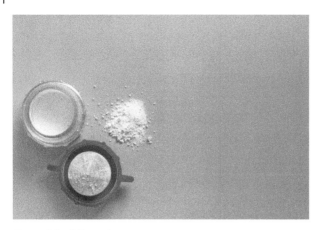

Figure 7.8   Pill crusher.

Sublingual Administration

Many drugs are designed for sublingual administration, including cardiovascular drugs, steroids, barbiturates, and analgesics. One of the best known drugs administered sublingually is nitroglycerin. Nitroglycerin sublingual tablets are vasodilators used to treat angina for patients with coronary artery disease.

Sublingual administration of sedatives can be considered a subcategory of oral administration because the sedative is delivered orally under the tongue and in a powdered form. However, there are significant differences in these two routes. As mentioned previously, sublingual drugs enter the circulatory system without significant absorption from the GI tract or metabolism in the liver. Sublingual administration results in faster onset and more profound effect when compared to oral administration.[25] Triazolam is a common benzodiazepine sedative hypnotic drug administered sublingually prior to dental procedures. Pills are crushed into fine powder that easily penetrates the thin sublingual mucosa. (See Figure 7.8.)

Berthold et al. compared the effects of sublingual vs oral administration of triazolam for premedication prior to oral surgery.[26] The double-blind, placebo-controlled study compared 0.25 mg sublingual triazolam, 0.25 mg oral triazolam, and placebo administered one hour before oral surgery. Sublingual administration of triazolam resulted in significantly less anxiety and pain at 15 minutes intra-operatively than both orally administered triazolam and placebo. No difference was demonstrated in the rate of recovery or incidence of side effects between the two drug groups. Plasma triazolam levels were higher after sublingual administration during and after the surgical procedure. These results indicate that sublingually administered triazolam results in greater sedation and less pain perception than orally administered triazolam.

Sublingual sedatives should be administered in the dental office under the supervision of trained office staff. Patient compliance is assured.

Intravenous Sedation

Intravenous sedation is a relatively new technique for the control of pain and anxiety in dentistry. Several scientific advancements preceded the use of intravenous sedation. Sterile technique, intravenous syringes, and new drugs were necessary before Niels Bjorn Jorgenson, the father of intravenous sedation, developed the Jorgenson technique in 1945. Dr. Jorgenson called his technique "intravenous premedication."[27]

The intravenous route for patient sedation has been used almost exclusively by oral and maxillofacial surgeons until recently. Today, the placement of dental implants is included in virtually every US dental school curriculum. Dental schools have begun to teach intravenous sedation to control the fear and anxiety of implant patients. In addition, there are many high-quality postgraduate IV sedation continuing education courses available today. Pulse oximetry and capnography are now available to monitor sedation and increase the margin of safety.

No drug administration route is perfect or without disadvantages. However, the IV route is considered the most predictable and effective sedation route due to the ability to easily titrate to the desired end point. The IV route, also known as parenteral, offers the ultimate control of drug administration. Sedative and analgesic drugs are rapidly titrated to the desired level of sedation. Benzodiazepines and narcotics can be reversed should a patient become more deeply sedated than intended. It is the most common route of drug administration used by oral and maxillofacial surgeons when removing impacted third molars.

Patient Selection

Moderate intravenous sedation is indicated for patients with moderate to severe anxiety. These patients may have had previous sedation with other techniques that were not successful. Moderate IV sedation is the logical next step.

The IV route is especially useful when removing impacted third molars. Opioids have analgesic properties and create euphoria. These characteristics help to mitigate the pressure, sound, and unpleasantness associated with impacted third molar surgery.

Although the IV route is very safe when properly administered, adverse events are more likely and serious when compared to N_2O/O_2 or oral sedation. The author recommends limiting IV sedation to ASA I and II patients.

Advantages and Disadvantages

There are several advantages to the IV route of administration.

1) There is no "first pass" hepatic metabolism and drugs reach the brain full strength.
2) Drugs are injected directly into the circulatory system and reach the brain within 20–25 seconds. The rapid onset of action of CNS-depressant drugs allows the dentist to easily titrate to the desired level of sedation.
3) Drug effects can be rapidly enhanced or reversed. The IV line offers a readily available route for the administration of emergency drugs if needed. This is one of the most important safety features of IV drug administration.
4) Recovery is more rapid than other routes with the exception of N_2O/O_2.
5) Nausea and vomiting are uncommon when drugs are administered intravenously.

The IV route of drug administration also has disadvantages.

1) Venipuncture is necessary and can be difficult, requiring multiple attempts. Apprehensive patients may not cooperate
2) Venipuncture site complications are rare, but possible. Complications include phlebitis, hematoma, and intra-arterial injection of a drug.
3) Drug overdose, allergic reaction, and associated problems are more likely when compared with other routes, due to the rapid onset of action of drugs administered intravenously.
4) Patients can be sedated deeper than intended if drugs are not titrated properly. Monitoring of patients must be more intensive and training more extensive in order to "rescue" patients who become more deeply sedated than intended.
5) Recovery is not complete as it is with N_2O/O_2. Patients sedated intravenously need an escort after the procedure.
6) IV sedation is not always successful. Patients with severe anxiety may require general anesthesia.

Equipment

IV sedation continuous infusion requires three sterile components: infusion solution, administration set, and catheter. (See Figures 7.9a, 7.9b, and 7.9c.) The most common infusion solution used in dental offices is 0.9% sodium chloride, also known as normal saline. Other options include 5% dextrose in water and Lactated Ringer's solution. The purpose of continuous infusion of fluid is to prevent blood clotting at the end of the catheter. The catheter is a short flexible tube that remains in the patient's vein during continuous infusion. The catheter is connected to larger diameter tubing, known as an IV administration set, which is connected to a the sterile solution. A basic IV administration set consists of sterile tubing 78 inches long with a plastic spike on one end and a male connector on the opposite end. The spike connects to the IV solution bag and the male connector connects to the catheter hub. The male connector is either Luer slip which is a friction connection or Luer lock which is a threaded connection. The Luer slip is used for short dental office procedures. The IV administration set has three components to control the flow of solution; a clamp to shut off flow, a roller clamp to control the rate of flow, and a drip chamber to view fluid dripping from the solution bag.

A catheter is recommended for venipuncture vs scalp vein needles. The catheter has a metal needle, a stylet within its lumen, and a plastic hub that connects to the administration set. The stylet is used to puncture the vein and introduce the catheter into the vein. Blood flow back into the stylet after venipuncture indicates the needle is within the vein. The catheter is slid off of the metal stylet and into the vein. The catheter is connected to the administration set. Many sizes and

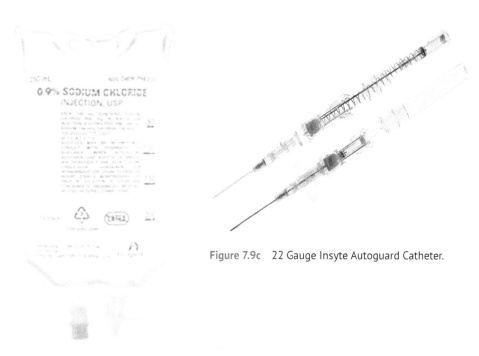

Figure 7.9c   22 Gauge Insyte Autoguard Catheter.

Figure 7.9a   IV Solution.

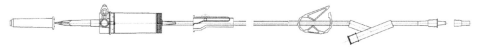

Figure 7.9b   IV Administration Set (Reproduced by permission of Excel International Co.).

designs are available. Most catheters are radiopaque when used in hospitals. Clear catheters (SureFlash, Terumo), 22 or 24 gauge, are recommended for dental office sedation due to the instant visibility of blood in the catheter once the catheter has entered a vein.

Ancillary equipment includes a tourniquet, alcohol gauze, medical adhesive tape, Velcro restraints, and a small bungee cord. A tourniquet is needed to engorge veins, making them more visible prior to venipuncture. Alcohol gauze is used to clean and prepared the venipuncture site. Once the venipuncture is complete, the catheter is connected to the administration set and secured with medical tape. The IV solution bag must be above the patient's heart. A small bungee cord can be used to attach the bag to the ceiling or operatory light's articulating arm. Solution is allowed to drip into the drip chamber and continue from the bag of solution into the patient's vein. Drugs are injected through a port in the administration set tubing. Velcro restraints can be used to prevent the patient's arm from bending while connected to the IV administration set.

Many alternatives exist for the equipment listed in this section. For example, an IV stand can be used instead of a bungee cord; a scalp vein needle can be used instead of a catheter. The myriad equipment available for sedation can be overwhelming and confusing to the beginner. The items listed provide simple and affordable options.

Venipuncture

The most common sites for venipuncture are the antecubital fossa and dorsum of the hand. The author recommends the antecubital fossa because the veins are large and relatively stable. Venipuncture of the dorsum of the hand is more painful and the veins are more likely to collapse or move. The median cubital vein connects the basilic and cephalic vein and is often used for venipuncture. (See Figures 7.10a and 7.10b.) It is also known as the median basilic vein. This vein is a

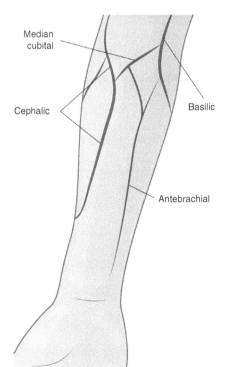

Figure 7.10a Antecubital fossa veins.

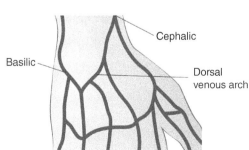

Figure 7.10b Dorsum of the hand veins.

superficial vein located close to the surface of the skin and away from nerves. The median cubital vein usually forms an H-pattern with the cephalic and basilic veins making up the legs of the H. Other forms include an M-pattern, where the vein branches to the cephalic and basilic veins.

Venipuncture steps for the antecubital fossa.

1) Apply a tourniquet 3–4 inches above the antecubital fossa.
2) Clean the site with 70% alcohol gauze, moving in an outward spiral from the site.
3) Hold the catheter above the vein at a 15- to 30-degree angle with the bevel facing up.
4) Place traction on the skin below the venipuncture site in the opposite direction of the venipuncture.
5) Puncture the skin and enter the vein a few millimeters in one smooth motion. Blood will be seen in the stylet chamber when the vein is entered. Blood will also be seen in the catheter before the stylet chamber if a clear catheter is used. This confirms that the catheter is in the vein lumen.
6) Immediately reduce the catheter angle to parallel the vein and advance the catheter a few more millimeters.
7) Slide the catheter off the stylet. The stylet should be held in place with one hand while the other hand slides the catheter off the stylet and into the vein. Dentists experienced with venipuncture can complete the venipuncture and slide the catheter off the stylet with one hand.
8) Place fingertip pressure on the skin above the catheter tip to prevent blood flow from the catheter hub when the stylet is removed.
9) The assistant holds the free end of the IV administration set close to the catheter hub and removes the stylet.
10) The dentist, while holding pressure above the catheter tip, immediately connects the IV administration set to the catheter hub. The IV set is secured with tape, the tourniquet removed, and the IV drip started.

Venipuncture steps for dorsum of the hand. These steps are essentially the same as the antecubital fossa steps with the following exceptions.

1) The patient's hand should be slightly flexed at the wrist to stabilize the vein.
2) Traction is placed on the skin below the patient's knuckles in a direction opposite to the venipuncture.
3) The catheter enters the vein from the side, not from above the vein. Veins of the hand tend to be more mobile than the superficial veins of the antecubital fossa.

Terminating IV infusion

1) Remove adhesive tape.
2) Place a sterile gauze pad over the puncture site, remove the catheter, and apply pressure.
3) Place a bandage or sterile gauze with tape over the puncture site.

Venipuncture is an art form that can only be learned through experience. Even phlebotomists and infusion nurses occasionally miss a vein. Obese patients with deep veins, elderly patients with fragile veins, and patients with small mobile veins are especially difficult.

Dental patients scheduled for the removal of impacted third molars with IV sedation have additional venipuncture challenges. Sedation patients should be NPO, with no fluids, for at least four hours prior the appointment. The resultant dehydration shrinks veins making successful venipuncture more difficult. Finally, patients scheduled for the removal of impacted third molars usually have anxiety and circulating catecholamines that cause peripheral vasoconstriction.

Table 7.3   Methods for finding veins.

Common Venipuncture Methods	Uncommon Venipuncture Methods
Take your time – be patient	Palpate with alcohol on skin
Check both arms	Use a BP cuff as tourniquet
Ask the patient for preferred site	Apply dry heat
Open and close fist	Use a trans-illumination device
Tap or rub the vein	Breathe nitrous oxide
Palpate, feel the vein "bounce"	

There are many methods that can help find a vein and increase successful venipuncture. (See Table 7.3.) Practitioners experienced in venipuncture typically spend significant time locating an appropriate vein to insure success on the first attempt. Look for the best vein on both arms. Patients with a difficult venipuncture history often remember the successful site. If veins are not obvious, ask the patient if they had difficulty in the past. Where is the best site for venipuncture? Placing a tourniquet, followed by opening and closing a fist, engorges the veins below the tourniquet and makes them more visible. Tapping or rubbing the vein may make the veins more prominent. If you can't see any veins, the best alternative is to palpate with your index finger before venipuncture. A "bouncy" sensation indicates a good vein.

Difficult venipuncture patients may require uncommon methods to find a good vein. A variation of palpating for vein bounce is to wet the palpating finger and venipuncture site with alcohol. It's a technique not found in textbooks, but the author has found it to be helpful. There's something about reducing friction on the skin that makes it easier to sense the curvature of a vein. Veins that are not visible and cannot be palpated may respond to a blood pressure cuff when used as a tourniquet. The cuff is inflated to a number near the patient's diastolic pressure. A third method for difficult veins involves heat. The application of heat increases blood flow and dilates veins. Fink et al. studied 136 patients randomly assigned to two groups using dry or moist heat. Warm towels were wrapped around each patient's arm for seven minutes prior to IV insertion. The dry heat group was 2.7 times more likely than the moist heat group to result in successful venipuncture on the first attempt.[28] The dry heat group was more comfortable and had significantly lower insertion times than the moist heat group. Another uncommon method is the use of a trans-illumination device. These devices use infrared LED lights to illuminate veins. They range from a few hundred dollars to several thousand. These vein finding devices work best in a darkened room. The final uncommon method for finding veins is unique to dentistry. Because nitrous oxide is a vasodilator, the use of N_2O can make veins more prominent while reducing the discomfort of venipuncture.

Once venipuncture is successful, the IV administration set is connected to the catheter and drugs can be added intravenously. Many IV drugs and administrative techniques are taught in dental schools, residencies, and postgraduate continuing education courses. This chapter focuses on the most common drugs and techniques used in dental offices when removing impacted third molars.

Administration

The IV route of administration provides superior control when compared with other routes. The ability to rapidly titrate to moderate sedation makes the IV route very desirable when removing impacted third molars. Drugs enter directly into the circulatory system at maximum strength, bypassing the GI tract and liver. The most common drugs used for moderate IV sedation are midazolam (Versed) and fentanyl (Sublimaze). Midazolam is a benzodiazepine. Fentanyl is an opioid. Benzodiazepines and opioids can be reversed using antagonistic drugs administered intravenously. This is an important safety feature of benzodiazepines and opioids when administered intravenously.

A review of the literature by Qi Chen et al. found the incidence of adverse events when midazolam was used during third molar removal was no higher than when a placebo was used. They concluded that midazolam can be used for ASA I and II patients as a safe and effective drug for anxiety control in third molar extraction surgery.[29] In spite of being relatively safe, intravenous midazolam should only be used with continuous monitoring of respiratory and cardiac function.

Direct monitoring of the patient is accomplished through verbal contact. Is the patient responsive? Other monitoring devices include pulse oximetry, capnography, precordial stethoscope, and ECG (see Chapter 8). Patients that are moderately sedated will respond purposefully to verbal commands and light tactile stimulation. They can breathe spontaneously without assistance. Signs of moderate sedation include Verrill sign, slurred speech, and delayed verbal response when questioned. Verrill sign is indicated by halfway ptosis of the upper eyelid. Patients that are moderately sedated have difficulty keeping their eyes open.

Midazolam is a sedative hypnotic that can create both sedation and amnesia. It can be used alone or with fentanyl. The intravenous administration of midazolam with fentanyl is not recommended for dentists new to moderate IV sedation. The author recommends at least 100 sedations using the single drug midazolam before adding another drug such as fentanyl.

The single drug midazolam technique illustrates the proper administration of IV drugs. Monitors consistent with state requirements are connected to the patient and baseline vital signs recorded. Following venipuncture, the IV line is opened and the patient is placed in a supine position. Opening the IV line allows a rapid flow of IV solution and decreases the possibility of local irritation at the venipuncture site when drugs are administered. Midazolam is administered in a concentration of 1 mg/ml. A 3 ml syringe containing 3 mg of midazolam is inserted into a port in the administration set and 1 ml (1 mg) of the drug is administered slowly. The patient is observed for hypersensitivity, allergic response, Verrill sign, slurred speech, or delayed verbal response. Additional midazolam is administered at 1 minute intervals until Verrill sign is observed (usually 5 mg or less) or 8 mg has been administered. Exceeding 8 mg of midazolam is not recommend for the dentist new to moderate sedation.[30] Patients who are not sedated sufficiently with 8 mg of midazolam may need a two drug technique or general anesthesia.

It has been the author's experience that virtually all impacted third molar surgery can be completed using fentanyl and midazolam to a level of moderate sedation. The following technique has been used successfully by the author for more than 30 years when removing impacted third molars.

This protocol is used for ASA I and II patients who are NPO for 6 hours prior to appointment. Patients arrive at the office one hour before the procedure. Informed consent is completed with the patient and/or parent and 0.5 mg of triazolam is administered sublingual. The sublingual sedative serves two purposes.

1) Sublingual administration increases safety. Administering a sublingual sedative prior to IV drug administration provides an indication of the patient's drug sensitivity. Most patients will be minimally sedated with 0.5 mg triazolam. However, this is not true for every patient. This phenomenon is illustrated by the normal distribution bell shaped curve. (See Figure 7.11.)

The slow onset of sublingual triazolam provides a margin of safety for the ultra-sensitive patient. Patients who are minimally sedated with sublingual triazolam may need reduced amounts of IV drugs. Fentanyl and midazolam are administered very slowly for these patients. Conversely, IV

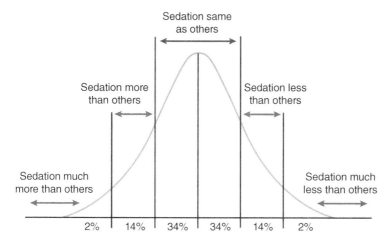

Figure 7.11 Patients vary in their response to drugs.

Fentanyl and midazolam can be safely administered faster and in larger amounts for patients who do not exhibit signs of minimal sedation following sublingual administration.

2) Sublingual administration increases patient venipuncture tolerance. Difficult venipuncture may require multiple attempts. Patients who are minimally sedated are more relaxed and venipuncture is more readily accepted.

Patients are seated in the operatory one hour after administration of triazolam. The patient is observed for signs of sedation. Some patients will appear normal while others will have difficulty walking and talking normally. Patients who are significantly sedated and exhibit Verrill's sign do not receive IV midazolam. Consistent with the normal distribution curve, about 2% of patients sedated with sublingual triazolam do not need IV midazolam. Most patients, about 2/3, receive 50 mcg of fentanyl and 3 mg midazolam. A very small percentage of patients require more midazolam titrated to a moderate level of sedation. All patients receive 8 mg dexamethasone intravenously to reduce swelling and postoperative nausea and vomiting.

Following patient sedation, local anesthetic is administered including maxillary PSA and pre-molar infiltration, mandibular and Gow Gates blocks, and palatal injections. The patient is observed during injections to assess the effectiveness of sedation. The palatal injection is especially noteworthy. This injection is universally acknowledged to be one of the most painful injections in dentistry. Patients who are adequately sedated will have no response or may ask, "What was that?" or "Did you just give me a shot?" Obviously, these patients are adequately sedated.

The palatal injection is also useful to differentiate between true pain and pressure. The removal of teeth often requires significant pressure. Most dentists have experienced patients who are tense and gripping the operatory chair when removing teeth with forceps and local anesthesia. When patients are questioned after the procedure, it is common to hear that the extraction was not painful, but the pressure was uncomfortable. No amount of sedation will completely eliminate the sensation of pressure.

It is important to note that no sedation technique will work 100% of the time. Safe sedation requires that patients remain responsive. A common mistake made by dentists who are new to IV sedation is to add more drug if a patient moves or complains. In most cases, these are patients with high anxiety who are responding to pressure. It is also possible that mandibular anesthesia is inadequate. Sedation is not a substitute for good local anesthesia.

Most surgeons and dentists removing impacted third molars will remove one side before the other. The author prefers to remove maxillary third molars before mandibular third molars. This sequence provides extra time for profound anesthesia of mandibular third molars. Also, maxillary third molars are usually easier to remove than mandibular third molars. The removal of maxillary third molars before mandibular third molars may increase patient confidence and the effectiveness of sedation. Patients with high anxiety are often more "relaxed" during removal of mandibular third molars when preceded by removal of maxillary third molars.

Many techniques and drugs are available for sedation. This chapter reviewed the most common techniques and drugs used by dentists for patient sedation. Regardless of the technique used, patient safety is paramount.

References

1 Kleinknecht RA, Thorndike RM, McGlynn FD, Harkavy J. Factor analysis of the dental fear survey with cross-validation. *J Am Dent Assoc*. 1984 Jan;108(1):59–61.

2 Getka EJ, Glass CR. Behavioral and cognitive-behavioral approaches to the reduction of dental anxiety. *Behav Ther*. 1992 Summer;23(3):433–48.

3 Milgrom P, Weinstein P, Getz T. *Treating fearful dental patients: a patient management handbook*, 2nd edition. Seattle, WA: University of Washington, Continuing Dental Education, 1995.

4 Gatchel RJ, Ingersoll BD, Bowman L, Robertson MC, Walker C. The prevalence of dental fear and avoidance: a recent survey study. *J Am Dent Assoc*. 1983 Oct;107(4):609–10.

5 Armfield JM, Stewart JF, Spencer AJ. The vicious cycle of dental fear: exploring the interplay between oral health, service utilization and dental fear. *BMC Oral Health*. 2007;7:1.

6 Dental Health Advisor. Our most common fears. 1987 Spring.

7 Gale EN. Fears of the dental situation. *J Dent Res*. 1972 Jul-Aug;51(4):964–6.

8 Sirin Y, Humphris G, Sencan S, Firat D. What is the most fearful intervention in ambulatory oral surgery? Analysis of an outpatient clinic. *Int J Oral Maxillofac Surg*. 2012 Oct;41(10):1284–90.

9 Enever G. The history of dental anaesthesia. In: *Oxford textbook of anaesthesia for oral and maxillofacial surgery*. Oxford University Press, 2010 Jun, 1–20.

10 Jorgensen NB, Hayden J. *Sedation, local and general anesthesia in dentistry*, 3rd edition. Philadelphia: Lea & Febiger, 1980.

11 Excerpted from continuum of depth of sedation: definition of general anesthesia and levels of sedation/ analgesia. American Society of Anesthesiologists (ASA), 2004.

12 American Dental Association. Guidelines for the use of sedation and general anesthesia by dentists. Guidelines Policy Statement Adopted by the ADA House of Delegates, 2012.

13 Becker DE, Haas DA. Management of complications during moderate and deep sedation: respiratory and cardiovascular considerations. *Anesth Prog*. 2007 Summer;54(2):59–69.

14 Harms RW. Antibiotics and pregnancy: what's safe? *Mayo Clin*. 2014 Oct 3.

15 Malamed SF. *Sedation a guide to patient management*, 5th edition. St. Louis Missouri 63146: Mosby Elsevier, 2010. Ch 3, 16.

16 Nusstein JM, Beck M. Effectiveness of 20% benzocaine as a topical anesthetic for intraoral injections. *Anesth Prog*. 2003;50(4):159–63.

17 Goodacre TE, Sanders R, Watts DA, Stoker M. Split skin grafting using topical local anaesthesia (EMLA): a comparison with infiltrated anaesthesia. *Br J Plast Surg*. 1988 Sep;41(5):533–8.

18 Becker DE. Pharmacodynamic considerations for moderate and deep sedation. *Anesth Prog*. 2012 Spring; 59(1):28–42. doi: 10.2344/0003-3006-59.1.28. PMID: 22428972; PMCID: PMC3309299.

19 Malamed SF. *Sedation a guide to patient management*, 5th edition. Mosby, 2010. Ch 3. 18.

20 ADA Council on Scientific Affairs. Nitrous oxide in the dental office. *JADA*. 1997;128(3):364–5.

21 Becker DE, Rosenberg M. Nitrous oxide and the inhalation anesthetics. *Anesth Prog*. 2008 Winter;55(4):124–31.

22 Howard WR. Nitrous oxide in the dental environment: assessing the risk, reducing the exposure. *JADA*. 1997;128(3):356–60.

23 School of Dentistry, University of Southern California. *Statistics from section of anesthesia and medicine*. Los Angeles: Mosby, 2006. unpublished.

24 Stoelting RK, Dierdorf SF. *Anesthesia and co-existing disease*, 4th edition. Philadelphia, PA: Churchill Livingstone, 2002. Diseases associated with aging, 740.

25 Narang N, Sharmna J. Sublingual mucosa as a route for systemic drug delivery. *Int J Pharm Pharm Sci*. 2011;3(Suppl 2): 18–22.ISSN- 0975-1491.

26 Berthold CW, Dionne RA, Corey SE. Comparison of sublingually and orally administered triazolam for premedication before oral surgery. *Oral Surg Oral Med Oral Pathol Oral Radiol Endod*. 1997 Aug;84(2):119–24.

27 Jorgenson NB, Leffingwell FB. Premedication in dentistry. *J South Calif Dent Assoc*. 1953;21:1.

28 Fink RM, et al. The impact of dryversus moist heat on peripheral IV catheter insertion in a hematology-oncology outpatient population. *Oncol Nurs Forum*. 2009 Jul;36(4):E198–204.

29 Chen Q, Wang L, Ge L, Gao Y, Wang H. The anxiolytic effect of midazolam in third molar extraction: a systematic review. *PLoS One*. 2015;10(4):e0121410.

30 Malamed SF. *Sedation a guide to patient management*, 5th edition. Mosby, 2010. Ch 26, 361.

8

Sedation Emergencies and Monitoring

The removal of third molars is one of the most feared surgical procedures in dentistry.[1] Third molars can be removed under local anesthesia alone, but most patients and dentists do not prefer this option. Conscious sedation options include nitrous oxide, oral sedation, and IV sedation. All of these options place the patient at some degree of risk for complications.

As stated previously in Chapter 7, the concept of sedation as a continuum is the foundation of patient safety. In 2004, the American Society of Anesthesiologists (ASA) made the following statement; "Because sedation and general anesthesia are a continuum, it is not always possible to predict how an individual patient will respond. Hence, practitioners intending to produce a given level of sedation should be able to diagnose and manage the physiologic consequences (rescue) for patients whose level of sedation becomes deeper than initially intended."[2] Dentists providing sedation must have the training, skills, drugs, and equipment necessary to manage patients that are more deeply sedated than intended until EMS arrives or the patient returns to the intended level of sedation. These attributes are the keys to patient safety.

Patient Safety and Sedation Law

In 2002 the Dental Board of California called for a review of anesthesia laws and patient outcomes to see if any improvements could be made to the existing regulatory program. The Board appointed the Blue Ribbon Panel on Anesthesia, an ad hoc committee composed of general dentists and dental specialists who were recognized experts in the field. The panel reviewed mortality data from the Dental Board, lawsuits from a major California malpractice insurance company, anesthesia regulations from other states, and the published scientific literature. The review found that in California, between 1991 and 2000, there were 12 deaths related to general anesthesia permits, 8 deaths related to non-permit holders (four deaths with oral sedation in children and four deaths with local anesthesia alone) and 0 deaths related to conscious sedation permits.[3] The California Dental Board Blue Ribbon Panel review clearly demonstrates the efficacy of conscious sedation.

The American Dental Association has published recommended guidelines for the use of sedation. California and the majority of states have adopted the American Dental Association's guidelines as state law. California sedation laws and permit requirements (2016) are discussed in this chapter with emphasis on intravenous sedation emergencies and monitoring. Although not required in California, capnography and EKG monitoring are briefly reviewed. A permit is not required in California for the administration of nitrous oxide and oxygen.

Impacted Third Molars, Second Edition. Edited by John Wayland.
© 2024 John Wiley & Sons, Inc. Published 2024 by John Wiley & Sons, Inc.

To obtain a California permit for the administration of oral (moderate) conscious sedation the applicant must have completed an approved post-doctoral or residency training program that includes sedation training; or, a board approved course that includes 25 hours of instruction and a clinical component utilizing at least one age-appropriate patient.

To obtain a California permit for IV (moderate) conscious sedation, the applicant must complete at least 60 hours of instruction and 20 clinical cases of administration of parenteral conscious sedation for a variety of dental procedures. The course must comply with the requirements of the Guidelines for Teaching the Comprehensive Control of Anxiety and Pain in Dentistry of the American Dental Association.

In California, a conscious sedation permit (IV sedation) is issued as a temporary permit for the first year. Within that time, the board conducts an onsite inspection and evaluation of the licentiate. Onsite inspections are required every six years. Fifteen units of continuing education related to conscious sedation and medical emergencies are required every two years.

All offices in which conscious sedation is conducted in California must complete an office inspection and applicant evaluation. The office inspection consists of three parts:

Office Facilities and Equipment

a) The following office facilities and equipment must be available and maintained in good operating condition:

1) An operating theatre large enough to adequately accommodate the patient on a table or in an operating chair and permit an operating team consisting of at least three individuals to freely move about the patient.
2) An operating table or chair which permits the patient to be positioned so the operating team can maintain the airway, quickly alter patient position in an emergency, and provide a firm platform for the management of cardiopulmonary resuscitation.
3) A lighting system which is adequate to permit evaluation of the patient's skin and mucosal color and a backup lighting system which is battery powered and of sufficient intensity to permit completion of any operation underway at the time of general power failure.
4) Suction equipment which permits aspiration of the oral and pharyngeal cavities. A backup suction device which can operate at the time of general power failure must also be available.
5) An oxygen delivery system with adequate full face masks and appropriate connectors that is capable of allowing the administration of greater than 90% oxygen at a 10 liter/minute flow for at least 60 minutes (650 liter "E" cylinder) to the patient under positive pressure, together with an adequate backup system which can operate at the time of general power failure.
6) A recovery area that has available oxygen, adequate lighting, suction, and electrical outlets. The recovery area can be the operating theatre.
7) Ancillary equipment:
    A) Emergency airway equipment (oral airways, laryngeal mask airways or Combitubes, and cricothyrotomy device).
    B) Tonsillar or pharyngeal type suction tip adaptable to all office outlets.
    C) Sphygmomanometer and stethoscope.
    D) Adequate equipment for the establishment of an intravenous infusion.
    E) Precordial/pretracheal stethoscope.
    F) Pulse oximeter.

Records

b) The following records must be maintained:

1) Adequate medical history and physical evaluation records updated prior to each administration of general anesthesia or conscious sedation. Such records must include, but are not limited to the recording of the age, sex, weight, physical status (American Society of Anesthesiologists Classification), medication use, any known or suspected medically compromising conditions, rationale for sedation of the patient, and visual examination of the airway, and for general anesthesia only, auscultation of the heart and lungs as medically required.
2) Conscious sedation records, which include a time-oriented record with preoperative, multiple intraoperative, and postoperative pulse oximetry (every 5 minutes intraoperative) and blood pressure and pulse readings, drugs, amounts administered and time administered, length of the procedure, any complications of anesthesia or sedation and a statement of the patient's condition at time of discharge.
3) Written informed consent of the patient or if the patient is a minor, his or her parent or guardian.

Drugs

c) Emergency drugs of the following types must be available:

1) Epinephrine
2) Vasopressor (other than epinephrine)
3) Bronchodilator
4) Appropriate drug antagonist
5) Antihistaminic
6) Anticholinergic
7) Coronary artery vasodilator
8) Anticonvulsant
9) Oxygen
10) 50% dextrose or other anti-hypoglycemic

The applicant evaluation consists of two parts:

Demonstration of Conscious Sedation

a) A dental procedure utilizing conscious sedation administered by the applicant must be observed and evaluated. Any conscious sedation technique that is routinely employed can be demonstrated. The patient must be monitored while sedated and during recovery from sedation. The applicant for a permit must demonstrate knowledge of the uses of emergency equipment and the capability of using that equipment.

Simulated Emergencies

b) Knowledge of and a method of treatment must be physically demonstrated by the dentist and his or her operating team for the emergencies shown in Box 8.1

Box 8.1 Simulated emergencies.

1) Airway obstruction
2) Respiratory depression
3) Allergic reaction
4) Bronchospasm
5) Emesis and aspiration
6) Angina pectoris
7) Myocardial infarction
8) Cardiac arrest
9) Hypotension
10) Hypertension
11) Seizures
12) Hypoglycemia

The 13 simulated emergencies evaluated in the state of California are representative of evaluations conducted in other states. The following section discusses recognition, treatment, and prevention of these emergencies.

Sedation Emergencies

When compared with local anesthesia alone, the two most significant negative variables introduced by any level of sedation are the added risks for either airway obstruction or respiratory depression (hypoventilation). Airway obstruction and respiratory depression are the most significant complications in deeply sedated or unconscious patients. Virtually all cardiovascular complications in healthy patients are preceded by airway complications.[4]

The management of any emergency begins with the ABC primary assessment taught in every basic life support course. Airway, breathing, and circulation are also the foundation of ACLS. Dr. Frank Grimaldi described this assessment in its simplest form: "air goes in and out and blood goes round and round."[5]

Airway Obstruction

Airway obstruction can be mechanical or pathological. Upper airway obstruction is caused by anatomical structures or foreign materials. The most common upper airway obstruction is the tongue. Common foreign materials include crowns, bridges, and teeth. Lower airway obstruction is caused by bronchospasm, laryngospasm, or allergic reaction. Airway obstruction leads to hypoventilation and hypoxemia. It can be prevented by titration of drugs and the use of a throat pack barrier. The treatment for airway obstruction begins with the triple maneuver; head tilt, chin lift, and jaw thrust (if unconscious). Supplemental oxygen should be administered with airway adjuncts added as needed. Possible airway adjuncts include oropharyngeal airways (OPA), non-rebreathing masks (NRB), and bag valve masks (BVM). Drug reversal should be considered. EMS should be called if oxygen saturation does not improve. (See Figure 8.1.)

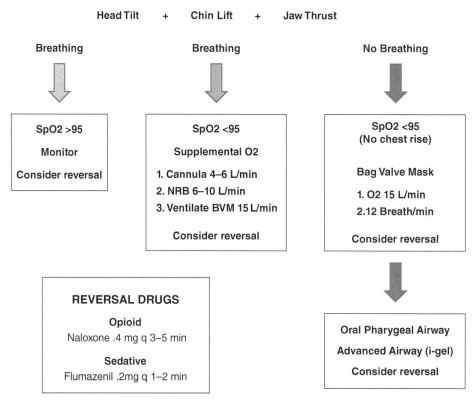

Figure 8.1   Airway obstruction / respiratory depression algorithm.

Respiratory Depression

Respiratory depression must be distinguished from airway obstruction. The risk of respiratory depression is low with moderate sedation when compared to anatomical airway obstruction (tongue, tonsils, adenoids). Patients with airway obstruction can't breathe. Patients with respiratory depression won't breathe. Respiratory depression is a side effect of CNS depressants. All opioids and sedatives have the potential to depress hypercapnic or hypoxemic drives. Opioids are the most powerful respiratory depressants. Treatment is the same as airway obstruction. (See Figure 8.1.)

Allergic Reaction

It's not uncommon for a patient's medical history to list adverse drug reactions. Generally, these are found to be drug sensitivities and not true allergic reactions. When the patient's history includes airway compromise or cutaneous reactions, allergy is more likely. In terms of cutaneous reactions, urticaria (hives) is most indicative of an IgE-mediated reaction.[5] Histories of compromised airway or difficulty breathing should be taken seriously. These reports indicate severe allergic reaction and anaphylaxis. A partial airway obstruction from anaphylaxis is characterized by a high pitched crowing sound.

Allergic reactions can be reduced by completing a thorough medical history and interview. Intravenous administration of a drug test dose and titration may provide an early warning of adverse reactions. Mild allergic reactions are treated by oral, intramuscular, or intravenous administration of diphenhydramine. Severe allergic reactions are treated with epinephrine.[6] (See Figure 8.2.)

Bronchospasm

Bronchospasm is a lower airway obstruction resulting from contraction or spasm of bronchial smooth muscle. Laryngeal edema is a common characteristic. Bronchospasm can result from an anaphylactic reaction or from a hyperactive airway as found with asthmatic patients. Dyspnea and wheezing are common characteristics of bronchospasm due to obstructions in the chest; not the throat or mouth.

Stress may trigger an asthmatic attack and bronchospasm. Sedation may decrease stress and help prevent bronchospasm in patients with asthma. Treatment includes use of a bronchodilator, such as albuterol, or epinephrine. (See Figure 8.2.)

Emesis and Aspiration

Emesis is possible following the administration of sedative drugs including nitrous oxide. Although, aspiration of vomitus is unlikely when airway protective reflexes are intact, dentists should be prepared for this emergency. Aspiration of liquids usually results in bronchospasm. Pulse oximeter values are usually under 90% and cannot be improved. EMS should be immediately activated. Patients should be placed in the Trendelenburg position with their head turned to the right to prevent vomitus from entering the left bronchus and lungs. The pharynx should be suctioned using pharyngeal suction. Oxygen should be administered and drugs reversed.

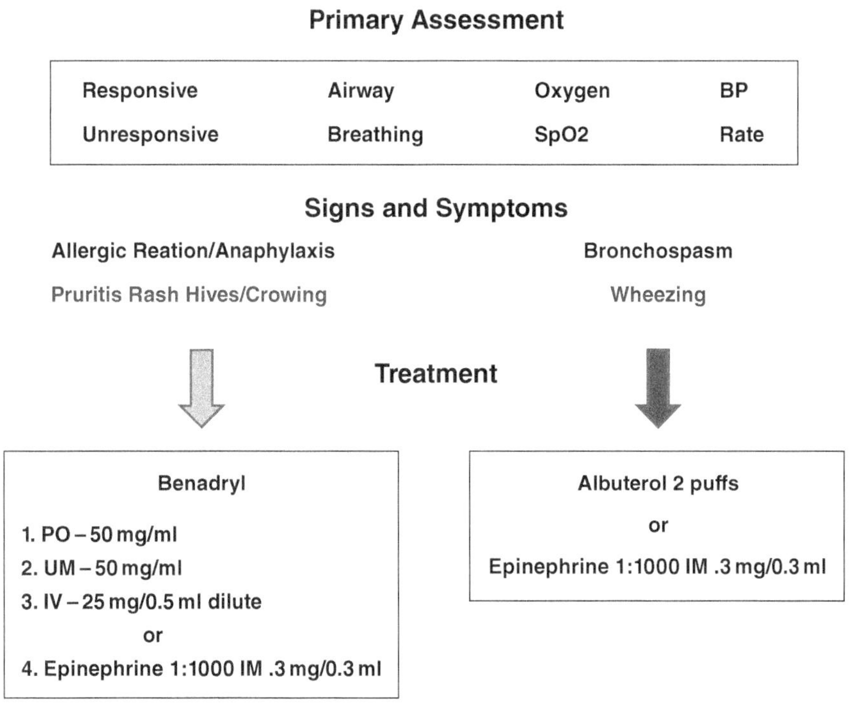

Primary Assessment

| Responsive | Airway | Oxygen | BP |
| Unresponsive | Breathing | SpO2 | Rate |

Signs and Symptoms

| Allergic Reation/Anaphylaxis | Bronchospasm |
| Pruritis Rash Hives/Crowing | Wheezing |

Treatment

Benadryl	Albuterol 2 puffs
1. PO – 50 mg/ml	or
2. UM – 50 mg/ml	Epinephrine 1:1000 IM .3 mg/0.3 ml
3. IV – 25 mg/0.5 ml dilute	
or	
4. Epinephrine 1:1000 IM .3 mg/0.3 ml	

Figure 8.2   Allergic reaction and bronchospasm algorithm.

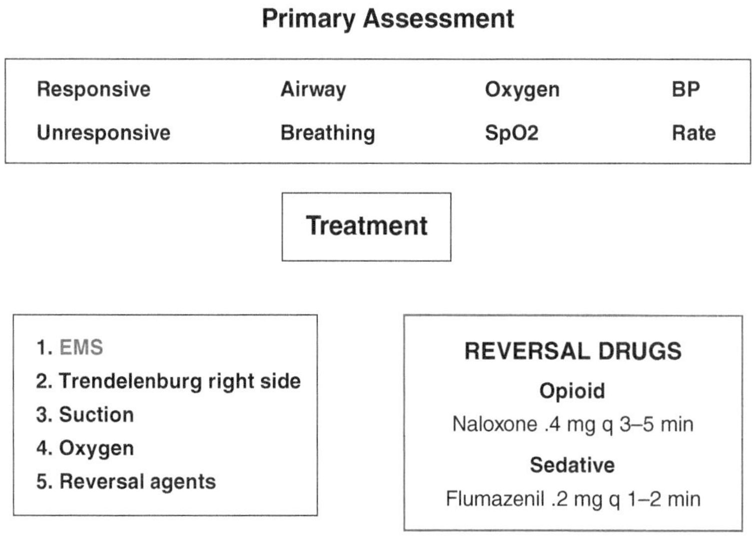

Primary Assessment

Responsive	Airway	Oxygen	BP
Unresponsive	Breathing	SpO2	Rate

Treatment

1. EMS	**REVERSAL DRUGS**
2. Trendelenburg right side	**Opioid**
3. Suction	Naloxone .4 mg q 3–5 min
4. Oxygen	**Sedative**
5. Reversal agents	Flumazenil .2 mg q 1–2 min

Figure 8.3 Emesis and aspiration algorithm.

A thorough patient interview may reveal a history of nausea and vomiting. Sedated patients should be NPO for 6 hours prior to the removal of third molars. Unfortunately, patients are not always compliant with this rule. Slow titration of drugs to light or moderate sedation reduces the possibility of nausea and vomiting. (See Figure 8.3.)

Angina Pectoris

Ischemic heart disease is a condition whereby coronary perfusion is inadequate for myocardial oxygen requirements. Angina pectoris is defined as chest pain caused by narrowing of coronary arteries and reduced oxygen to the heart. Inadequate oxygen supply precipitates angina and myocardial infarctions. Patients with a history of angina whose chest pain is provoked by stress, anxiety, or inadequate local anesthesia are treated with nitroglycerin. Unprovoked chest pain may be a myocardial infarction. (See Figure 8.4.)

Myocardial Infarction (MI)

Myocardial infarction is the death of myocardium caused by ischemia. Myocardial infarction should be suspected in patients with unprovoked chest pain and no prior history of angina. Angina patients that do not get relief from nitroglycerin may also be having an MI. An MI is a serious complication requiring EMS intervention. Treatment includes fentanyl for pain, oxygen to increase coronary perfusion, nitroglycerin for vasodilation, and chewed aspirin to prevent clot formation by decreasing platelet aggregation (FONA). Adverse cardiovascular events are reduced when stress, pain, and myocardial oxygen demand are decreased. (See Figure 8.4.)

Cardiac Arrest

Cardiac arrest is confirmed by absence of a pulse. Immediate actions include EMS activation, CPR, and AED deployment. Deep sedation, general anesthesia, and treatment of medically compromised patients will increase the likelihood of this emergency. (See Figure 8.5.)

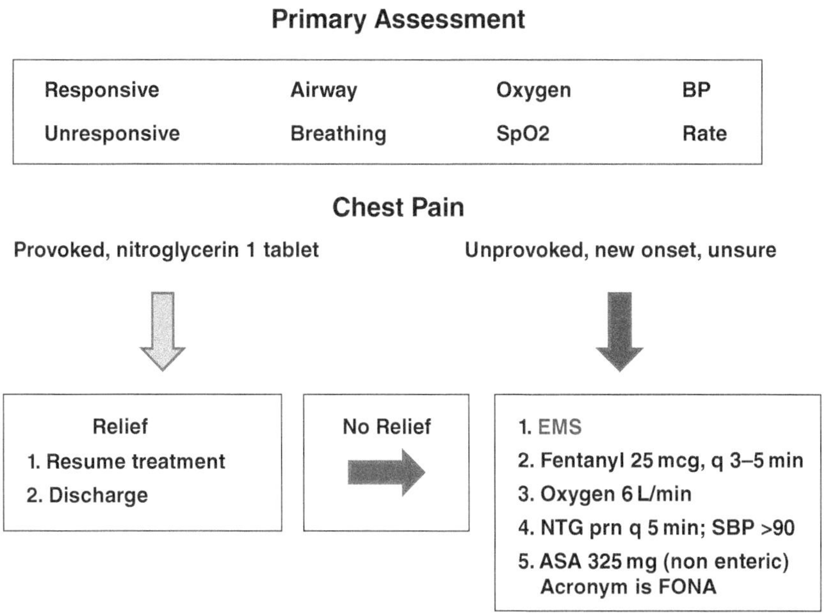

Primary Assessment

Responsive	Airway	Oxygen	BP
Unresponsive	Breathing	SpO2	Rate

Chest Pain

Provoked, nitroglycerin 1 tablet

Unprovoked, new onset, unsure

Relief
1. Resume treatment
2. Discharge

No Relief

1. EMS
2. Fentanyl 25 mcg, q 3–5 min
3. Oxygen 6 L/min
4. NTG prn q 5 min; SBP >90
5. ASA 325 mg (non enteric)
   Acronym is FONA

Figure 8.4   Angina pectoris / myocardial infarction algorithm.

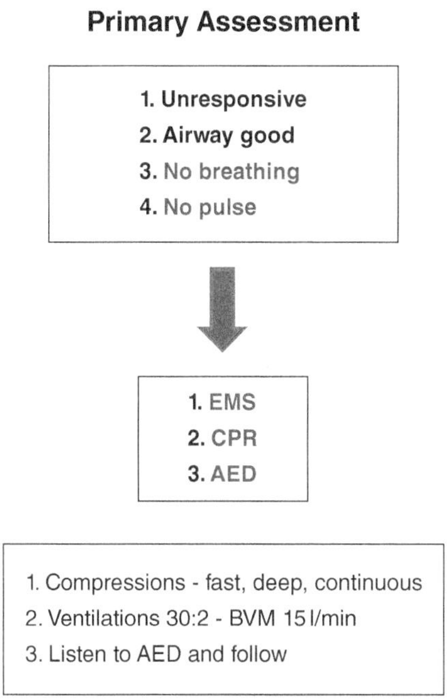

Primary Assessment

1. Unresponsive
2. Airway good
3. No breathing
4. No pulse

1. EMS
2. CPR
3. AED

1. Compressions - fast, deep, continuous
2. Ventilations 30:2 - BVM 15 l/min
3. Listen to AED and follow

Figure 8.5   Cardiac arrest algorithm.

Hypotension

Hypotension during sedation is defined as 30 mm Hg below systolic baseline. It is prevented by slow titration of fentanyl and sedatives. Treatment includes the Trendelenburg position and the rapid administration of 500 ml of IV solution. Atropine is the drug of choice for hypotension

Primary Assessment

Responsive	Airway	Oxygen	BP
Unresponsive	Breathing	SpO2	Rate

Treatment

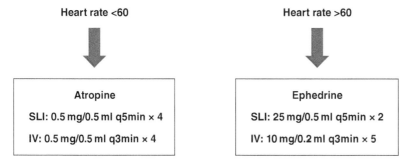

Persistent Hypotension

IV Fluids/Elevate Legs

Heart rate <60

Heart rate >60

Atropine
SLI: 0.5 mg/0.5 ml q5min × 4
IV: 0.5 mg/0.5 ml q3min × 4

Ephedrine
SLI: 25 mg/0.5 ml q5min × 2
IV: 10 mg/0.2 ml q3min × 5

Figure 8.6   Hypotension algorithm.

accompanied by bradycardia (pulse rate less than 60 bpm). Ephedrine is recommended when the heart rate is normal. (See Figure 8.6.)

Hypertension

A hypertensive crisis is often described as diastolic blood pressure greater than 120 mm Hg. The most common cause is pain and anxiety. A "time out" is often all that is need to restore normal blood pressure. In some cases, additional local anesthetic will correct the problem. Hypertension is considered an emergency when it is accompanied with signs or symptoms. Headache, chest pain, and visual disturbances are all indications of a hypertensive emergency. Treatment includes the administration of nitroglycerin and activation of EMS. (See Figure 8.7.)

Seizure

The patient will usually present with a history of seizures. A seizure is usually preceded by an aura. The aura is unique to each individual. Examples of auras include unusual odors, headaches, and changes in vision. The aura can serve as a warning of an impending seizure allowing time to prepare the patient. The patient should be on 100% oxygen in a supine position and objects removed from the mouth.

Seizure patients lose consciousness and are unaware of their surroundings during the seizure. They should be gently protected from injuring themselves. A seizure can be tonic or tonic-clonic. During the tonic seizure the patient's body assumes a ridged, arched position. Tonic-clonic seizures involve flexion and extension of the arms and legs.

Primary Assessment

Responsive	Airway	Oxygen	BP
Unresponsive	Breathing	SpO2	Rate

Treatment

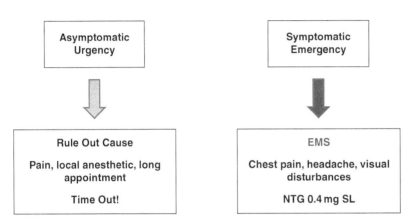

Asymptomatic Urgency	Symptomatic Emergency
Rule Out Cause Pain, local anesthetic, long appointment **Time Out!**	EMS Chest pain, headache, visual disturbances NTG 0.4 mg SL

Figure 8.7   Hypertension algorithm.

Recognize Problem

1. History of seizures
2. Aura warning
3. Loss of consciousness
4. Tonic-clonic or clonic

Treatment

	Intravenous Access	Post Seizure
1. Empty mouth 2. Supine position 3. Protect patient 4. 100% oxygen	1. Midazolam 2 mg bolus 2. Midazolam 1 mg/min 3. 50% dextrose	1. Patient on side 2. Airway adjuncts?

1. Recurring seizure
2. Seizure >5 min

EMS

Figure 8.8   Seizure algorithm.

Seizures are very unusual in the patient sedated with midazolam since this drug is used to treat seizures. Fifty percent dextrose should be administered if an IV line is available. Airway adjuncts may be useful to help breathing during recovery after the seizure. The patient should be turned on their right side to prevent aspiration of vomitus post seizure. Recurring seizures or seizures lasting longer than 5 minutes require EMS. (See Figure 8.8.)

Hypoglycemia

Hypoglycemia is defined as blood glucose levels below 60 mg/dL. Signs and symptoms include diaphoresis, confusion, convulsions, and loss of consciousness. Prevention includes a thorough medical history, short appointments, and early morning appointments. Blood glucose should be checked before appointments. Dextrose 5% IV fluid is recommended for diabetic patients in lieu of normal saline when IV sedation is planned.

All patients with symptoms should receive 100% oxygen. Conscious patients should be given sugar such as cake frosting. Unconscious patients should be given glucagon IM or 50% glucose IV. EMS should be activated if blood glucose level does not improve. (See Figure 8.9.)

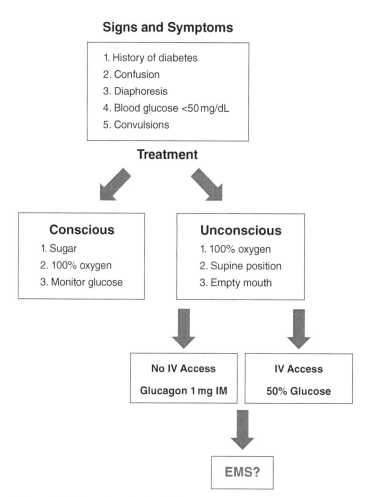

Signs and Symptoms

1. History of diabetes
2. Confusion
3. Diaphoresis
4. Blood glucose <50 mg/dL
5. Convulsions

Treatment

Conscious
1. Sugar
2. 100% oxygen
3. Monitor glucose

Unconscious
1. 100% oxygen
2. Supine position
3. Empty mouth

No IV Access

Glucagon 1 mg IM

IV Access

50% Glucose

EMS?

Figure 8.9   Hypoglycemia algorithm.

Syncope

Syncope is the most common medical complication in dentistry. It is triggered by fear or pain. Vasovagal reactions decrease oxygen/glucose to the brain causing loss of consciousness. A brief convulsive period is possible. Patients may appear pale and exhibit diaphoresis. They may feel cold or dizzy. Treatment includes emptying the patient's mouth, triple airway maneuver, and assessment. More serious complications should be suspected if this emergency does not resolve quickly. (See Figure 8.10.)

Monitors

The most reliable monitor of patients who are moderately sedated is verbal communication. Patients who are aware of their surroundings and can respond to verbal commands are able to maintain their airway. Other monitors include the pulse oximeter, precordial stethoscope, capnometer, and electrocardiogram.

Pulse Oximeter

Pulse oximetry measures the saturation of oxygen in blood. It monitors a patient's peripheral oxygen saturation (SpO_2). A fingertip sensor compares red and infrared wavelengths of light

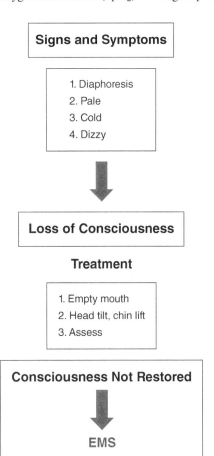

Figure 8.10 Syncope algorithm.

passing through the fingertip. (See Figure 8.11.) The ratio of R/IR is expressed as a percentage of oxygen in the hemoglobin molecule. Most pulse oximeters consist of a monitor, blood pressure cuff, sensor, and printer. (See Figure 8.12.) The Edan M3 pulse oximeter has an adjustable audible alarm and measures blood pressure, pulse rate, and mean arterial pressure in addition to oxygen saturation.

Pulse oximetry monitors oxygenation, the process of getting oxygen to blood and tissue. Capnography monitors the mechanical process of breathing, spontaneously or with help. This is important because pulse oximetry may indicate 99% oxygenation even when a patient is not breathing.

The oxygen dissociation curve is also an important factor for pulse oximetry. (See Figure 8.13.)

The vertical axis is SaO_2, the amount of hemoglobin saturated with oxygen. The horizontal axis is PaO_2, the partial pressure of oxygen in the alveolus. The oxygen dissociation curve is important because it shows that oxygen saturation at the sensor is not equal to available oxygen in the lungs.

A SpO_2 of 90 reflects a PaO_2 of ~60 mm Hg. An oxygen saturation of 90% indicates that available oxygen is at the "edge of a cliff" and is a warning to aggressively reestablish adequate ventilation. By definition, this is hypoxemia. Saturation that repeatedly drops below 95% requires action, i.e., "Take a slow deep breath," head tilt/chin lift, or nasal cannula.

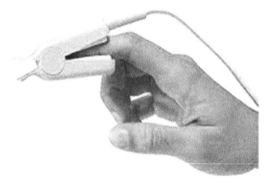

Figure 8.11   Finger sensor. (Reproduced with permission of Mediaid, Inc.)

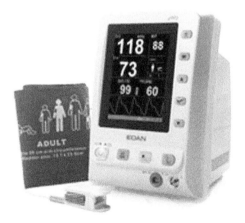

Figure 8.12   Edan M3 pulse oximeter. (Reproduced with permission of Edan Diagnostics, Inc).

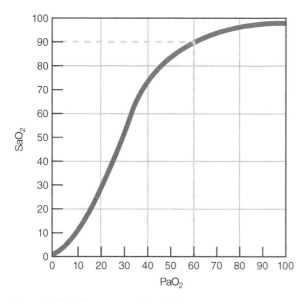

Figure 8.13   The oxygen dissociation curve.

Capnometer

Capnography monitors ventilation and the partial pressure (concentration) of carbon dioxide (CO_2) in exhaled air. It consists of a number and a graph. (See Figure 8.14.) Infrared technology is used to analyze carbon dioxide in exhaled gas. Exhaled air enters a nasal cannula and passes between a light and a detector plate. (See Figure 8.15.) More light is absorbed by concentrated CO_2 and less light is transmitted to the detector plate. The amount of light absorbed reflects the partial pressure of CO_2 at the end of exhalation. This is called end-tidal CO_2 ($ETCO_2$) which is normally 35–45 mm HG.

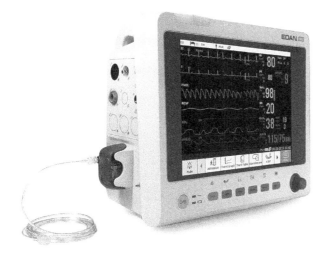

Figure 8.14   Capnometer. (Reproduced with permission of Edan Diagnostics, Inc.)

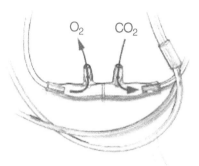

Figure 8.15 CO_2 sampling nasal cannula. (Reproduced by permission of Salter Labs, Inc.)

Capnography provides three important parameters. (See Figure 8.16.)

1) Waveform tracing for every breath
2) Respiratory rate (AwRR)
3) End tidal CO_2 value ($ETCO_2$) – normal 35–45 mm Hg

Capnography provides an earlier warning of airway obstruction or apnea when compared to pulse oximetry with supplemental oxygen. At the time of this writing, capnography is not required by most states. However, it is recommended by the American Dental Association and is likely to become the standard of care for moderate sedation.

Precordial Stethoscope

A precordial stethoscope is an affordable and effective way to monitor ventilations. It consists of a weighted stethoscope bell, rubber tubing, and an earpiece. The weighted pretracheal stethoscope

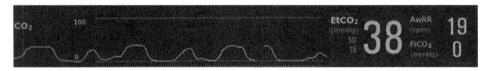

Figure 8.16   Capnography parameters. (Reproduced with permission of Edan Diagnostics, Inc.)

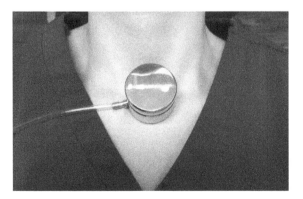

Figure 8.17a   Pretracheal stethoscope bell. (Reproduced with permission of Sedation Resource).

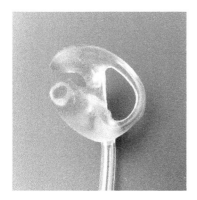

Figure 8.17b Custom earpiece.

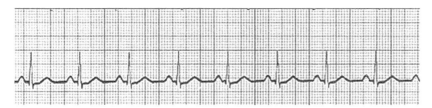

Figure 8.18 Normal sinus rhythm.

bell, placed over the suprasternal notch, monitors airway patency and ventilation. Double-sided adhesive disks stabilize its position. (See Figures 8.17a and 8.17b.)

A normal open airway produces a whooshing sound. Gurgling indicates liquid in the airway. Wheezing is the hallmark of bronchospasm. A high-pitched crowing sound can be heard when partial laryngospasm is present. All of these conditions can be detected when using a simple pretracheal stethoscope.

Electrocardiogram (EKG)

The electrocardiogram is a graphic representation of the cardiac cycle. Each event has a distinctive waveform. (See Figure 8.18.) The cardiac cycle refers to a complete heartbeat from its generation to the beginning of the next beat. The cardiac cycle is coordinated by a series of electrical impulses that are produced by specialized pacemaker cells found within the (SA) sinoatrial node and the (AV) atrioventricular node of the heart. Conduction of the electrical impulses produces a waveform. EKG is not required by most states for patient monitoring during moderate sedation.

The removal of impacted third molars can be done in relative comfort with moderate sedation. Patient safety is paramount when sedation is used. Monitoring patients during sedation alerts the dentist of impending sedation complications. Dentists employing sedation must have the training and knowledge to manage sedation emergencies.

The American Dental Society of Anesthesia (ADSA) provides a forum for education, research, and recognition of achievement in order to provide safe and effective patient care for all dentists who have an interest in anesthesiology, sedation, and the control of anxiety and pain. Membership in this organization is recommended for dentists providing sedation when removing impacted third molars.

References

1 Sirin Y, Humphris G, Sencan S, Firat D. What is the most fearful intervention in ambulatory oral surgery? Analysis of an outpatient clinic. *Int J Oral Maxillofac Surg.* 2012 Oct;41(10):1284–90.

2 Excerpted from continuum of depth of sedation: definition of general anesthesia and levels of sedation/ analgesia. American Society of Anesthesiologists (ASA), 2004.

3 Merin RL. Summary of the California blue ribbon panel report on anesthesia. *J West Soc Periodontol Periodontal Abstr.* 2005;53(2):37–9.

4 Becker DE, Haas DA. Recognition and management of complications during moderate and deep sedation Part 1: respiratory considerations. *Anesth Prog.* 2011 Summer;58(2):82–92.

5 Grimaldi F. Course director ACLS certification course. San Francisco, CA, 2016 Oct.

6 Becker DE. Drug allergies and implications for dental practice. *Anesth Prog.* 2013 Winter;60(4):188–97.

9

Documentation

A dentist in the United States is sued, on average, once in his or her career (more or less depending on location and scope of practice).[1] In other words, a dentist whose scope of practice includes high-risk procedures such as reconstruction, cosmetic dentistry, implants, or the removal of impacted third molars will, on average, be sued more than once in his or her career. (See Figure 9.1.)

The dental record, also referred to as the patient's chart, is the official legal document that records all of the treatment done and all patient related communications that occur in the dental office. State and federal laws and regulations determine how it is handled, how long it is kept, and who may have access to the information. The dental record provides for continuity of care for the patient and is critical in the event of a malpractice insurance claim.[2] Incomplete documentation leaves dentists vulnerable to liability.

Informed Consent

Dr. Crystal Baxter, DMD, MDS, evaluated 242 medical legal cases for dental negligence. The majority of the 242 cases were filed against general dentists, and of these cases, most were filed in the disciplines of oral surgery (extractions) and endodontics. In the oral surgery category, all general dentists who were alleged negligent were sued due to extraction complications. The majority of alleged cases also lacked proper informed consent and referral protocol.[3] Informed consent and complete progress notes are vital documents when litigation is an issue. This is especially true when sedation is used for the removal of impacted third molars.

State laws and court decisions determine the criteria for informed consent.[4] In 1914, a New York state court ruled that "every human being of adult years and sound mind has a right to determine what shall be done with his own body."[5] Another ruling from the Supreme Court of North Dakota found that laws pertaining to a physician's duty to obtain informed consent also pertained to dentists.[6] Although most cases have involved other health professionals, oral health care providers should follow the rulings established by these cases.

Informed consent is not well understood by most dentists. Consent is a process, not just a form. It is a process that includes a written document and a discussion with the patient that include the risks, benefits, and alternatives of third molar removal. The informed consent conversation should be completed by the doctor performing the procedure. Overly broad statements such as "any and

Impacted Third Molars, Second Edition. Edited by John Wayland.
© 2024 John Wiley & Sons, Inc. Published 2024 by John Wiley & Sons, Inc.

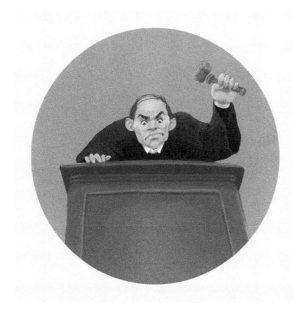

Figure 9.1   Malpractice trial judge.

all treatment deemed necessary..." or "all treatment which the doctor in his/her best medical judgment deems necessary, including but not limited to..." should be avoided. Courts have determined generalized statements to be so broad and unspecific that they do not satisfy the duty of informed consent. The dentist should also avoid downplaying the risks involved with impacted third molar surgery. The discussion should be completed at a consultation appointment, not on the day of surgery.[7] Booklets or videos may be helpful to the patient in understanding a proposed procedure. Time should be provided for the patient to review the consent in the privacy of their home. Otherwise, in court, the plaintiff's attorney will argue that their client did not have time to make a correct decision. The plaintiff will claim they were "coerced" into treatment.

Informed consent is governed by the statutes and case laws of individual states; dentists should review the applicable laws and regulations of their state.[8] Risks of nerve injury, broken teeth, displacement of teeth or roots, infection, TMJ injury, and infection are examples of risks when removing third molars. See Figures 9.2 and 9.3 for examples of impacted third molar and IV sedation consent forms.

A recurrent theme throughout this book is the recommendation for the early removal of third molars. The ideal time for removal, to decrease surgical complications, is when third molar roots are ½ – ¾ formed.[9] Many of these patients are teenagers under the age of 18. In most states, this means the informed consent should be given to a parent or guardian.

Dentists should be aware that the adult accompanying the patient may not be a legal guardian allowed by law to consent to medical procedures. Examples of such an adult include a grandparent, step-parent, noncustodial parent in instances of divorce, babysitter, or friend of the family.[8]

Another option for obtaining authorization for treatment is a telephone conversation with the parent. The parent should be told there are two people on the telephone and asked to verify the patient's name, date of birth, and address and to confirm he/she has responsibility for the patient.[10] Informed consent via phone should include all elements of a valid informed consent. The conversation must be documented in the patient's chart. Consent forms are signed by the treating dentist and witnessed by the staff member who participated in the phone discussion.

Surgical Consent

WHAT IS AN IMPACTED TOOTH?

An impacted tooth is a tooth that has not erupted normally. It may be covered by bone as well as gum tissue. Impacted teeth that press against other teeth may cause damage to those teeth. They may also cause crowding, infections, swelling, pain, cysts, earaches, headaches, generalized head and neck pain, and even tumors. Surgical removal of impacted and erupted third molars can correct and prevent future problems. However, as is the case with all surgical procedures, the removal of third molars involves risk. The benefit of removing third molars must be weighed against the risk.

WHAT IS A SURGICAL EXTRACTION?

Since impacted teeth are partially or completely beneath the surface of the gum tissue or bone, their removal is a surgical procedure. A surgical extraction requires the removal of bone, soft tissue incisions, or sectioning of teeth. Pain medication and instructions will control post-operative pain, swelling, bleeding, and discomfort.

DISCOMFORT, SWELLING, LIMITED OPENING, AND BLEEDING ARE NORMAL FOLLOWING SURGICAL EXTRACTIONS.

Slight bleeding may continue until the morning following surgery. The corners of the mouth may be irritated. Curved and thin root tips can fracture during extraction. They are usually removed, but may be left in place if they are near vital structures. Post-operative infections occasionally occur and are treated with antibiotics. Because of the close proximity of impacted teeth to adjacent teeth, occasionally a tooth or dental restoration may be damaged. VERY RARELY, post-operative complications include sinus opening, displacement of a tooth into the sinus or infra temporal fossa, lip or tongue numbness which can be temporary or permanent, damage to other oral structures, severe infections, jaw joint problems and broken jaws. In extremely rare circumstances even death may occur. A CT scan radiograph (xray) may be recommended when a wisdom tooth is near a nerve.

We will do our very best to make this a comfortable experience. If you have any questions please ask for clarification.

 I UNDERSTAND THAT DR. JANE DOE IS <u>NOT </u>AN ORAL SURGEON. I HAVE READ AND UNDERSTAND THE ABOVE ENTIRELY AND HEREBY CONSENT TO THE PERFORMANCE OF SURGERY AS PRESENTED TO ME.

Patient's or Guardian's Signature_____Date_____

Witness Signature_____Date_____

Doctor's Signature_____Date_____

Figure 9.2   Third molar impaction consent form.

INTRAVENOUS SEDATION CONSENT

WHAT IS IV SEDATION?

Intravenous sedation is a form of anesthesia. Anesthesia can create light, moderate, or deep sleep. IV sedation, administered properly, creates a light sleep. Patients are conscious and are able to respond to verbal commands, but have decreased awareness of their surroundings. Patients have little or no memory of the procedure because of the amnesia produced by the sedative agents. Intravenous sedation is not general anesthesia which creates a deep sleep and an unconscious state.

Oral sedation may be used prior to injection of small amounts of medications into a vein in the arm. Sedative agents are not completely eliminated from the body for several hours afterwards. Therefore, patients who have intravenous sedation need an escort home.

The risks and complications associated with any sedation include nausea, vomiting, allergic reaction, pain, inflammation and/or infection at the intravenous site. In extremely rare circumstances even death may occur.

MEDICAL HISTORY: Any personal illness, weakness, or allergy must be reported. Also, details of any drugs being taken – especially sleeping drugs, tranquilizers, or cortisone medications, must be reported to us. This includes over the counter drugs, street drugs, or prescription drugs.

PREPARATIONS: No food or drink within six (6) hours of the appointment time and the previous meal should be light and easily digestible. A small amount of water may be used to take any medications prescribed for your appointment. Loose clothing should be worn and sleeves should be easily drawn up past the elbow. Also, comfortable flat-heeled shoes that are easy to walk in should be worn. Dentures, glasses, and/or contact lenses should be removed prior to the appointment.

FOLLOWING SEDATION: A responsible adult (friend or family member) must accompany the patient home.

NO WARRANTY OR GUARRANTEE: No warranty or guarantee is implied or given regarding the success of sedation.

ANY PATIENT ACCEPTING A SEDATION APPOINTMENT MUST SPECIFICALLY AGREE TO THE FOLLOWING:

- NOT to drive a vehicle or operate any machinery after sedation for the rest of the day

- NOT to undertake any responsible business matters

- NOT to drink alcohol for 24 hours after sedation

I HAVE READ AND UNDERSTAND THE ABOVE ENTIRELY AND HEREBY CONSENT TO THE PERFORMANCE OF SEDATION AS PRESENTED TO ME.

_____   _____

Patient's or Guardian's Signature   Date

_____   _____

Witness Signature   Date

_____   _____

Doctor's Signature   Date

Figure 9.3   Intravenous sedation consent form.

Informed refusal occurs when the patient/parent refuses the proposed and alternative treatments. It is recommended by the ADA that informed refusal is documented in the chart and that the dentist informs the patient/parent about the consequences of not accepting the proposed treatment. The dentist should attempt to obtain an informed refusal signed by the parent for retention in the patient record. An informed refusal, however, does not release the dentist from the responsibility of providing a standard of care. If the dentist believes the informed refusal violates proper standards of care, he/she should recommend the patient seek another opinion and/or dismiss the patient from the practice.[7]

Progress Notes

Progress notes record clinical details of each patient visit. Progress notes document patient treatment and provide written communication between health care professionals. They are legal documents that protect the interests of both patient and dentist. Adequate documentation of patient treatment is also essential information for billing and reimbursement from third-party insurance carriers.

The biggest challenge for adequate documentation is consistent and thorough progress notes. Every dentist has experienced stressful days when things don't go as planned. A staff member calls in sick, 3 patients are late for their appointment, the compressor stops functioning, and 2 patients arrive for emergency treatment. Stress and multitasking are not conducive to detailed and complete progress notes. One solution to this problem is "SOAP" progress notes.

Dr. Lawrence Weed, MD, introduced the concept of SOAP progress notes in an article published in 1964.[11] SOAP notes begin with the patient's chief complaint and history followed by objective data (tests, observations, radiographs, etc.), assessment, and plan. The SOAP note is an acronym for subjective, objective, assessment, and plan or procedure. (See Box 9.1.) The soap format virtually guarantees comprehensive notes.

Box 9.1 SOAP progress notes.

S: Subjective is the patient's chief complaint
O: Objective is what the clinician sees or elicits with tests
A: Assessment is the diagnosis
P: Procedure is treatment rendered or planned

Digitized progress notes are often included in dental office management software. Custom progress note templates can be created for different procedures. An impacted third molar template is shown in Box 9.2.

Box 9.2 SOAP impacted third molar notes example.

S: Pain lower left and lower right
O: Roots 1/2 – 3/4 developed, good access, 17 and 32 mesioangular
A: Impactions, pericoronitis
P: Informed consent for mother and patient, risks, alternatives, and benefits discussed, see IV record, 1, 16, 17, 32 flap, remove buccal, occlusal, and distal bone, 1 and 16 elevator delivery, 17 and 32 section, elevator delivery, bone file, irrigate, one 3.0 polyglycolic acid suture used distal #17 and #32, post-operative instructions written and oral for mother and patient, no complications

---

Abbreviations are useful to document repetitive procedures when notes are hand written. The removal of impacted third molars is a repetitive and predictable procedure. The abbreviated notes shown in Box 9.3 are as valid as the notes in Box 9.2 Abbreviations are acceptable legal documentation when standardized and used by all staff. Excessive use of abbreviations should be avoided. This can make the dentist appear rushed and impersonal which would not bode well in the defense of a malpractice suit. A key for frequently used abbreviations should be included in the patient's chart and posted in an office manual.

Box 9.3 SOAP impacted third molar notes example abbreviated

S: Pain LL and LR
O: Roots 1/2 – 3/4, good access, 17 and 32 MA
A: Impactions, pericoronitis
P: ICMP, RAB, CIVR, 1, 16, 17, 32 flap, RBODB, 1 / 16 ED, 17 / 32 section, ED, BF, I, 1 × 3.0 PGA, PO/WO/MP, n/c.

Malpractice Cases

Dental malpractice lawsuits contain four essential elements: duty, breach of duty, proximate cause, and damage. A dentist may successfully defend a suit by proving no duty existed, no breach of duty occurred, that the dentist's conduct was not the cause of damage, or that no damage exists.[12]

A professional duty is created when a professional relationship is established between a patient and dentist. It is the dentist's duty to provide care for the patient. A breach of duty occurs when the dentist's care is not similar to how other dentists would have acted under similar circumstances. This is often referred to as "standard of care". Dentists are judged by a national standard of care. This standard, when removing impacted third molars, is usually the care given by an oral surgeon. The plaintiff's attorney must show that damage or injury occurred to the plaintiff. They must prove that the dentist's actions caused the patient's injury and that the patient's injury was foreseeable and not extraordinary.

The Dentist's Advantage Insurance Company has provided medical malpractice coverage for dentists for more than 50 years. They are endorsed by the American Academy of General Dentistry. The Dentists Advantage published dental malpractice case studies occurring from 2012 to 2015. Seven cases involving the removal of third molars are presented here. (Reproduced by permission of The Dentist's Advantage Insurance Co.)

1. **June 2012 – Jaw Fractured During Wisdom Tooth Extraction – Additional Surgery Required and Woman Claims Fibromyalgia From Trauma – defense verdict**

The plaintiff, age 29, went to a dental office in August 2007 for oral surgery which was performed by the defendant dentist. The plaintiff was to have three impacted wisdom teeth pulled. The plaintiff claimed that she had requested that the defendant dentist not perform the procedure, but he did.

The plaintiff claimed that the defendant dentist failed to section an impacted wisdom tooth in her lower jaw before pulling it, resulting in greater removal of bone from her jaw than necessary, which led to a fractured jaw. The plaintiff also claimed that it was ten days before she was referred to an oral surgeon. The plaintiff underwent open reduction and internal fixation of the left jaw and later underwent removal of an infected bone plate.

The plaintiff claimed that she developed fibromyalgia due to the trauma from the extraction. The plaintiff alleged battery, lack of informed consent, and negligence in the performance of the extraction.

The defendant claimed that proper consent was obtained and that jaw fracture was a risk of the procedure which was included in the consent form. The defendant claimed that the extraction was performed without complications and that the bone was thin on the left side of her jaw and that she was informed that she should avoid putting pressure on that side of her face.

The defendant also claimed that the plaintiff was given instructions to call or return to the office if she had any change in her condition. The defendant claimed that the plaintiff's follow-up visit, six days later, included complaints of swelling and tenderness on the left side of her face and she returned the next day for an X-ray, which revealed a mandible fracture.

The defendant dentist claimed that the plaintiff was informed of this and indicated that she was feeling better and had little pain and swelling. The plaintiff was told to return in three days, at which time there was good improvement. The defendant then referred the plaintiff to an oral and maxillofacial surgeon and gave her a list of surgeons and a letter detailing his treatment.

According to a published account a defense verdict was returned.

2. **August 2012 – Lingual Nerve Damage From Wisdom Tooth Extraction – Microsurgical Repair, But Some Numbness Continues – $187,500 settlement**

"The plaintiff, age twenty-nine, had a wisdom tooth extracted from his lower jaw in January 2009 by the dentist. The plaintiff suffered numbness to the anterior two-thirds of the right half of his tongue, the floor of the mouth on the right side and the lingual gingiva of the lower right side after the procedure.

He underwent a microsurgical repair to the lingual nerve in April 2009. The repair surgery returned fifty percent of sensation to the affected part of the tongue. The plaintiff claimed that the defendant dentist severed the right lingual nerve during the extraction, perforating through the lower right lingual plate of bone and into the soft gum tissue where the right lingual nerve is located. Photographs and a visit to an oral surgeon who finished the extraction confirmed that there was damage to the soft gum tissue.

The defendant dentist denied any negligence. According to a published account a $187,500 settlement was reached in mediation."

3. **Drill Bit Breaks During Wisdom Tooth Extraction and Part is Retained in Jaw – Attempt to Extract Drill Bit Tip Causes Nerve Injury – $2.69 Million Verdict Reduced to $300,000 Under High/Low Agreement.**

The plaintiff, age 37, went to the defendant dentist for treatment of mouth pain. The defendant dentist diagnosed an impacted wisdom tooth and recommended extraction. The plaintiff was referred to a contractor for the procedure. The contractor, an oral surgery resident, performed the extraction in November 2007. During the procedure the burr tip of the drill fractured in the plaintiff's mouth and was retained in her jaw.

The plaintiff returned to the defendant dentist with complaints of oral pain and was referred back to the oral surgery resident. An X-ray revealed the drill bit. An attempt was made to remove the drill bit a week after the extraction, but the bit was actually pushed into the inferior alveolar nerve canal, resulting in a nerve injury.

The plaintiff claimed permanent numbness, hypersensitivity and pain in her left, lower lip and chin. The plaintiff alleged lack of informed consent regarding the referral to an oral surgery resident, rather than an oral surgeon. The plaintiff claimed that she would have declined the extraction if she had known she was being referred to a resident.

The defendant claimed that nerve damage was listed as a possible complication of wisdom tooth extraction on the informed consent document. The defendant dentist also maintained that there was no requirement on him to inform the plaintiff that the contractor was a resident.

According to a published account a $2,690,000 verdict was returned, which was reduced to $300,000 under a high/low agreement.

4. **Extraction of Wisdom Teeth Alleged to Sever Lingual Nerve – Numbness and Loss of Taste – Defendant Claims Nerve Not Damaged and Nerve Injury Was a Known Risk – $25,000 Verdict.**

The plaintiff, age fourteen, underwent extraction of wisdom teeth in 2005. The procedure was performed by the defendant dentist. The plaintiff claimed that a high-speed drill severed her lingual nerve, leading to residual numbness of the left side of her mouth and tongue. The plaintiff particularly claimed a loss of her sense of taste. The plaintiff underwent surgery for the lingual nerve, but her condition continued. The plaintiff alleged negligence in the performance of the extractions.

The defendant claimed that images of the lingual nerve did not show any damage to the nerve and that the plaintiff's post-extraction symptoms quickly improved, which would not have occurred if there was a significant injury of the lingual nerve. The defendant additionally claimed that the plaintiff and her parents were informed of the possibility of an injury to the lingual nerve.

The defendant also claimed that the plaintiff's surgery had restored most of her sense of taste and sensation and that the injury did not affect the right side of the tongue.

According to a published account a $25,000 verdict was returned.

5. **Man Dies Following Wisdom Tooth Extraction- Necrotizing Mediastinitis, Septic Shock, Ludwig's Angina – $2.6 Million Net Verdict.**

The plaintiff's decedent went to the defendant dental practice in March 2011 for routine dental work. The decedent returned in April for extraction of tooth number 32 (wisdom tooth), which was performed by the defendant dentist. The plaintiff suffered severe pain in the extraction area on the right side of his face, with swelling and difficulty swallowing. The decedent contacted the defendant dental practice two days after the extraction and was told to call again if his symptoms did not subside in four or five days. The decedent began vomiting and having difficulty breathing, and was transported by ambulance to a hospital five days later. Antibiotics were administered and drainage of the neck was performed. The man had developed necrotizing mediastinitis and septic shock, then Ludwig's angina from the dental abscess. The man died at the age of forty-two four days later.

The plaintiff alleged lack of informed consent regarding use of antibiotics to prevent infection, and a failure to provide proper advice in the telephone call after the procedure. The defendants denied any negligence and maintained that the decedent was given instructions verbally and in writing to contact the office or go to an emergency department if he had severe or unexpected complications. The defendant dentist claimed that she was not contacted and was not aware of the decedent's condition and that she did not give any employee of the defendant dental practice any advice or instructions for the decedent.

According to the trial reports, a jury returned $985,000 in damages for the surviving spouse and $2,485,000 in damages to the decedent's minor son. The decedent was found 25% at fault, the defendant dentist 50% at fault, and the defendant dental practice 25% at fault. The net verdict was $2,602,500.

6. Lingual Nerve Injury During Wisdom Tooth Extraction – $875,000 Settlement

The plaintiff, age 28, went to the office of the defendant dentist in 2005 for the removal of the lower left wisdom tooth. During the procedure the plaintiff's lingual nerve was severed. The plaintiff was referred to an oral surgeon to repair the nerve damage. Despite multiple subsequent surgeries, the plaintiff's injury was irreparable, resulting in severe and chronic pain. The plaintiff claimed negligence by the defendant dentist in using a surgical technique which was unnecessarily invasive and also claimed that the method used for the extraction was not appropriate.

The plaintiff argued that the technique used by the defendant dentist was not taught by any dental school. The defendant dentist claimed that the technique he used was proper and had been taught to him by the head of a college oral surgery department. The defendant dentist also claimed that the nerve injury was from the use of an elevator to extract the tooth, which was a common practice.

The plaintiff was able to present the person referenced by the defendant dentist as having taught him his technique (whom the defendant dentist had claimed was deceased). This individual testified that neither he nor any other instructor at the college would have taught such a surgical technique.

The matter was initially tried to a defense verdict, which was set aside on appeal and remanded for a new trial. Prior to retrial, the parties entered a high/low agreement of $875,000/$195,000. The matter was subsequently settled for $875,000 four hours after the jury announced having reached a verdict on liability, but needed more time to deliberate the issue of damages.

7. Trigeminal Nerve Injury From Wisdom Tooth Extraction – $1,000,000 Settlement

The plaintiff, age thirty-three, went to the defendant dentist for evaluation. At the plaintiff's next visit to the defendant, three of the plaintiff's wisdom teeth were extracted. The procedure took six hours.

The plaintiff claimed that she suffered injury to the trigeminal nerve, causing permanent trigeminal neuropathic pain. The plaintiff claimed that the defendant dentist failed to appreciate the significance of the bony involvement of her third molars and the proximity of the third molars to the inferior alveolar canal. The plaintiff argued that a specialist in complex third molar removal should have been consulted. The plaintiff also claimed that she was not informed of the complexity of the third molar extraction and the risk of nerve injury.

The defendant dentist argued that the nerve injury was a known risk of the extraction and denied any negligence. According to reports, a $1 million policy-limits settlement was reached.

Malpractice Case Summary

The seven cases cited represent The Dentist Advantage third molar suits published between 2012 and 2015. Each case illustrates the need for documentation.

Patient # 1 claimed that she had requested that the defendant dentist not perform the procedure. However, **informed consent was completed** by the defendant dentist. The court ruled in favor of the defendant.

Patient# 2 proved that damage was done to the right lingual plate and soft tissue (oral surgeon photos). The injured tissue was outside the surgical field. In this case, negligence was proven and **informed consent became irrelevant**. The court ruled in favor of the plaintiff.

Patient #3 alleged **lack of informed consent** regarding the referral to an oral surgery resident. The defendant dentist argued that there was no requirement for him to inform the plaintiff that the contractor was a resident. This case highlights the need for a thorough discussion with patients. The fact that the contractor dentist was not an oral surgeon was not discussed or documented. The court ruled in favor of the plaintiff.

Patient #4 alleged negligence in the removal of her lower left third molar. Subsequent images of the lingual nerve did not show damage. The plaintiff failed to prove negligence. **Informed consent stated** that lingual nerve injury was a possible surgical complication. A minimal award of $25,000 was given to the plaintiff.

Patient #5's descendent claimed that the patient contacted the defendant dental practice two days after the removal of # 32. The defendant dentist instructed the patient to call back if symptoms did not improve. The defendant dentist argued that she was not aware of a phone call or the patient's condition. In this case, the plaintiff's attorney likely argued that the dentist's conduct contributed to the plaintiff's injury. Antibiotics were **not discussed** or prescribed. Antibiotics may be indicated for difficult extractions or medically compromised patients. Although not required, the dentist did not make a postoperative phone call to follow up. The author recommends a postoperative phone call within 24 hours following the removal of impacted third molars. The phone call should be documented in progress notes. Verdict ruled in favor of the plaintiff.

Patient #6 claimed negligence due to a lower left severed lingual nerve. This injury was verified with a CT scan. In this case the defendant's character was questionable due to his statement that he was taught the surgical technique by an instructor in dental school. This was found to be untrue. The defendant's **duplicitous character** may have led the jury to believe the dentist's conduct caused the injury. The verdict was ruled for the plaintiff.

Patient #7 claimed that she was **not properly informed** of the complexity involved with the removal of her wisdom teeth. The amount of time required to remove 3 third molars calls into question the dentist's competence. The procedure was not completed within the standard of care. The case was settled for $1,000,000.

Summary

Informed consent and progress note documentation will not help if negligence is proven. Dentists removing impacted third molars should practice within the scope of their training and experience to avoid the appearance of negligence. Age appears to have been a significant factor in most of The Dentist Advantage cases. Only one patient was younger than 28 years old. Surgical complications and the appearance of negligence increase with patient age.

The importance of the patient's relationship with the dentist, office, and staff cannot be overstated. The following quote from Wilhemina Leeuw, MS, CDA, illuminates the importance of this relationship. "Cases have been reported in which patients decided not to file a claim against the dentist simply because they liked a staff member or felt that the dental team was polite. Patients do not expect their dentists to be perfect, but they do expect them to show compassion and honesty rather than indifference. Most medical and dental malpractice claims arise from an unfavorable interaction with the dentist and not necessarily from a poor treatment outcome."[13]

Since the 1960s the frequency of medical malpractice claims filed in the United States has increased. Today, malpractice claims are relatively common.[14] Dentists should take steps to protect themselves from malpractice suits. Documentation, including informed consent and SOAP progress notes, should be an essential part of every dental practice.

References

1 Medical Protective Insurance. Closed claims analysis. 2003–2012.

2 Council on Dental Practice Division of Legal Affairs. Dental records. ADA, 2007.

3 Baxter C. A review of dental negligence. Dentistry IQ. http://www.dentistryiq.com/articles/wdj/print/volume-2/issue-8/you-and-your-practice/a-review-of-dental-negligence.html. Accessed 2016 Nov 24.

4 Sfikis P. A duty to disclose: issues to consider in securing informed consent. *J Am Dent Assoc.* 2003;134(10):1329–33.

5 Schloendorffer v Society of New York Hospital (105N.E. 92). 1914.

6 Koapke v Herfendal, 660 NW 2d 206 (ND 2003).

7 American Dental Association, Division of Legal Affairs. Dental records. Chicago, IL: American Dental Association, 2007, 16.

8 Council on Clinical Affairs, American Academy of Pediatric Dentistry. Guideline on informed consent. Revised 2009.

9 Reznick JB. The wonderful world of oral surgery. Dental Town 2nd Annual Gathering, Las Vegas, Nevada, 2004 Mar 27.

10 Watterson DG. Informed consent and informed refusal in dentistry. Registered Dental Hygienist. 2012 Sept.

11 Wachter B. Time to tackle an epic problem. Wachters World: http://community.the-hospitalist.org/2012/09/03.

12 Malamed SF. *Sedation a guide to patient management*, 5th edition. St. Louis, Missouri 63146: Mosby Elsevier, 2010. Ch 40, 562.

13 Leeuw W. Maintaining proper dental records. Crest® Oral-B® at dentalcare.com Continuing Education Course. Revised 2013 Jul 11.

14 Sonny Bal B. An introduction to medical malpractice in the United States. *Clin Orthop Relat Res.* 2009 Feb;467(2):339–47.

10

Local Anesthesia

Many patients have anxiety when going to the dentist. One of the most feared dental procedures is the removal of third molars.[1] Intravenous and oral sedation can help mitigate this fear, but local anesthesia is needed to eliminate pain.

History

Nitrous oxide anesthesia was discovered in 1844, before local anesthesia. This notable discovery was made by a dentist, Horace Wells. Forty years later cocaine became the first local anesthetic. Prior to local anesthesia all surgical procedures were completed with general anesthesia using ether. Ether was discovered by another dentist, William T. G. Morton.

Cocaine played a major role in the evolution of local anesthesia (see Table 10.1). In July 1884, Sigmund Freud published a review on cocaine and his experiments, noting the alkaloid's anesthetic effect on mucous membranes. Freud's colleague and friend, ophthalmologist Carl Koller (1857–1944), took part in a series of cocaine experiments with Freud during the spring and summer of 1884. Koller noted the deadening effect on his tongue when he swallowed cocaine and grasped the surgical importance of cocaine's anesthetic effect.[2]

Table 10.1 Rapid development in 1884 of cocaine use as a local anesthetic.

1884
July
● Freud cocaine paper published
September
● Koller performs eye surgery using cocaine as a local anesthetic
October
● Koller publishes his cocaine local anesthetic paper
December
● Richard Hall reports the first application of local anesthesia in dentistry
● William S. Halsted conducts local anesthetic mandibular nerve block

Impacted Third Molars, Second Edition. Edited by John Wayland.
© 2024 John Wiley & Sons, Inc. Published 2024 by John Wiley & Sons, Inc.

Table 10.2   Maximum recommended dose of local anesthetic for a healthy 150 lb patient.

Drug	mg/lb	MRD/150 lb	Max Cartridge
Lidocaine 2% + 1:100,000 epinephrine	33.2	480 mg	13
Articaine 4% + 1:100,000 epinephrine	33.2	480 mg	7
Bupivacaine 0.5% + 1:200,000 epinephrine	00.6	90 mg	10

German chemist Alfred Einhorn invented the dental anesthetic novocaine (procaine). Novocaine appeared in a publication for the first time in 1905 in an article written by the German surgeon Heinrich Braun. Compared to other promising local anesthetics, novocaine was found to be safe and quickly became the standard local anesthesia in dentistry. Many new and improved local anesthetics have now replaced novocaine.

The most common local anesthetics used for inferior alveolar and mandibular nerve blocks in the United States include lidocaine, articaine, and bupivacaine. (See Table 10.2.) Estimates of pulp anesthesia duration following block anesthesia with epinephrine vary widely depending on the study. Lidocaine and articaine have similar duration of 1–2 hours. Articaine pulpal anesthesia usually lasts a little longer than lidocaine. Bupivacaine is a long duration local anesthetic that provides pulpal anesthesia for at least 6–8 hours with epinephrine 1:200,000. If oral or IV sedation is used with these local anesthetics, synergy will increase the duration of each anesthetic.

The lowest dosage needed to provide effective anesthesia should be administered.[3] (See Table 10.2.)

Allergic Reaction

Patients often claim that they are allergic to local anesthetic. They may experience tachycardia or syncope during an injection. These reactions are usually related to epinephrine in the solution or anxiety. True local anesthetic allergies are very unusual and are caused by methylparaben preservative or sulfite antioxidant in the local anesthetic cartridge.

Compounded topical anesthetic (e.g., EMLA), slow injections, and frequent aspiration can decrease or eliminate these reactions.

Toxicity – Overdose

Many factors may contribute to local anesthetic overdose.[4]

1) Medically Compromised Patients
   Liver and kidney dysfunction increase the blood local anesthetic level. Congestive heart failure can increase local anesthetic overdose. A consistent theme in this book is the recommendation to refer medically compromised patients.
2) Medications
   Medications can increase local anesthetic concentration causing toxic reactions. Caution should be used with patients on existing medication.
3) Age
   Absorption, metabolism, and excretion are underdeveloped or diminished with young and old patients resulting in increased anesthetic blood levels.

4) <u>Weight</u>

Large patients have a larger blood volume than small patients. Large patients will have a lower concentration of drug per area than lighter patients. The maximum recommended dose (MRD) of a drug is calculated as the number of milligrams of a drug per kilograms (lbs) of body weight.

5) <u>Pregnancy</u>

During pregnancy renal function may be impaired increasing the risk of local anesthetic overdose.

6) <u>Vascularity</u>

Increased vascularity of the injection site will increase absorption into the circulation. This is one advantage of the Gow-Gates injection site since it is less vascular and well perfused.

Local Anesthetic Potency

Local anesthetics vary in potency allowing for concentrations that typically range from 0.5% to 4%. This is largely the result of differences in lipid solubility, which enhances diffusion through nerve sheaths and neural membranes.

Bupivacaine is more lipid soluble and potent than articaine, allowing it to be formulated as a 0.5% concentration (5 mg/mL) rather than a 4% concentration (40 mg/mL).[3] See Table 10.3.

Local anesthetics should be respected as CNS depressants. They potentiate any respiratory depression associated with sedatives and opioids.

Articaine

Though articaine is classified as an amide local anesthetic, it possesses chemical characteristics of both the amide and ester groups. It has become an extremely popular local anesthetic wherever it has been made available.[5] As a result of it undergoing metabolism in the plasma (as well as in the liver) articaine is a preferred local anesthetic during pregnancy, nursing and in lighter-weight patients.

For normal healthy adults, the Septodont product insert states the maximum recommended dose (MRD) of articaine administered by submucosal infiltration and/or nerve block should not exceed 3.2 mg/lb of body weight. This equals seven cartridges for a 150 lb. patient.[6]

Articaine deserves a closer look due to claims of increased IAN paresthesia. Two anesthesia icons, Stanley Malamed and Anthony Pogrel, have studied articaine local anesthesia.

Malamed's 2001 study included 1,325 subjects, 882 of whom received articaine 4% with epinephrine 1:100,000 and 443 of whom received lidocaine 2% with epinephrine 1:100,000. The overall

Table 10.3 Local anesthetics commonly used for the removal of impacted third molars.

Anesthetic Agent	Agent/Formulation	Duration of Pulp Anesthesia	Pregnancy Category
Articaine (Septocaine)	4% articaine / 1:100,000 epinephrine	1–2 hours	C
Bupivacaine (Marcaine)	0.5% bupivacaine / 1:200,000 epinephrine	6–8 hours	C
Lidocaine (Xylocaine)	2% lidocaine / 1:100,000 epinephrine	1–2 hours	B

incidence of adverse events in the combined studies was 22% for the articaine group and 20% for the lidocaine group. The study concluded that articaine is a well-tolerated, safe, and effective local anesthetic for use in clinical dentistry.[6]

Malamed also wrote an article published in *Oral Health* in 2016. Malamed's *Oral Health* article conclude,s "All reports claiming an increased risk of paresthesia with articaine are anecdotal. There is no scientific evidence demonstrating an increased risk of paresthesia following the administration of articaine compared with other local anesthetics."[7]

According to Dr. Pogrel's article published in 2007, permanent nerve involvement following inferior alveolar nerve blocks may occur from 1 in 20,000 to 850,000 patients with little information on the local anesthetic used. Patients with permanent nerve damage from blocks were recorded. Lidocaine was associated with 35%, with articaine used in approximately 30% of the cases. Nerve blocks can cause permanent damage to nerves, independent of the local anesthetic used. Pogrel concluded that articaine is associated with this phenomenon in proportion to its usage.[8] Other studies have done unbiased database searches that show articaine is equivalent to lidocaine regarding block paresthesia.

E. Martin, et al performed database searches in Medline Ovid, Medline Pubmed, Scopus, Emcare, Proquest, and the Cochrane Central Register of Controlled Trials.[9] Inclusion criteria were all existing English, human, randomized controlled trials of interventions involving 4% articaine and 2% lidocaine in routine dental treatment. Twelve studies were included for meta-analysis using Cochrane Review Manager software. Anesthetic success odds ratios were calculated using a random-effects model.

The review of 12 studies concluded articaine is a safe and efficacious local anesthetic for all routine dental procedures in patients of all ages and more likely to achieve successful anesthesia than lidocaine in routine dental treatment. Neither anesthetic has a higher association with anesthetic-related adverse effects. Further studies on articaine are indicated.

Adverse events due to anxiety are the most common phenomena associated with local anesthetic injection.

Nerve Block Local Anesthesia in Dentistry

Three nerve block anesthesia techniques are commonly used when removing impacted third molars; the Halstead (inferior alveolar), Gow-Gates, and Vazirani-Akinosi. The Halstead and Vazirani-Akinosi injections target the inferior alveolar nerve. The Gow-Gates injection targets the mandibular nerve and its terminal branches; the inferior alveolar, lingual, mylohyoid, auriculo-temporal, and buccal nerve. The author prefers a combination of the inferior alveolar and Gow-Gates injections when removing third molars. The combination technique is virtually 100% effective and will be discussed later in the practical application section of this chapter.

A 25-gauge needle is recommended for all block anesthesia. The larger needle will not deflect as it passes through tissue. Injections with a 25 – gauge needle are no more painful than injections with a smaller needle.[10] The larger needle results in fewer intravascular injections since positive aspirations are more clearly seen. Short needles should be avoided. A short needle will generally not reach the target area without the risk of advancing to the hub of the needle. The stress on the hub could cause the needle to break, as the hub-needle interface is the weakest part of the needle.

During manufacturing, a barb is sometimes created at the end of the needle. The barb causes drag through patient tissue and increases pain. It's recommended that every needle is checked for barbs prior to injection. Manufacturing defects can be felt when the needle is wiped from hub to needle tip with sterile gauze. Defective needles should be discarded.

Inferior Alveolar Nerve Block (Halstead)

In the traditional (Halstead) technique for the inferior alveolar nerve block the dentist approaches the injection site with the barrel of the syringe over the contralateral second premolar.[11] (See Figures 10.1 and 10.2.)

Bony landmarks and needle insertion depth should be observed when performing an inferior alveolar nerve block.[11] (See Figure 10.2.)

Vertical plane needle insertion. The needle is placed at or slightly below the mandibular occlusal plane. The coronoid notch is a helpful landmark for vertical positioning of this injection. To use this landmark the thumb of the free hand is placed in the middle of the coronoid notch. The needle should parallel the mandibular occlusal plane and bisect the thumb in a vertical plane. The mandibular foramen is usually found slightly below the level of the deepest concavity of the coronoid notch.

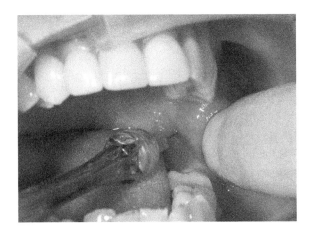

Figure 10.1   Injection site for inferior alveolar nerve block. Healthjade.net.

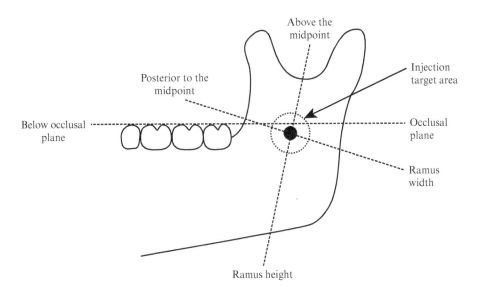

Figure 10.2   Landmarks for inferior alveolar nerve block. Wolters Kluwer https://aeronline.org/temp/AnesthEssaysRes813-3435552_093235.pdf / last accessed February 02, 2023.

Horizontal plane needle insertion. The bony landmarks for needle insertion in the horizontal plane are the anterior and posterior surface of the ramus. By placing the thumb in the coronoid notch and the index finger on the posterior surface of the ramus, one can feel the front and back of the ramus. The needle should bisect the anterior and posterior ramus, slightly posterior to the midpoint.

Depth of needle insertion. The operator inserts the needle about three-quarters (20–25 mm) of the length of a long needle, or until bone is touched. At this point the operator will aspirate, and inject a full cartridge of local anesthetic solution.

Mandibular Nerve Block (Gow-Gates)

Dr. Gow-Gates initially described what became known as the "Gow-Gates mandibular nerve block" in 1973. A wide opening is essential for success with this technique. Just before needle insertion, ask the patient to open his or her mouth as widely as possible. Once the needle is inserted, advance it slowly until it contacts the neck of the condyle.[12] (See Figure 10.3.)

This contact should occur at a depth of 25 millimeters, although a greater depth may be required for larger patients or those with a markedly flaring ramus. If bone is not contacted, do not administer the injection but instead redirect the needle until you feel the neck of the condyle.

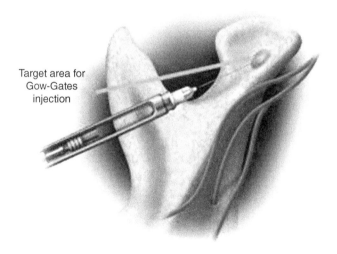

Target area for Gow-Gates injection

Figure 10.3   Target area of the Gow-Gates injection. Jaypee Brothers Medical Publishers https://www.codsjod.com/doi/CODS/pdf/10.5005/cods-6-1-35 / last accessed February 01, 2023.

Gow-Gates Extraoral Landmarks

Figure 10.4 shows an imaginary line drawn from the corner of the patient's mouth to the intertragic notch.[12] Align the syringe parallel to this plane during insertion. The objective of the technique is to place the needle tip and administer the local anesthetic at the neck of the condyle. This position is in proximity to the mandibular branch of the trigeminal nerve after it exits the foramen ovale.

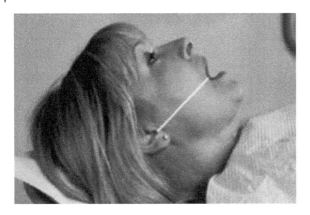

Figure 10.4 An imaginary line is drawn from the corner of the patient's mouth to the intertragic notch. Reproduced with permission of Elsevier.

Gow-Gates Intraoral Landmarks

The superior boundary of the insertion point is the maxillary occlusal plane. The intraoral insertion point is lateral and superior compared with that of the inferior alveolar nerve block. Usually, the needle lies just below the mesiopalatal cusp of the maxillary second molar, which can be a reliable landmark, provided that this tooth has not drifted or rotated.[13] (See Figure 10.5.) The barrel of the syringe usually is over the contralateral mandibular canine or premolars.

The time for onset of anesthesia is greater than the alveolar nerve block because the anesthetic is deposited about 10 mm from the mandibular nerve. Patients should keep their mouths open following the injection to improve anesthesia onset.

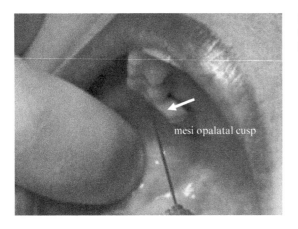

mesi opalatal cusp

Figure 10.5 Insertion below the mesiopalatal cusp of the second molar. Reproduced with permission of Elsevier.

Vazirani-Akinosi Nerve Block (VA)

The intraoral landmarks for the VA block are the bone of the medial surface of the mandibular ramus, maxillary tuberosity, and mucogingival junction of the maxillary third or second molar. The Vazirani-Akinosi nerve block requires lining up the syringe parallel with the occlusal table of the maxillary teeth at the height of the mucogingival junction of the upper teeth.[14] (See Figure 10.6.) The injection site is at the same height as the mucogingival junction of the maxillary second molar directly across from the tooth.

Figure 10.6 Syringe parallel with the maxillary occlusal table and the ramus at the height of the mucogingival junction. SlideShare https://www.slideshare.net/ / last accessed February 01, 2023.

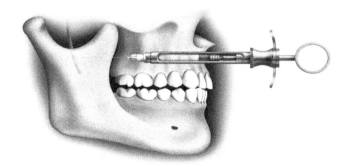

Figure 10.7 Injection site at the mucogingival junction, opposite the second molar, depth of 18 mm. Endeavor Business Media, LLC.

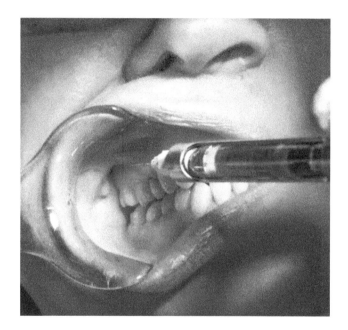

Inject parallel to the ramus, at the depth of 18 mm. The target for this injection is below that of the Gow-Gates injection, but above that of the Halstead injection (see Figure 10.7).[14]

This injection has the added advantage of being able to be performed with the patient's mouth closed.

Facial Nerve Injury

In cases of maxillary third molar surgery, facial nerve paralysis may develop after local dental block anesthesia or even after tooth extraction. The mechanism of this nerve injury after dental procedures is unknown, but there are three possible explanations for its occurrence.[15]

One possibility is direct trauma to the nerve from the needle. Hematoma formation with facial nerve compression is another possible explanation. This is very unlikely when PSA block injections are done properly with aspiration. Finally, facial nerve injury can result from local anesthetic toxicity.

Practical Application and Summary

The removal of third molars is one of the most feared procedures in dentistry. If done painlessly it can build your practice. Patients talk with family members, neighbors, and friends before and after this procedure. Profound local anesthesia is a practice builder; especially, when combined with IV sedation.

1) Third molar removal without sedation.

Every local anesthetic injection can be done painlessly with compounded topical anesthetic. EMLA is a brand name compounded topical anesthetic cream used in medicine for skin grafts. It is a combination of lidocaine and prilocaine. The Best Topical Ever is another compounded topical anesthetic that can be used in dentistry. Instructions for oral use must be followed. Compounded topical anesthetics must be ordered by prescription from a compounding pharmacy.[16]

2) Third molar removal with sedation.

When third molars are removed with sedation, most patients prefer to remove all third molars in one appointment. Topical anesthetic is not needed when using sedation.

The author follows a protocol using articaine and bupivacaine when administering local anesthetic for removal of 4 third molars. One cartridge is 1.8 ml of anesthetic solution. Maxillary third molars are anesthetized with articaine 4% and removed first since profound maxillary anesthesia is normally fast and very predicable when compared with mandibular anesthesia. The local anesthesia begins with maxillary posterior superior alveolar block (PSA), premolar infiltration, and greater palatine block injection for the maxillary right third molar. This is repeated for the maxillary left third molar. Total articaine used is two cartridges for maxillary third molars; one for the right and one for the left (144 mg).

Continuing with articaine in a clockwise direction, mandibular third molars are anesthetized. An inferior alveolar nerve block with one cartridge articaine is used for the lower left third molar. The IAN block is followed by a long buccal injection and vestibular infiltration with ½ cartridge articaine. A long buccal block and vestibular infiltration eliminates any accessory nerves. Total articaine used is 1.5 cartridges (108 mg).

To insure profound anesthesia a Gow-Gates injection is added with bupivacaine 0.5%. Total bupivacaine used is one cartridge (9 mg). This is repeated for the right mandibular third molar. This protocol virtually guarantees painless dentistry when done properly.

Local Anesthetic MRD

The maximum recommended dose for articaine and bupivacaine is shown below in Table 10.3.

The systemic effects when using different local anesthetics follows the principle of summation. Through at least 2010, product inserts for 4% articaine, 1:100,000 epinephrine list an absolute MRD of seven cartridges, which is approximately **500 mg**. The MRD for bupivacaine is 10 cartridges, which is approximately **90 mg**. The summation of all anesthetic used in this protocol is 18 mg for bupivacaine and 360 mg for articaine; well below the summed total MRD of 590 mg.

Table 10.3 A local anesthetic protocol for the removal of 4 third molars in one appointment.

ARTICAINE – 5 cartridges (360 mg Septocaine 4% + epinephrine 1:100,000)

1) PSA and infiltration near premolars – 3/4 cartridge, right and left

2) Palatal – 1/4 cartridge, right and left

3) IAN block – 1 cartridge, right and left

4) Long buccal block – 1/4 cartridge, right and left

5) Mandible vestibular infiltration – 1/4 cartridge, right and left

BUPIVACAINE – 2 cartridges (18 mg Marcaine 0.5% + epinephrine 1:200,000)

6) Gow-Gates mandibular nerve block – 1 cartridge bupivacaine, right and left

TOTAL LOCAL ANESTHETIC 7 cartridges (378 mg)

Vasopressor MRD

Maximum permissible doses of vasopressors have not been established. A sensible protocol is to record baseline heart rate and blood pressure preoperatively and again following every 20–40 μg administered. This would equate to 1–2 cartridges containing a 1 : 100,000 epinephrine concentration. Virtually any patient can tolerate the cardiovascular influences of this amount. If the patient remains stable, additional doses may be administered and followed by a similar pattern of reassessing vital signs.[16]

References

1 Sirin Y, Humphris G, Sencan S, Firat D. What is the most fearful intervention in ambulatory oral surgery? Analysis of an outpatient clinic. *Int J Oral Maxillofac Surg*. 2012 Oct;41(10):1284–90.

2 Calatayud J, González Á. History of the development and evolution of local anesthesia since the coca leaf. *Anesthesiology*. 2003 Jun;98:1503–8.

3 Moore PA, Hersh EV. Local anesthetics for dentistry chapter 7. 2020 Feb 15.

4 Becker DE, Reed KL. Local anesthetics: review of pharmacological considerations. *Anesth Prog*. 2012 Summer;59(2):90–101.

5 Dental local anesthetic market share, United States, Calendar year 2014. Septodont Inc. Lancaster PA, Malamed SF, Gagnon S, Leblanc D. Articaine hydrochloride: a study of the safety of a new amide local anesthetic. *J Am Dent Assoc*. 2001 Feb;132(2):177–85.

6 Drugs.com Articaine / epinephrine dosage, medically reviewed by Drugs.com. Last updated on 2021 Sep 20.

7 Malamed S. Oral health, articaine 30 years later. 2016 Feb 4.

8 Pogrel MA. Permanent nerve damage from inferior alveolar nerve blocks--an update to include articaine. *J Calif Dent Assoc*. 2007 Apr;35(4):271–3. PMID: 17612365.

9 Martin E, Nimmo A, Lee A, Jennings E. Articaine in dentistry: an overview of the evidence and meta-analysis of the latest randomised controlled trials on articaine safety and efficacy compared to lidocaine for routine dental treatment. *BDJ Open*. 2021 Jul 17;7(1):27. doi: 10.1038/s41405-021-00082-5. Erratum in: BDJ Open. 2021 Aug 11;7(1):29. PMID: 34274944; PMCID: PMC8286260.

10 Flanagan T, Wahl MJ, Schmitt MM, Wahl JA. Size doesn't matter: needle gauge and injection pain. *Gen Dent*. 2007 May-Jun;55(3):216–7. PMID: 17511363.

11 Khalil H. A basic review on the inferior alveolar nerve block techniques. *Anesth Essays Res.* 2014;8:3–8.

12 Haas DA. Alternative mandibular nerve block techniques: a review of the Gow-Gates and Akinosi-Vazirani closed-mouth mandibular nerve block techniques. *J Am Dent Assoc.* 2011 Sep;142 (Suppl 3):8S-12S. doi: 10.14219/jada.archive.2011.0341. PMID: 21881056.

13 Seth R, Anuradha M, Yashavanth Kumar D, Babji HV. Variants of inferior alveolar nerve block: a review. *CODS J Dent.* 2014;6(1):35–39.

14 Kiran BSR, et al. Comparison of efficacy of Halstead, Vazirani Akinosi and Gow Gates techniques for mandibular anesthesia. *J Maxillofac Oral Surg.* 2018 Dec;17(4):570–5.

15 Cakarer S, Can T, Cankaya B, Erdem MA, Yazici S, Ayintap E, Özden AV, Keskin C. Peripheral facial nerve paralysis after upper third molar extraction. *J Craniofacial Surg.* 2010 Nov;21(6):1825–7.

16 Becker DE, Reed KL. Local anesthetics: review of pharmacological considerations. *Anesth Prog.* 2012 Summer;59(2):90–102.

11

Imaging

It's hard to imagine third molar surgery without imaging. The discovery of X-rays in 1895 by Sir Wilhelm Conrad Roentgen was an incredible era in the history of medicine. The first dental radiograph was made in 1896.[1] See Figure 11.1 In 1903 Kells opened the first dental-ray lab in the United States. The year 1948 witnessed the introduction of panoramic radiography. This is significant because a panoramic X-ray is still considered "standard of care" for the removal of third molars. Tomography became available in 1978 followed by intraoral scanners in 1989. It was not until 2001 that Kodak introduced cone beam computed tomography (CBCT) in the United States.

CBCT scanners changed the way oral and maxillofacial radiology is practiced. Dentistry embraced CBCT very rapidly due to its compact size, low cost, and low radiation exposure when compared to medical computed tomography.

Medical CT scanners are large and expensive. Patients lay flat on a table surrounded by X-ray beam detectors. The X-ray tube moves around the patient taking a series of 2D image slices. 3D images are created by stacking the 2D slices together. (See Figures 11.1a and 11.1b)

CBCT is a variation of the traditional medical computed tomography (CT) system. During a cone beam CT examination, patients are standing or sitting. (See Figure 11.2a.) The C-arm or gantry rotates around the head in a complete 360-degree rotation while capturing multiple 2D images from different angles that are reconstructed to create a single 3-D image. CBCT hardware is compact in size when compared to medical devices. CBCT size is similar to panoramic size and produces 2D and 3D images. CBCT machines are rapidly replacing panoramic equipment. (See Figure 11.2b)

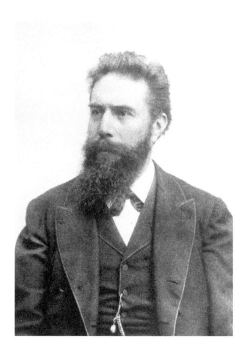

Figure 11.1   Sir Wilhelm Conrad Roentgen. *Source:* Unknown Source / Wikimedia Commons / Public domain.

Impacted Third Molars, Second Edition. Edited by John Wayland.
© 2024 John Wiley & Sons, Inc. Published 2024 by John Wiley & Sons, Inc.

(a)

(b)

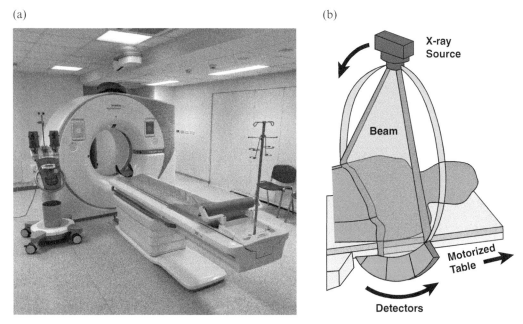

Figure 11.1a and 11.1b   Medical computed tomography (CT). *Source:* Tomáš Vendiš / Wikimedia Commons / CC BY-SA 4.0.

(a)

(b)

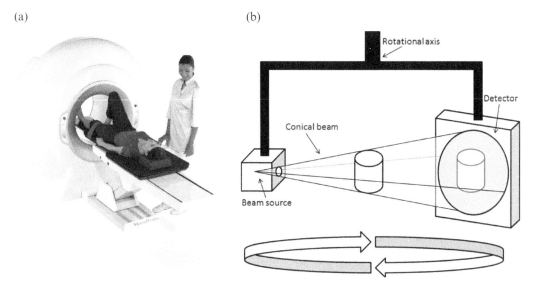

Figure 11.2a and 11.2b   CBCT size is similar to panoramic size and produces 2D and 3D images. Wikipedia Commons.

Radiation

Radiation is cumulative and is always a concern. We are all exposed to background radiation every day from natural sources such as minerals in the ground, and man-made sources such as medical/dental X-rays. Putting it in perspective, the daily background radiation dose for

Table 11.1   Average dental radiation doses for a medium field of view, in microsieverts.

DENTAL	Procedure	Approximate effective radiation dose in microsieverts	Comparable to natural background radiation for:
	Dental X-ray	5	1 day
	Panoramic X-ray	25	3 days
	Cone beam CT	180	22 days

Source: Radiology Info.org.

everyone is about 10 microsieverts (μSv). A flight from New York to LA is about 35 microsieverts. Smoking 1 pack a day is about 1 microsievert. According to the US Nuclear Regulatory Commission Sources of Radiation, the average annual radiation dose per person in the US is 6200 microsieverts.[2]

Advances in digital technology have permitted significant reductions in exposure compared to conventional film. However, users of CBCT and panoramic technology should balance scan needs with radiation risk. Dentists should think about why the scan is needed and consider how to get that information with as low a dose as possible.

The radiation dose from CBCT and panoramic scans can vary with field of view, image resolution, X-ray beam energy, filtration, exposure time, receptor technology, and human factors including the patient's size and age. Not all CBCT units are created equal. The effective dose in some CBCT units can be as low as 27 microsieverts. Also, images can be enhanced and manipulated with software which can reduce radiation exposure.

Average dental radiation doses for a medium field of view, in microsieverts, are shown in Table 11.1

The ionizing radiation and free radicals created with medical/dental imaging causes a tiny amount of tissue damage. A rough estimate of the risk of fatal cancer from a panoramic radiograph is about 1 in 20,000,000. The age of the person being imaged also alters the risk. The risk is doubled for young patients age 1–10.[2]

The conical beam used in CBCT machines reduces radiation exposure when compared to medical tomography. However, the CBCT radiation is more than a panoramic X-ray. CBCT for third molars are indicated only when high risk radiographic markers are found on a quality panoramic X-ray

CBCT vs Panoramic X-ray

Many studies have compared the ability of CBCT and panoramic imaging to predict IAN injury when removing third molars.

Guidelines for the use of CBCT scanning for examination of mandibular third molars before surgical intervention have suggested that CBCT can be used in cases where the conventional image displays a close interrelation between the third molar and the mandibular canal. A review on radiographic examination of mandibular third molars reported that there is little evidence that CBCT will change either the treatment or the post-operative patient outcome.[3] A report prepared by the SEDENTEXCT project concluded that the evidence for the use of CBCT is sparse.[4] Also, it has been documented that the use of CBCT is connected with higher costs and radiation to the patient than conventional methods.[5] New and up-to-date evidence-based recommendations

(a) (b) (c)

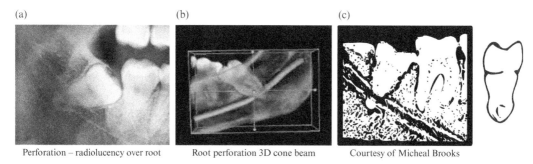

Perforation – radiolucency over root   Root perforation 3D cone beam   Courtesy of Micheal Brooks

Figure 11.3 a,b,c   Cone beam tomography and panoramic X-rays predict nerve injury. *Source:* Aron Saar / Wikipedia Commons / CC BY 3.0.

advocate that CBCT imaging of the mandibular third molar should not be applied as a routine method before removal of mandibular third molars. CBCT imaging should only be applied when the surgeon has a very specific clinical question in an individual patient case that cannot be answered by conventional (panoramic and/or intraoral) imaging.[6]

In very rare cases the inferior alveolar nerve perforates the third molar root. In Figure 11.3, the cinematic CBCT rendering clearly shows penetration of the third molar root. The 2D pano is also a very reliable indicator of root perforation. The panoramic radiograph drawing shows narrowing of the inferior alveolar canal and a radiolucent band where the canal perforates the third molar root. In this case, a CBCT would be indicated.

The panoramic radiograph in Figure 11.4 shows an important radiographic inferior alveolar nerve marker. This useful radiographic marker is called superimposition. In this image, the inferior alveolar nerve canal cortical bone is superimposed over the third molar root. This means that the IAN is buccal or lingual to the third molar root.

The American Association of Maxillofacial Oral Surgeons (AAMOS) published a third molar white paper in 2007. As part of their third molar research, they asked the following question: "Among patients with impacted mandibular third molars, do those who have preoperative computerized tomographic (CT) imaging, when compared to those who do not, have a decreased frequency of inferior alveolar nerve (IAN) injury after third molar removal"?

A thorough review of the literature failed to provide substantive answers to the clinical question posed above. At face value, one might imagine that the routine use of CBCT imaging would decrease the risk for nerve injury. An alternative hypothesis is that it may increase the risk of nerve injury.

Knowing the three-dimensional relationships between the third molar and IAN may tempt some clinicians to remove teeth that ordinarily they may elect to refer or monitor, due to concerns regarding IAN injury. CT data provides no information regarding lingual nerve position; as such, lingual nerve injury risk is unchanged.

Matzen and Berkhout concluded that "CBCT imaging of the mandibular third molar should not be applied as a routine method before removal of mandibular third molars and therefore, CBCT imaging should only be applied when the surgeon has a very specific clinical question in an individual patient case that cannot be answered by conventional (panoramic or intraoral) imaging."[7]

Panoramic imaging has a long history beginning well before CBCT machines. Panoramic images have been used in oral surgery to evaluate third molars for half a century; more than 50 years before CBCT was introduced in the United States.

Panoramic imaging advantages

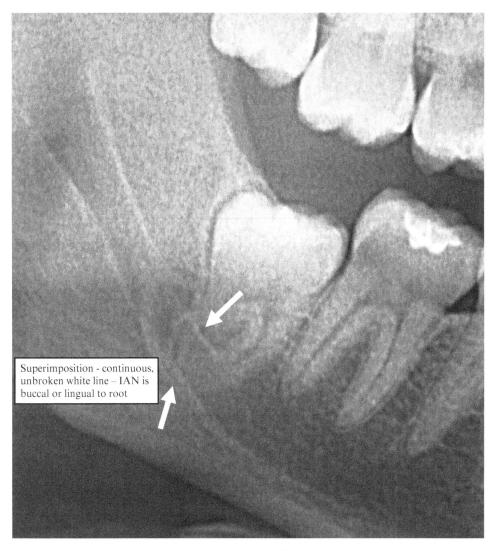

Superimposition - continuous, unbroken white line – IAN is buccal or lingual to root

Figure 11.4 Superimpositiona continuous, unbroken white line (canal cortical bone) indicates that the IAN is buccal or lingual to the third molar root. Assessment of and Surgery for Impacted Third Molars, Hooley and Whitacre

- Broad coverage of facial bone and teeth
- Low patient radiation dose
- Convenience of examination for the patient (no intraoral films)
- Can be used in patients who cannot open their mouth or when the opening is restricted
- Short time required for making the image
- Patients understand panoramic films, making them a useful visual aid in patient education and third molar case presentation.
- Easy to store compared to intraoral X-rays.

Many panoramic radiographic signs (markers) are associated with an increased risk for IAN injury. These include root distance from the IAN canal, loss of the cortical (white) lines of the canal, darkening of the third molar root, root deflection, canal deflection, narrowing of the canal where it passes the third molar root and a dark or bifid root apex. Considering all factors associated with IAN injury after third molar removal is more predictive than any individual panoramic finding.

At the time of this publication, panoramic radiography is the standard of care for evaluating third molars.

Practical Application and Summary

Patient selection is critical to surgical success.

Panoramic radiographic markers can reliably predict IAN injuries. Studies have shown that CBCT imaging does not decrease IAN injuries. Panoramic imaging is currently the standard of care when removing impacted third molars. A CBCT is recommended only if you decide to do a high-risk case or the CBCT becomes the standard of care for the removal of impacted third molars. A conservative approach would be referral to a maxillofacial surgeon when panoramic X-rays indicate high risk for complications.

Several companies offer reasonably priced panoramic machines that can be upgraded to cone beam when you are ready. For example, at the time of this publication, Carestream and Panoramic Corporation offer upgradeable machines for less than $15,000.

The following panoramic radiographic markers are discussed in Chapter 2 – Case Selection.

1) Position
2) Depth
3) Angulation
4) Combined root width
5) Root length, size, and shape
6) Periodontal ligament and follicle
7) Bone elasticity and density

Radiographic markers are essential to learn for case selection. In addition, many other factors play a role in patient selection and are discussed in Chapter 2.

References

1 Wikipedia Commons – Sir Wilhelm Röntgen.

2 U.S. Nuclear Regulatory Commission. Sources of Radiation. 2009. www.nrc.gov/about-nrc/radiation/around-us/sources.html.

3 Matzen LH, Wenzel A. Efficacy of CBCT for assessment of impacted mandibular third molars: a review – based on a hierarchical model of evidence. *Dentomaxillofac Radiol*. 2015 Jan;44(1):20140189.

4 Sedentexct Project. *Radiation protection no 172: cone beam CT for dental and maxillofacial radiology*. Luxembourg: European Commission Directorate-General for Energy, 2012.

5 Lorenzoni DC, et al. Cone-beam computed tomography and radiographs in dentistry: aspects related to radiation dose. *Int J Dent.* 2012;2012:813768.

6 Petersen LB, Olsen KR, Christensen J, Wenzel A. Image and surgery-related costs comparing cone beam CT and panoramic imaging before removal of impacted mandibular third molars. *Dentomaxillofac Radiol.* 2014;43:20140001.

7 Matzen LH, Berkhout E. Cone beam CT imaging of the mandibular third molar: a position paper prepared by the European Academy of DentoMaxilloFacial Radiology (EADMFR). *Dentomaxillofac Radiol.* 2019 Jul;48(5):20190039.

12

Patient Management

The removal of impacted third molars may cause postoperative swelling, pain, and bleeding. Infection is also possible. These issues can be minimized or eliminated with good patient management.

Every patient is different, both physically and emotionally. The dentist's surgical experience is also variable. These issues have a profound effect on the patient's experience. Third molar patients usually have no idea what to expect on surgery day. They may have misinformation from friends, family, or the internet. It's crucial that patient expectations are in agreement with the actual procedure. Good communication is paramount. See Figure 12.1.

Sedation is recommended when 4 third molars are removed at the same appointment. Sedation may also be best when patients are very apprehensive with a history of anxiety or depression. Discuss the benefits and risks of each type of sedation; oral and IV sedation. Sedated patients usually have profound amnesia and no memory of the procedure. Local anesthetic patients are fully conscious and will remember everything.

The sedation continuum should be discussed with all sedation patients. It's crucial that patients understand the difference between sedation and general anesthesia. The following illustration is helpful when communicating with sedation patients. Draw a line on a blank piece of paper with an X midway on the line. See Figure 12.2.

The following dialogue is recommended.

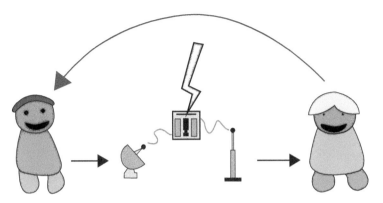

Figure 12.1   Communication. Einar Faanes / Wikipedia Commons / CC BY 3.0.

Impacted Third Molars, Second Edition. Edited by John Wayland.
© 2024 John Wiley & Sons, Inc. Published 2024 by John Wiley & Sons, Inc.

This line represents different levels of sleep from wide awake to unconscious. Sedated patients can be lightly asleep, medium asleep, or deeply asleep. You will be in medium sleep (point to the X). Medium sleep patients, moderately sedated, are usually snoring during the surgery and have little or no memory of the procedure. You can feel things and hear conversation, but have <u>no pain</u>. Pain is controlled with local anesthesia.

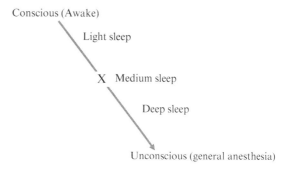

Figure 12.2 The sedation continuum.

At this point, you can demonstrate pressure by holding and squeezing the patient's hand or arm. "Do you feel this? Do you feel pain?" They can feel pressure, but not pain. "General anesthesia is much more dangerous than sedation. General anesthesia should be administered by an anesthesiologist in a hospital." This short conversation will improve your sedation.

Anxiety and Depression

Many people who experience the symptoms of mental health disorders, such as anxiety and depression, turn to drugs and alcohol to cope.[1] There is a strong link between mental illnesses and substance abuse. Some patients self-medicate before their third molar appointment due to anxiety. Dentist removing third molars must be aware of potential drug interactions for these patients.

In 2019 the National Center for Health Statistics reported that 20% of young adults had anxiety symptoms and 21% had depression symptoms.[2] These numbers increased dramatically with the onset of the Covid epidemic.

Selective serotonin reuptake inhibitors (SSRIs) are frequently prescribed for depression and anxiety disorders.[3] They can ease symptoms of moderate to severe depression, are relatively safe, and typically cause few side effects. FDA-approved SSRIs include brand names Celexa, Lexapro, Prozac, Luvox, Paxil, Zoloft, and Viibry. Patients taking these drugs may react unpredictably when sedated.

SSRIs treat depression and anxiety by increasing levels of serotonin in the brain. Serotonin is one of the chemical messengers that carry signals between brain nerve cells (neurons). SSRIs block the reabsorption (reuptake) of serotonin into neurons. This makes more serotonin available to improve transmission of messages between neurons. Serotonin syndrome develops when too much serotonin accumulates in the brain.

Rarely, an antidepressant can cause high levels of serotonin to accumulate. This usually happens when two medications act together to raise the level of serotonin. For example, the co-administration of SSRIs and narcotics may precipitate serotonin toxicity. There must be consideration of this unusual interaction when administering fentanyl to patients on SSRIs Dentists should be vigilant of the features of serotonin toxicity developing in such patients.

The number of cases of serotonin syndrome reported has increased over the past several years due to increased use of SSRIs and more diagnosis of the syndrome.[4] Serotonin syndrome can be self-limiting or life-threatening.

Signs and symptoms of serotonin syndrome include anxiety, agitation, high fever, sweating, confusion, tremors, restlessness, lack of coordination, major changes in blood pressure, and a rapid heart rate.

Benzodiazepines are often used in oral and IV sedation. They are also used to manage mild hypertension and tachycardia. Common benzodiazepines used in dentistry to sedate and control anxiety include diazepam, triazolam, lorazepam, and midazolam. Diazepam has been shown to blunt symptoms of serotonin syndrome.[5]

Other drug interactions are possible. Epinephrine used with local anesthetics can increase the side effects of antidepressants.[6] The mood stabilizer Abilify can boost the effect of an antidepressant.[7]

Tricyclic antidepressants (TCAs) are another class of medication used primarily for the management of depression. TCAs were discovered in the early 1950s.[8] TCAs are used in the clinical treatment of mood disorders.[9] TCAs can cause sedation, respiratory depression, and hypotension. Caution is advised when TCAs are used with other central nervous system depressants.[10] The FDA has approved these brand-name TCAs for the treatment of depression: Vivactil, Pamelor and Aventyl, Norpramin, Amoxapine, Surmontil, Tofranil, and Sinequan.

Another class of medications used to treat depression and anxiety is monoamine oxidase inhibitors (MAOIs). Monoamine oxidase inhibitors were the first type of antidepressant developed. MAOIs are also used to treat panic attacks, Parkinson's disease, and several other disorders.[11] Like SSRIs, MAOIs can cause dangerously high levels of serotonin when two medications that raise serotonin are combined. MAOIs have been shown to be significantly superior to placebo in the treatment of anxiety.[12] FDA-approved MAOIs for depression include Marplan, Nardil, Emsam, and Parnate.

Swelling and Pain

Postoperative swelling is in direct proportion to surgical difficulty and patient compliance. Deeply impacted third molars and poor surgical access increase pain and swelling. Bony impaction surgery for older patients is generally more difficult than surgery for teens due to bone density. This results in more swelling and postoperative pain. Removal in the teenage years is recommended.

Patient compliance is also important. Proper application of ice and timely salt water rinse will decrease swelling and improve recovery. Immediate application of ice will cut down on long-term swelling and potentially lessen recovery time. Icing immediately can decrease inflammation and numb pain in the surgical area. Ideally, patients should use ice for 20 minutes at a time, with a 20-minute break between sessions. Icing is effective at reducing pain and swelling because the cold constricts blood vessels and decreases circulation to the area.

Ibikunle and Adeyemo found that quality of life after the surgical extraction of third molars was improved when ice was used postoperatively.[13] Subjects who required surgical extraction of lower third molars were randomly allocated into two groups. Subjects in group A were instructed to apply ice when at home every one and a half hours on postoperative days 0–1. Group B subjects did not apply ice packs.

The study found that the quality of life after third molar surgery was significantly better in subjects who use ice after third molar removal than those who did not use ice. The study concluded that cryotherapy is a viable adjunct to other established modes of improving the quality of life of patients following surgical extraction of third molars.

Hands-free facial compresses are recommended to reduce pain and swelling. They should be adjustable to accommodate different sizes and shapes. There are many companies offering these devices. The author uses Rester's compress which includes 4 gel packs. (See Figure 12.3.)

Patients leave the office after surgery with ice in place. Hands are not needed which is very helpful when patients are sedated. Patients and parents appreciate the extra care that this device shows. Also, the compress and ice are reusable for the family.

JAW PAIN RELIEVER - CHIN AND JAW WRAP
COMFORTABLE AND SOFT ADJUSTABLE STRAP

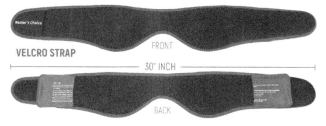

4 HOT & COLD GEL PACKS INCLUDED

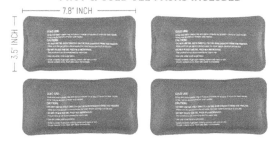

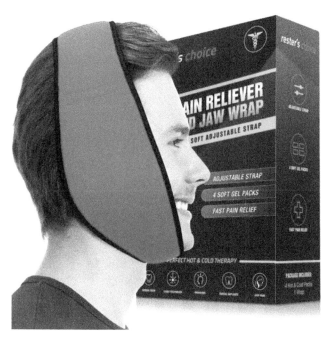

Figure 12.3 Rester's choice facial compress (RESTER'S CHOICE).

Pain is expected following the removal of impacted third molars. This can be minimized when patients use ice and take appropriate medication. Many studies have shown that ibuprofen combined with acetaminophen is more effective for pain than narcotics. On a scale of 1–10, post-operative pain should be 4–5 when medication is used. Narcotics are not needed to control pain. Many studies have verified this point.

A study published in the *Journal of the American Dental Association* in 2013 found that using a combination of ibuprofen-acetaminophen may be a more effective analgesic than many of the opioid-containing formulations. When making recommendations for the management of acute postoperative third molar pain, dentists should consider including ibuprofen-acetaminophen combination therapy. The adverse effects associated with the combination were similar to those of the individual component drugs.[14]

Postoperative instructions for swelling and pain:

- ICE for 24 hours. Swelling normally increases for three to four days following surgery and then gradually decreases. Ice may be applied for 20 minutes and removed for 20 minutes, alternating on and off.
- RINSE AFTER 2 DAYS. Use ½ teaspoon of salt per cup of warm water. Rinse for one minute 5–6 times per day for four days.
- TAKE IBUPROFEN AND AMOXICILLIN 1 HOUR BEFORE APPOINTMENT AND 3 TIMES A DAY AFTER APPOINTMENT. Medication should be "by the clock" until all medication is gone. For example, take both medications upon wakening, at bedtime, and once in between. Two Extra Strength Tylenol (500 mg) can be taken with ibuprofen 4 times a day if pain exceeds 4–5 on a 10 scale. Do not exceed 8 Tylenol Extra Strength tablets per day.

Bleeding

Bleeding is normal following the removal of impacted third molars. Local anesthetic with 1:50,000 epinephrine can be used in office if needed.

Patients should expect bleeding. Postoperative bleeding is typically controlled with gauze and pressure on the surgical site. When sutures are used for surgical extractions, patients should carefully change gauze if needed to avoid opening the surgical flap. Excessive bleeding can also be controlled at home by biting softly on a moist tea bag. Walking, talking, and movement of the mouth and tongue will increase bleeding. Sleep will lower blood pressure and is recommended after surgery.

Uncontrollable bleeding after tooth extraction usually occurs in patients with coagulation diseases, including hemophilia, von Willebrand's disease, vitamin K deficiency, platelet deficiency, and anti-coagulant drugs. Hemophilia A is an X-linked recessive disorder caused by insufficiency of coagulation factor VIII. Mild hemophilia is characterized by uncontrollable bleeding after invasive operations.

Table 12.1   Post-extraction bleeding – normal, primary, reactionary, and secondary.

	Post-extraction Bleeding		
Normal	**Primary**	**Reactionary**	**Secondary**
• Normally persists for half an hour • Oozing and blood-tinged saliva for up to 8 hours • Controlled with pressure	• During and after extraction • Typically presents as blood filling up the mouth • Controlled with pressure and tea bags	• 2–3 hours after extraction when vasoconstrictor effect wears off • Usually due to bleeding disorders • May require a blood test	• Begins 7 to 10 days after extraction • Due to secondary infection • Rare

Some mild hemophiliacs may remain undiagnosed until late adulthood. Post-extraction bleeding usually stops 30 minutes after surgery, followed by blood-tinged saliva.[15] (See Table 12.1.)

Patients that have experienced bleeding that won't stop following small incisions, punctures, or cuts need a bleeding time test before third molar surgery. A bleeding time test determines how quickly blood clots. The test is a basic assessment of how well blood platelets work to form clots. Most people will never need a bleeding time test.

Abnormal results from a bleeding time test can mean that the patient needs more in-depth testing to find the cause of prolonged bleeding. It could mean the patient has an acquired platelet function defect. Acquired platelet function defect is a condition that develops after birth and affects how well blood platelets work. The body may produce too many or too few platelets, or platelets may not work properly.[16]

Abnormal results could also indicate the following conditions:

- A blood vessel defect that affects how well blood vessels transport blood.
- A genetic platelet function defect that affects how well platelets function. Hemophilia is an example of this type of defect.
- Primary thrombocythemia that causes bone marrow to create too many platelets.
- Thrombocytopenia that causes the body to produce too few platelets.
- Von Willebrand's disease is a hereditary condition that affects how blood coagulates. The author has had one patient with undiagnosed Von Willebrand's disease. This case will be discussed further in Chapter 14, "Case Studies."

Normal bleeding test time is between 1 and 8 minutes. Results outside of that range could indicate a platelet defect and require further testing.

SSRIs directly increase the risk of abnormal bleeding by lowering platelet serotonin levels, which are essential to hemostasis. SSRIs interact with anticoagulants, like warfarin, and antiplatelet drugs, like aspirin. This includes an increased risk of GI bleeding, and postoperative bleeding.[17]

Infection

Third molar patients can be divided into two groups: (1) third molar patients with pain and (2) third molar patients without pain. Patients with erupting third molars typically have pain from pericoronitis. Pericoronitis is an infectious disease often associated with the eruption of a third molar. It can be either acute or chronic. Pain is usually the predominant symptom in acute stages, whereas chronic forms of infection may display very few symptoms. The infection is predominantly caused by anaerobic microorganisms. Treatment measures are symptomatic, antimicrobial, and surgical.

Antimicrobial treatment is indicated for preoperative prophylaxis when surgically removing impacted third molars and during the acute stages of suppurative pericoronitis when surgery must be postponed. First-line treatment in this case consists of amoxicillin and pain medication. The treatment of pericoronitis presenting at the third molar is the most common indication for extraction of a retained third molar.[18]

Maxillary infections after third molar extraction surgery are very rare. Infection mainly occurs in the mandible. The risk factors for postoperative infection in the mandibular are related to the depth of tooth extraction, surgical technique, and patient compliance. Chewing on day 1 and 2 will increase the chances for a delayed infection due to food in the surgical site. Delayed-onset infections after third molar extractions are rare.[19]

A certain type of delayed onset infection, subperiosteal, may occur several weeks after an apparently uneventful healing of a mandibular third molar wound. The infection may migrate from the original third molar surgical site. This may present itself as swelling in the mucoperiosteal tissue as far forward as the first molar or second premolar. When the diagnosis is made, antibiotic therapy should be initiated.[20]

A study of 307 patients by Brunello found that delayed subperiosteal infections, after third-molar extractions, tend to occur about a month after the surgical procedure.[21] Other studies concerning secondary infections are less clear about the timing of their onset, but it usually occurs between 10 and 30 days after surgery. In the Brunello study, patients who developed a delayed onset infection were slightly younger than others at a mean age of 18 years. This finding is consistent with a report from Osborn et al. that found a majority of secondary infections occurring in a group of patients between 12 and 24 years old.

The Brunello study included 209 extracted mandibular third molars. The results show that partial bony impactions of lower right third molars with fully developed roots and a mesioangular position are most likely to develop a subperiosteal infection.

Antibiotic treatment is indicated when patients have subperiosteal infections. The author has successfully treated subperiosteal infections with amoxicillin 500 mg and metronidazole 500 mg, three times a day for 10 days. When the antibiotic treatment is ineffective, surgical debridement of the extraction site becomes necessary. Careful monitoring is very important since this infection can spread to neck and chest spaces. Patients should call the office if the infection has not improved within 3 days of the antibiotic regimen.

Patient management is an integral part of third molar surgery. Prevention of complications through patient management is always preferable to treatment.

References

1 Quello SB, Brady KT, Sonne SC. Mood disorders and substance use disorder: a complex comorbidity. *Sci Pract Perspect*. 2005 Dec;3(1):13–21.
2 Vahratian A, Terlizzi EP, Villarroel MA, et al. Mental health in the United States: new estimates from the National Center for Health Statistics. 2020. webinar–2020–508.
3 Rang ST, Field J, Irving C. Serotonin toxicity caused by an interaction between fentanyl and paroxetine. *Can J Anaesth*. 2008 Aug;55(8):521–5.
4 Volpi-Abadie J, Kaye AM, Kaye AD. Serotonin syndrome. *Ochsner J*. 2013 Winter;13(4):533–40.
5 Boyer EW, Shannon M. The serotonin syndrome. *N Engl J Med*. 2005 Mar 17;352(11):1112–20. Erratum in: *N Engl J Med*. 2007 Jun 7;356(23):2437.
6 Chioca LR, et al. Antidepressants and local anesthetics: drug interactions of interest to dentistry. *RSBO*. 2010 Oct.
7 Bhandari S. WebMD. Drugs used to treat mental disorders. 2022 Oct 25.
8 Carson VB. *Mental health nursing: the nurse-patient journey*. Philidelphia: W.B. Saunders, 2000, 423. ISBN 978-0-7216-8053-8. 2000, 423.
9 Broquet K. Status of treatment of depression. *South Med J*. 1999;92(9):846–56.
10 Tricyclic antidepressants (TCAS). Mental and behavioral health. 2012 Jan 30.
11 Tyrer P, Shawcross C. Monoamine oxidase inhibitors in anxiety disorders. *J Psychiatr Res*. 1988;22(Suppl 1):87–98.
12 Cristancho MA. Atypical depression in the 21st century: diagnostic and treatment issues. Psychiatric Times. Archived from the original on 2 December 2013. 2012 Nov 20.

13 Ibikunle AA, Adeyem WL. Oral health-related quality of life following third molar surgery with or without application of ice pack therapy. *Oral Maxillofac Surg*. 2016 Sep;20(3):239–47.

14 Moore PA, Hersh EV. Combining ibuprofen and acetaminophen for acute pain management after third-molar extractions. *J Am Dent Assoc*. 2013 Aug;144(8):898–908.

15 Kumbargere Nagraj S, Prashanti E, Aggarwal H, Lingappa A, Muthu MS, Kiran Kumar Krishanappa S, Hassan H. Interventions for treating post-extraction bleeding. *Cochrane Database Syst Rev*. 2018 Mar 4;3(3):CD011930.

16 Fan G, Shen Y, Cai Y, Zhao JH, Wu Y. Uncontrollable bleeding after tooth extraction from asymptomatic mild hemophilia patients: two case reports. *Oral Health*. 2022 Mar 13;22(1):69.

17 Andrade C, Sandarsh S, Chethan KB, Nagesh KS. Serotonin reuptake inhibitor antidepressants and abnormal bleeding: a review for clinicians and reconsideration of mechanisms. *J Clin Psychiatry*. 2010 Dec;71(12):1565–75.

18 Gutiérrez-Pérez JL. Third molar infections. *Med Oral Patol Oral Cir Bucal*. 2004;9(Suppl 9):122–5; 120–2.

19 Sukegawa S, Yokota K, Kanno T, Manabe Y, Sukegawa-Takahashi Y, Masui M, Furuki Y. What are the risk factors for postoperative infections of third molar extraction surgery: a retrospective clinical study? *Med Oral Patol Oral Cir Bucal*. 2019 Jan 1;24(1):e123–9.

20 Wei M, Mahdey HM. Dissecting subperiosteal abscess after surgical removal of mandibular third molar. *On J Dent & Oral Health*. 2019;1(4). OJDOH.MS.ID.000518.

21 Brunello G, et al. An observational cohort study on delayed-onset infections after mandibular third-molar extractions. *Int J Dent*. 2017;2017:1435348.

13

PRF

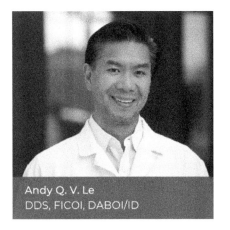

Andy Q. V. Le
DDS, FICOI, DABOI/ID

A patient's own blood can be used to enhance wound healing. A small amount of the patient's blood is placed in a centrifuge to create platelet rich plasma (PRP). Platelets contain more than 1100 different proteins, with numerous post-translational modifications, resulting in over 1500 protein-based bioactive factors.[1] Platelet-rich fibrin (PRF) began as platelet-rich plasma. PRP and PRF include immune system messengers, growth factors, enzymes and their inhibitors and other factors which can participate in tissue repair and wound healing.

The use of this blood collection technique is constantly changing and additional growth factors are being incorporated into the PRF. Many factors such as centrifugal force, spin times and removing anticoagulants are changing the amount of growth factors within PRF. This chapter will focus on the techniques and science behind the use of PRF in the wound healing process for wisdom teeth extractions.

History of PRF

The use of concentrated platelets as a fibrin mesh has been documented since the 1990s. Robert Marx in 1998 documented the use of PRP (platelet-rich plasma) in surgeries to promote hemostasis and enhanced wound healing.[2] See Figure 13.1.

PRP is concentrated autogenous blood consisting of platelets and plasma that has the potential to release growth factors. PRP blood draw tubes have an anticoagulant in them; usually bovine thrombin which keeps the blood from clumping together. Liquid PRP needs a scaffold such as bone graft material in order to create a solid matrix that can be used to regenerate wound sites.

Platelets are derived from megakaryocytes which have a lifespan of 7–10 days. The concentration of platelets can be 1,000,000 platelets/ul in a 5 ml volume of plasma. Alpha granules can form fibrinogen and release growth factors. Platelets also release cytokines which aid in cell

Impacted Third Molars, Second Edition. Edited by John Wayland.
© 2024 John Wiley & Sons, Inc. Published 2024 by John Wiley & Sons, Inc.

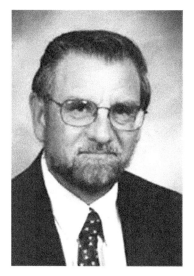

Figure 13.1   Robert E. Marx.

modulation, regulation, and differentiation of leukocytes. These cells are white blood cells that are involved in wound healing and infection control. The first generation PRP, used by Dr. Marx, did not form a fibrin glue; the PRP layer consisted of a liquid substance. This liquid layer was applied on top of grafts, mixed with bone graft material, and layered onto wound sites.

In 2006 PRP eventually evolved into PRGF (plasma rich in growth factors). A new preparation technique consisting of blood tubes that had zero bovine thrombin thus inhibiting the coagulation cascade. The idea behind PRGF technology started with drawing blood from patients with a tube that lacked an anticoagulant. The unique thing about PRGF is that it lacked leukocytes in its preparation; it only contained plasma enriched platelets. The blood goes through a centrifugal process and a fibrin clot is collected that can be applied to wound sites that need regeneration.

L- PRF was developed in 2012 and is now the standard bio active modifier used for wisdom teeth enhanced healing. Fibrin is an insoluble protein that is produced in response to bleeding and is the major component of the blood clot. Fibrin provides a thick matrix of cells that aid in the migration of healing cells such as fibroblasts and endothelial cells. These cells increase blood flow to a site which enhances wound healing. The high density of the fibrin clot is greater than the past forms of PRP and PRGF. Cells such as fibroblasts and endothelial cells are incorporated into this fibrin matrix which helps with healing. The tight fibrin mesh that is formed captures more platelets and lymphocytes. This matrix of cells slowly releases the growth factors that enhance wound healing over the next 7–10 days.

The major cell type in L-PRF is the leukocytes. L-PRF is a dense natural fibrin matrix full of platelets and growth factors. These cells play a major role in wound healing and can regulate the immune response which leads to less infection. Science on leukocytes shows that these cells make growth factors and fight infection. The cells promote wound healing, reduce swelling and pain, and regulate cells to inhibit infection. This matrix also has cytokines which can signal cells that promote healing and growth to a wound site. The proteins from this fibrin matrix enhance healing within the first 7 days. L-PRF has more growth factors than its previous creations due to the fact that it is more natural. No anticoagulant means no bovine thrombin (which is an anticoagulant), no heating, and no pipetting. L-PRF blood collection tubes have no chemical additives and are 100% autogenous meaning the concentration of growth hormones is better than its previous ancestors. We refer to the new L-PRF in this chapter as PRF.

The new PRF is considered the 2nd Generation of blood borne bioactive modifiers. This new generation platelet gel is known for not having artificial biochemical modifiers. The centrifugal process times were reduced 10 fold. Old generation PRP required multiple centrifugal spins that could last up to an hour. Spins were also very technique sensitive in which certain blood layers had to be removed and centrifuged again. The old PRP was a liquid form that had limited applications in the regenerative process.

A centrifuge is needed to create PRF. See Figure 13.2. New PRF centrifugal times are around 10 minutes with only natural blood in the tubes. New centrifuge time and speed combined with natural blood creates a fibrin matrix that is full of platelets and leukocytes. The result leads to seven to ten days of cytokines released by these leukocytes which has an anti-inflammatory and anti-infection effect. The leukocytes produce cytokines. The cytokines contribute to the

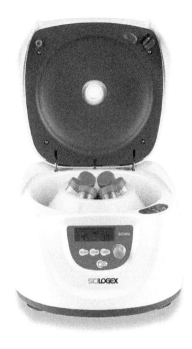

Figure 13.2   SCILOGEX clinical centrifuge.

anti-inflammatory effects of the PRF. Leukocytes have a key role in the wound healing process through their ability to fight infection and regulate the release of cytokines which aid in wound healing.

Many growth factors are derived from PRF. These growth factors have a role in speeding up the wound healing process. Each of these growth factors contributes to healing in a specific way. The following growth factors are contained in PRF:

1) VEGF
2) TGF-B
3) PDGF
4) TSP-1

The growth factor VEGF is known for angiogenesis. Angiogenesis is the increase in blood supply to a site through the creation of new blood vessels in the tissues. This increase brings many more healing cells to the site. With an increase in rich blood filled with nutrients; wound healing is increased. Another growth factor, TGF-B, is known for its ability to increase bone formation by signaling a plethora of cells to the site, especially osteoblasts and fibroblasts. PDGF is known for its ability to aid in soft tissue healing. TSP-1 is the growth factor that is involved in the coagulation pathway which forms a cellular matrix that aids in the migration of the healing cells.

PRF and Third Molars

What happens after a tooth is extracted? How does wound healing occur and what are the cascade of events that happen? Blood is our friend. Seeing blood at a site is a good sign that a site may heal well. For areas that lack blood supply; PRF is a good substitute to incorporate in these areas. The blood supply to a surgical site brings many cells that begin the healing process. The growth factors will initiate wound healing by bringing in cells such as osteoblasts, epithelial cells, leukocytes, and connective tissue cells.

Third molar surgical sites can heal by repair or regeneration depending on how many bony walls are present after the trauma. The amount of periodontal disease and granulation tissue at an infected site can determine if the site will heal through repair or regeneration. For example: a simple extraction that allows a 5-wall bony defect will heal through the process of regeneration. Atraumatic extractions regenerate through the process of inflammation, cell proliferation and differentiation, then bone remodeling.

Third Molar Healing Stages

What are the stages of wound healing? The first 3 weeks are mainly involved with soft tissue healing. The first stage is the formation of a blood clot. Angiogenesis begins from the blood vessels of the bony walls. The blood supply from the bony walls fill the extraction site. Within this blood clot are lymphocytes and neutrophils that begin the healing process. White blood cells fight off the bacteria and begin to dissolve all foreign material. Healing occurs from the bottom of extraction sockets first; this area seems to have the highest amount of blood vessels that are not injured from the extraction. After 1 week fibroblast cells develop immature capillaries, new blood vessels, and granulation tissue to begin the soft tissue healing process.

Bone formation usually begins at 4 weeks. Bone begins forming at the bottom of the socket. Bone cells work together to repair existing bone and regenerate new bone. Woven bone is formed first which slowly develops to form lamellar bone. Woven bone is weak and immature bone that lacks a matrix rich in minerals. It is essential in early wound healing. Woven bone is not normally found in the human skeleton. It will remodel during the wound healing process to form a strong and mature lamellar bone. Osteoblast and osteoclast cells are involved in growing bone. Osteoclasts are bone cells that break down or resorb bone. Osteoblasts are bone cells that lay down the matrix for bone formation. Bone needs to be broken down first in order to create new bone.

Lamellar bone is rich in a mineral matrix is present in most of the human body's bones. Lamelar bone forms after woven bone and is much more organized cellularly. Osteoblast cells are mainly responsible for lamellar bone formation. New bony walls, regeneration, are slowly being formed from the outside and apical regions of the socket towards the center.

At the 5–6 week period bone will go through the remodeling and modeling process. Bone remodeling involves the change in bone density and bone turnover rate as woven bone is transformed to lamellar bone. Bone remodeling will continue for the next 4 to 6 months. Bone formation depends on the size of the site. Third molar sites will take more time than smaller anterior teeth sites to form bone. Bone remodeling can be observed on a microscopic scale where changes in bone density at a cellular level occur.

Bone modeling is the change in the size and shape of bone as it repairs or regenerates. Bone modeling is most predictable when all bony walls are intact. Loss of bone height and width is minimized when more walls are intact. As bony walls, such as buccal bone, are lost during an extraction, the modeling may lead to a loss of buccal bone including the width and height. Bone repair instead of bone regeneration is more common in these situations where bony walls are lost. For example some wisdom teeth extractions in the mandible may lead to traumatic loss of buccal bone. In these cases bone repair may occur more than the process of bone regeneration. In simple terms, this means that an atraumatic third molar extraction will heal with more bone than an extraction that removes the buccal plate. This may help maintain the bone distal to second molars.

Bone regeneration depends on an individual's age, health, and genetic history. Patient's older than 25 will have more bone defects following third molar removal.[3] Patients who have osteoporosis or are on bisphosphonate therapy have bone cells that are not working properly.

These patients can have delayed bone healing. Bone can be replaced (regeneration) instead of repaired in these situations when PRF is used.

Bone Density

Remodeling is the change in bone density and bone turnover. Bone density is categorized into 4 types of bone according to Hounsfeld units.[4] These units are based on the number of pixels present in a segment of bone on a CT image. D1 bone is greater than 1000 Hounsfield units. D2 bone is between 650 to 1000 Hounsfield units. D3 bone is 250 to 650 Hounsfield units. D4 bone is less than 250 Hounsfield units. D1 bone is considered the most dense bone, while D4 bone is the least dense bone.

D1 dense bone is made up of cortical bone. Cortical bone is solid and has no porosity or spacing. D2 bone has a layer of solid cortical bone around it and the center is composed of porous bone with

Table 13.1 Misch bone density classification.

Bone Density	Description	Tactile Analogue	Typical Anatomic Location	Hounsfield Units
D1	Dense cortical	Oak/maple	Anterior mandible	>1250
D2	Porous cortical & coarse trabecular	White pine/ spruce	Anterior and posterior mandible, anterior maxilla	850–1250
D3	Porous cortical (thin) & fine trabecular	Balsa wood	Posterior mandible, anterior and posterior maxilla	350–850
D4	Fine trabecular	Styrofoam	Posterior maxilla	150–350

spacing. D3 bone is made up of trabecular bone which is less dense with more porous bone spaces. D4 bone is considered very soft bone which has large porous spaces made of trabecular bone. Cortical bone is very dense with little porous spacing while trabecular bone is quite soft with large spacing and porosities.

Bone density is a major factor that needs to be considered when removing third molars. Denser bone may be harder to manage during wisdom teeth extractions. Bone density can change from soft to hard bone depending on location in the oral cavity.[5] Maxillary bone is usually not as dense as mandibular bone. Commonly the mandibular anterior area has D1 bone with the most density. The posterior mandible is composed of bone that is considered D2 and D3 bone. The anterior or premaxillary region has D2 and D3 bone as well. Finally the posterior maxillary is known for D4 bone; the area in the oral cavity with the softest or least dense bone. See Table 13.1

Many other factors will contribute to bone density such as gender, genetics, race, and age. Generally maxillary 3rd molars are embedded in D4 soft bone and can be elevated out fairly quickly if accessible. Wisdom teeth in the mandible are in denser bone and may require bone removal in order to extract. Age also plays a major role in the density of bone. Patients under 25 years old will have softer maxillary and mandibular bones than patients who are older. Males generally have more dense bones than females. Race, gender, and genetics can vary the bone densities that are observed among each individual.

PRF can be used in traditional dentistry in situations where extractions, tissue healing, and bone augmentation procedures can benefit from the growth factors. This can aid in faster healing with extractions as well as bone growth. Bone grafts with all types of bone from human allograft to bovine cow bone can be enhanced with the use of PRF. Nowadays the use of PRF has become a lot more efficient. Spin times are down to 10 minutes vs an hour. Single spins are a benefit now instead of multiple spins. Spin tubes are natural with zero additives such as an anticoagulant which makes growth factors even more potent. PRF is a fibrin matrix that can be manipulated into wound sites more easily than liquid PRP. The applications for the solid matrix form of PRF can be mixed with other sources to enhance many different aspects of surgical dentistry.

Bone Grafting and PRF

Bone grafting materials can be used with PRF to graft extraction sites in order to grow bone or pre-serve the size and shape of a site. Grafting materials include synthetic (alloplast), human (allo-graft), animal (xenograft), and the patient's own bone (autograft). These grafted sites can aid in maintaining bone levels around teeth to minimize periodontal defects that can lead to tooth loss. Grafting with PRF can reduce periodontal defects distal to second molars after third molar removal.

An **alloplast** is a synthetic grafting material made up of minerals found in bone such as calcium and phosphate. Alloplast is synthesized in a lab environment using precursors of bone such as hydroxyapatite, bioactive materials, and B tricalcium phosphate minerals. Alloplasts grow bone through osteoconductive pathways. The synthetic bone material maintains a space or a matrix in which bone cells can lay down bone and grow. Alloplasts are the least popular of bone grafting materials but can be used in patients who are not comfortable with the use of human and animal bone grafts in their body. Augma is an example of an alloplast graft material made up of calcium sulfate and hydroxyapatite bone matrix. The material is compacted into a cylinder to control accurate particle size distribution. Alloplasts are usually not combined with other bone grafting materials such as allograft and xenografts. A PRF membrane placed over this graft can improve the bone augmentation process. This graft material is not popular but in the right hands can be a great bone regenerative alternative.[6]

Allograft is grafting material that comes from human cadaver bone that has gone through a process of sterilization and ground down to micron particles. This allograft bone comes in cortical and cancellous particles ranging from microns to 1 mm size particles. Cortical bone is harder and does not resorb as fast while the cancellous bone is more porous and allows for better vascular blood flow. The combination of cortical/ cancellous bone in an allograft mix is very popular to promote bone growth.

Allograft also comes in mineralized and demineralized particle forms. Mineralized cadaver bone is formed with the calcium and phosphate still in the bone which allows bone to form by osteoconduction. This mineralized bone does not resorb quickly and forms a matrix and scaffold in which bone growth cells can grow bone. Demineralized bone is processed so that the minerals calcium and phosphate are removed from the cadaver bone particles. This bone will have only BMP's (bone morphogenic proteins) left in the particulate. BMP's will allow bone to grow through a process called osteoinduction. This process forms bone cells (osteoclasts and osteoblasts) to grow new bone. BMP's have a chemotactic signal which causes cells to differentiate into bone forming cells. Allografts are the most popular bone grafting materials in the United States. They are used in over 60 percent of bone grafting procedures and can be combined with PRF to increase their bone regenerative potential.[6]

Xenografts are bone particles that are derived from animal bone sources such as pig and cow. The sterilization process of this bone creates particles that can grow bone through the osteoconductive pathway. This type of bone, when placed into an extraction site, will create a scaffold in which bone can grow. Xenografts resorb very slowly and sometimes do not even resorb at all. It may stay at a site and bone will form in and around it. Xenografts are often combined with other bone sources such as PRF when large bone graft volumes are needed. Xenografts unique resorption characteristics can create large amounts of space for bone to grow.

Autografts are the gold standard for bone growth. This type of bone is autogenous bone which comes from the patient. Sources of autografts can be harvested from a patient's mandible and maxilla. The hip bone is also another source of autogenous bone. Harvesting autogenous bone is technique sensitive and if not done properly can lead to morbidity. Autogenous grafts need a good blood supply in order to survive. Growth hormone in PRF is a good source of angiogenesis for bone grafting. The posterior mandible buccal shelf is the most common site for autogenous bone grafts. Bone can be scraped from this site or a larger block graft can be harvested. Autogenous bone has osteogenic properties meaning bone cells (osteoblasts and osteoclasts) are already present at the site and directly grow bone. Bone cells are already there and do not have to be recruited to the site. Autogenous bone is the only type of bone that is osteogenic, osteoinductive, and osteoconductive. It has bone cells present, it can recruit more bone cells, and it can maintain the space and matrix for bone growth. The only hard part is obtaining the autogenous bone from a patient. It requires advanced bone grafting skills and is technique sensitive. Autogenous bone can be combined with all other bone types and PRF to enhance bone regeneration.[6]

PRF, as a fibrin matrix, traps more platelets and growth factors inside which allows for a consistent and slower release of growth factors over 7–10 days. The old liquid form of PRP released growth factors too quickly so the healing effects were not as potent. 2nd generation PRF can be incorporated into dentistry because of its new form which is a 3D fibrin matrix that is easily handled. It comes from an autogenous source in the patient's blood. Lastly it has bio active modified growth factors which can recruit healing cells and make cells differentiate into cells that enhance wound healing.

PRF is also known to regenerate tissue. More blood vessels are created because of the growth hormone VEGF contained in PRF. The amount of growth factor is not important. It is now known that the slow release of growth factors over a 7- to 10-day period is more important than the amount of growth factors to regenerate tissue and bone.

The clinical applications of PRF have increased since the discovery of PRP. The medical and dental field use PRF to regenerate tissue and bone. The dental field uses PRF in the regenerative process because it is cost effective and efficient. The technique of drawing blood and spinning it in a centrifuge has become easier. PRF is used in wisdom teeth extraction sites and for socket grafting. It is also combined with bone grafting materials for guided bone regenerative procedures. PRF membranes have been placed for wound closures, gingival recession procedures, and sinus lifts. Periodontal defects have also been aided with the use of PRF. Dental surgery has thrived with the use of PRF because of its ability to increase blood supply to tissue defects and the fibrin matrix with growth factors that increases the process of wound healing.

PRF is used every day in my dental implant and extraction practice. It is used in all the scenarios that have been discussed. The armamentarium for the use of PRF needs to be discussed. There are many companies that make centrifuges. Many different companies will claim that their machine and PRF techniques are superior to others based on the way their centrifuge spins the blood tubes. It is really up to the practitioner to decide which equipment is best for them.

Blood Collection and Centrifuge

The important equipment needed for PRF is mainly the centrifuge, a butterfly needle to draw the blood, and 10 ml red blood collection tubes without any anticoagulants. See Figures 13.3a, 13.3b, 13.3c.

Venipuncture has been discussed in previous chapters relating to IV sedation. The most common place for me to begin my PRF blood draw is the antecubital area of the right or left arm. Depending on different skin and mass types, blood draws may lead to venipuncture in other areas such as the forearm and hand.

There are many different ways and set ups to connect the butterfly and collection tubes. Many adaptors are available to create a blood collection system. If the practitioner is doing IV sedation; many protocols exist for getting a PRF blood draw and then switching to the IV setup where drugs can be administered to the patient. Knowing the different equipment and parts will aid the practitioner in creating an efficient workflow for IV sedation and PRF blood draw.

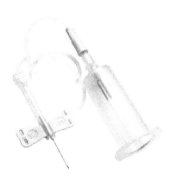
Figure 13.3a BectonDickenson Vacutainer and butterfly needle.

The hardest part is getting a proper venipuncture. Without a proper blood draw there is no moving forward with the procedure. Proper selection of butterflies is also key. Some blood draw butterflies make it easy to see a flash of blood to let the practitioner know that they have a good vein. I prefer to use butterflies with this flash perk but they are a bit more expensive. Once the flash of blood is indicated; insert the 10 ml red blood collection tube into the vacutainer collection tube. These tubes are manufactured with a certain amount of vacuum air in them that allows for the blood to draw. Done properly, blood will start to fill in the red blood collection tube. These red tubes are specifically designed this way in order to collect blood. Once the tube is filled or blood is no longer being drawn, pull out the red tube and insert another 10 ml red blood collection tube. Depending on the number of sites or size of the regenerative process; keep collecting blood.

Most centrifuges have 6 slots for a maximum of 6 red 10 ml tubes. These tubes have to be placed in a balanced order in the centrifuge or the machine will start to vibrate and shake. If only one 10 ml red tube of blood is drawn and placed in the centrifuge, another empty 10 ml red tube needs to be placed exactly opposite of this tube to counter the weight and balance. Don't try just spinning 1 red tube without balancing it. The centrifuge will not work properly. No tubes should be placed in the centrifuge next to each other. Red tubes always need to be countered with other red tubes. An even number of tubes is recommended to avoid vibration and imbalance. See Figures 13.4a and 13.4b.

A key factor that affects creating PRF is the amount of time that passes from when the blood is drawn and the placement of the red tube into the centrifuge to begin spinning. There are zero anticoagulants in the 10 ml red tubes. This means that the process of blood collection to centrifugation needs to happen quickly. If too much time passes, the PRF may not form properly.

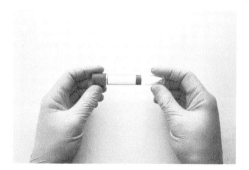

Figure 13.3b   Red blood collection tube.

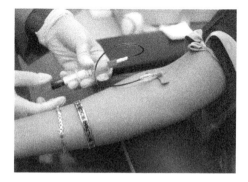

Figure 13.3c   Blood draw with collection tube in vacutainer (U.S. Navy / Wikimedia Commons / Public Domain).

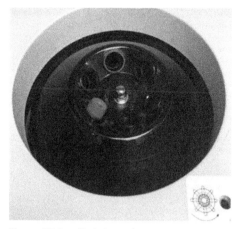

Figure 13.4a   Unbalanced.

I use the centrifuge manufactured by Salvin Dental. Many centrifuges exist and every company will tell you why their centrifuge is the best. It is primarily up to the practitioner to decide which centrifuge is best for them. The Salvin centrifuge protocol spins the 10 ml red blood collection tubes at 3100 rpm for 12 minutes. The end of the 12 minute spin cycle will be signaled by a bell or an alarm. Be aware of this time because it is also critical to evaluate the PRF.

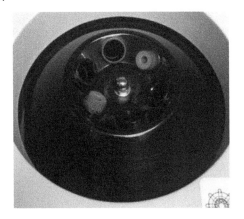

Figure 13.4b   Balanced.

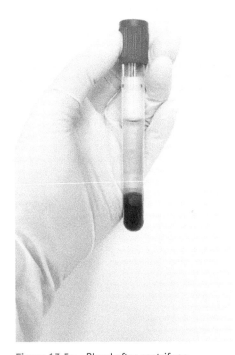

Figure 13.5a   Blood after centrifuge.

The PRF will have 3 layers once the 12 minute spin cycle is over. The upper most layer will be the PPP (plasma poor protein), the middle will be the PRF clot, and the bottom layer is a red blood cell layer. See Figures 13.5a and 13.5b and 13.5c.

Carefully use a dental tweezer to extract the PRF layer out and place it in a metal sterile dish or a separation tray that is also available from Salvin Dental. Other companies will have PRF trays as well. These trays can help manipulate the PRF into different fibrin matrices depending on the surgeon's needs. PRF can be flattened using these trays to create barrier membranes that can be placed over bone grafts and other bone deficiencies to promote healing. PRF clots can be placed into the cylinders of these trays to produce small PRF plugs that can be placed into extraction sockets. The metal pistons will condense the PRF clots into small plugs that are easier to handle. See Figure 13.5c

How to treat wisdom teeth extraction sites with PRF?[7] It depends on which wisdom tooth is extracted. Wisdom teeth extraction sites must be curetted and debrided thoroughly. I prefer to remove all granulation tissue and infected tissue without causing any damage to the inferior alveolar nerve or maxillary sinus. Careful attention to the flap must be considered. I like to suction and irrigate mandibular flaps to decrease the possibility of subperiosteal infections.

After thoroughly cleansing the wisdom teeth extraction sites, I use the PRF plug as a whole fibrin clot. I do not flatten or make a small plug out of the PRF. I take the large yellowish clot that has been removed from the 10 ml red tubes and placed in a metal dish or tray. I push the clot into the extraction site with my fingers or the end of my surgical tweezers. A lot of acellular fluid such as the PPP layer will gush out of the extraction socket as the PRF is being condensed. Careful attention must be made to not use a high-speed surgical suction in the area during PRF application because the high-speed suction can suck away the clot full of growth factors. In that case you better hope you have another PRF clot waiting. Instead use a small slow speed suction to remove excess fluid when condensing the PRF.

Once the PRF clot is thoroughly condensed into the wisdom tooth extraction site; flap closure is indicated. Sometimes extraction sites may be larger than usual and this may require extra PRF clots. This is a judgment call that is up to the surgeon. I usually just put 1 PRF clot per extraction site no matter the size of the extraction site. For lower wisdom teeth extraction sockets; 1 suture is usually needed for the site to heal. This suture technique has been discussed in earlier chapters. I use a 3.0 chromic gut suture that will resorb on its own within 10–14 days or a PGA suture for longer resorbable period

Maxillary wisdom teeth extraction sites will get the same PRF treatment. Condense the large, yellowish clot and suction any excess acellular fluids that come out of the PRF. Make sure to use a slow speed suction. The only difference with the maxillary wisdom teeth is the suturing technique may be a bit more difficult. An X-shaped suturing technique is needed on upper wisdom teeth extraction sites to keep the PRF in the socket. Sometimes it is too hard to access the area so I may not use the PRF plug in wisdom teeth extraction sites for maxillary teeth.

The postoperative appointment for patients with wisdom teeth extractions is usually 1 week for me. During this appointment, the patient is interviewed on how the procedure went. This is also the moment of truth to see how the PRF has healed the patient. Usually there is significant healing of the wisdom tooth extraction site after 1 week. The healing that occurs in 3 weeks after wisdom teeth extractions usually occurs in 1 week with PRF wisdom teeth extraction therapy.

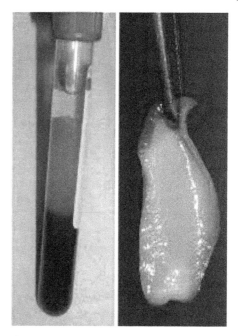

Figure 13.5b   Fibrin clot removed.

Shorter healing periods are usually observed with wisdom teeth extractions that receive PRF. Complications such as dry socket, bleeding, and infection are usually not observed as well. Patient pain and sensitivity thresholds are also decreased with PRF therapy. The controlled studies involving groups of extractions receiving PRF therapy after extractions and groups not receiving any PRF seem to prove that PRF significantly reduces complications with wisdom teeth extractions.

In one clinical study, ten patients underwent surgical wisdom tooth extraction with PRF, while the other ten underwent the procedure without PRF use. Following surgery, 69% of PRF

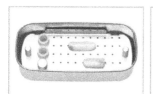
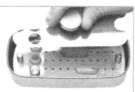
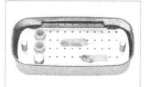

Form Fibrin Membrane Shape From Clot

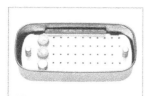
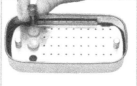
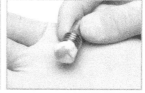

Form Fibrin Plug Shape From Clot

Figure 13.5c   Metal trays for shaping fibrin clot. *Source:* Salvin Dental Specialties, Inc. / https://salvin.com/product/salvin-prf-box last accessed Jan 28, 2022.

participants reported having a comfortable night's sleep on the first postoperative day compared to 31% in the control group (Table 13.2).

Reviewing patient medical history before treatment is important. Conditions such as anticoagulant therapy can increase bleeding complications. Patients with a history of diabetes that is uncontrolled have poor wound healing and are more prone to infection. Patients with liver issues may have increased bleeding issues due to the lack of coagulation factors that are created by a healthy liver. Surgical experience by the operator is also important. Proper surgical technique and experience can help decrease complications and increase wound healing. Proper suturing techniques can decrease surgical complications as well. Iatrogenic factors such as patients smoking and lacking proper home care can also lead to complications.

PRF can help decrease all these complications. The literature and science support the application of PRF in wisdom teeth extraction sockets. Discussion has been made about the importance of angiogenesis which increases the blood supply to a site which minimizes the chance of dry socket. Bone repair, soft tissue, and hard tissue healing is increased significantly with PRF therapy.

Granulation tissue should be debrided before placing the PRF. Patients with incomplete debridement may end up experiencing postoperative pain and infection. In this case, postoperative appointments may include further socket debridement with saline irrigation. PRF therapy can be repeated but this is a surgeon's judgment call. I usually allow the patient to heal with a natural blood clot if this rare situation arises.

Patients who are on anticoagulation therapies for blood clots may have trouble with PRF therapy. This includes patients who are taking Plavix, warfarin (Coumadin), Xarelto, and patients who have missing blood factors that cause blood to coagulate properly. These patients are not candidates for PRF therapy because their blood will not coagulate to form the fibrin clot. Once the venipuncture is completed and the blood is done spinning for 12 minutes, the operator will notice that there is not a PRF blood clot present in the 10 ml red tube. Accurate medical history and patient conditions must be considered before performing PRF therapy.

The complication of tough venipunctures in which no blood collection is possible will eliminate PRF therapy automatically. Some patients are just too tough to perform proper venipuncture. Sometimes it is up to the surgeon's judgment to decide if further attempts at getting a blood draw is possible. After multiple attempts of venipuncture from the antecubital fossa or hand are unsuccessful, I usually call it a day. Some operators may choose to go to the legs, neck, and other body parts depending on skill level to achieve a blood collection. Sometimes PRF therapy is just not possible.

Surgical extractions of wisdom teeth usually require the patient to be sedated. PRF can be incorporated with the IV sedation set up in order to comfortably achieve both under one venipuncture. Patients do not have to go through multiple venipunctures that could lead to complications such as hematomas. PRF and IV sedation all starts with an accurate venipuncture using a blue 22 gauge or yellow 24 gauge catheter.

Table 13.2 Comfort between the study and control groups during the first postoperative night.

Degree of comfort	First night's sleep	
	Study	Control
	N (%)	N (%)
Comfortable	9 (69.2)	4 (30.8)
Uncomfortable	1 (14.3)	6 (85.7)

My IV wisdom teeth extractions with PRF protocol that I use daily will be discussed. Patient will arrive at the office at 9 AM. Patient medical history is reviewed and confirmation that the patient did not eat for 6 hours before the surgery is confirmed. Patient vitals are monitored throughout the procedure and 0.5 mg of crushed triazolam is administered sublingually. Treatment plans and final treatment discussions are reviewed with the patient while waiting for the triazolam to take effect.

A 22 gauge catheter is used for venipuncture and the extension is used to draw four 10 ml red tubes with blood. Then the IV line is set up to the extension and securely taped. 1 assistant will take the red blood tubes to the centrifuge. It takes 12 minutes for the red tubes to spin to form the PRF. During these 12 minutes, IV medications are administered and the wisdom teeth extractions are completed. Sometimes the surgery will take more or less than 12 minutes. After surgery, the PRF is usually ready to be placed into the sockets and suturing is completed shortly after. Postop instructions are given and the patient is usually dismissed within hour.

Based on my personal experience and the results of published studies, I recommend the use of PRF after removing third molars.

References

1 Boswell SG, Cole BJ, Sundman EA, Karas V, Fortier LA. Platelet-rich plasma: a milieu of bioactive factors. *Arthroscopy*. 2012;28:429–39.

2 Marx RE, Carlson ER, Eichstaedt RM, Schimmele SR, Strauss JE, Georgeff KR. Platelet-rich plasma: growth factor enhancement for bone grafts. *Oral Surg Oral Med Oral Pathol Oral Radiol Endod*. 1998;85(6):638–46.

3 Leventis M, Tsetsenekou E, Kalyvas D. Treatment of osseous defects after mandibular third molar removal with a resorbable alloplastic grafting material: a case series with 1- to 2-year follow-up. *Materials (Basel)*. 2020 Oct 21;13(20):4688.

4 Chugh T, Jain AK, Jaiswal RK, Mehrotra P, Mehrotra R. Bone density and its importance in orthodontics. *J Oral Biol Craniofac Res*. 2013 May-Aug;3(2):92–7.

5 Premnath K, Sridevi J, Kalavathy N, Nagaranjani P, Sharmila MR. Evaluation of stress distribution in bone of different densities using different implant designs: a three-dimensional finite element analysis. doi: 10.1007/s13191-012-0189-7.

6 Patil N, Vaze S, Patil S, Patil P, Madhura K, Mahamuni A. Alloplastic bone graft for pocket reduction after third molar surgery. *Int J Curr Res*. 2016 June;8(06):33487–92.

7 Nourwali I. The effects of platelet-rich fibrin on post-surgical complications following removal of impacted wisdom teeth: a pilot study. *J Taibah Univ Med Sci*. 2021 Mar 13;16(4):521–8.

14

Case Studies – Lessons Learned

This chapter includes real-life cases. As mentioned previously, case selection is critical to the successful removal of third molars. The cases mentioned in this chapter did not proceed as planned. Most of the problems encountered could have been avoided with proper case selection. Hopefully, sharing these cases with you will help you to avoid similar complications.

Age

Age is everything when deciding to proceed or refer. Teenage bone is like Styrofoam. Adult bone is like concrete. Studies have shown that surgical complications increase after age 25. Age is only one factor, but it is an important one.

Fully developed roots may be divergent, thin, bulbous, or curved. A periodontal ligament may not be visible on a panoramic X-ray or CBCT. The removal of these third molars may be easy or nearly impossible. Surgical removal of third molars for older patients with dense bone and fully developed roots is unpredictable.

Surgical skills are constantly improving with every patient treated. The case described below was done after I had removed more than 30,000 third molars. Overconfidence led to poor case selection.

A 48-year-old male patient complained of intermittent lower left and right pain. He was scheduled for the removal of 4 full bony third molars with IV sedation. Dense bone was visible on the panoramic X-ray (ground glass appearance). See Figure 14.1

The maxillary right third molar did not move. My 46R elevator broke attempting to elevate #1. The maxillary third molars were finally extracted after bone removal and sectioning.

Axiom – maxillary third molars are easier to remove than mandibular thirds.
Corollary – a difficult maxillary third molar is much more difficult than a difficult mandibular third molar.

This case was done with IV sedation and took 1 ½ hours to complete. My normal time to remove 4 third molars is less than ½ hour.

Lesson learned: over confidence can lead to poor case selection.

Impacted Third Molars, Second Edition. Edited by John Wayland.
© 2024 John Wiley & Sons, Inc. Published 2024 by John Wiley & Sons, Inc.

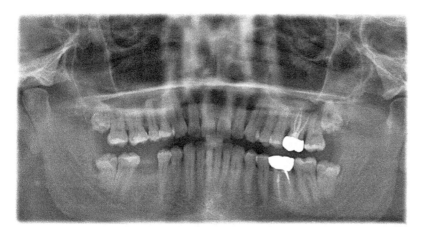

Figure 14.1   Preop panoramic X-ray.

Mental and Emotional Health

A 19-year-old female patient was referred by her pediatric dentist for 4 full bony third molars. The patient arrived, with her father, dressed similar to the photo in Figure 14.2. Her father told me that she was auditioning for a movie role in Los Angeles.

Since my practice is mobile, I had not met the patient before her appointment. All medical records and imaging were reviewed and approved prior to scheduling. Unfortunately, it was not possible to assess the patient's mental/emotional state or parent child relationship before scheduling.

Figure 14.2   Not the actual patient.

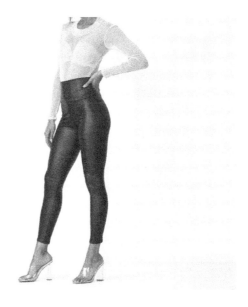

Several red flags were warning caution in this case. The inappropriate dress was exacerbated by her father's approval. In cases where the patient's mental/emotional status is questionable, sedation is not always successful.

After the IV medication (fentanyl and midazolam) was administered, the patient became agitated; crying, and moving. The procedure was stopped and the patient was referred for surgery with general anesthesia.

Third molar patients with questionable mental/emotional status are best treated with general anesthesia. This paradoxical reaction is not always easy to predict.

Lesson learned: Some patients need GA with an anesthesiologist.

Bleeding after Surgery

A 16-year-old male patient presented for the removal of impacted third molars. See Figure 14.3 His medical and dental history was unremarkable and the procedure was uneventful. The patient's father was given postoperative instructions, verbal and written, and the patient was dismissed.

The patient's father called that evening and stated that his son was still bleeding. Postoperative instructions were reviewed and biting on a tea bag was recommended. The patient's father was instructed to call again if there was no improvement within two hours. A phone call was received at 11:30 pm stating that there was no improvement and the patient was still bleeding. The patient was instructed to drink lots of water, continue to bite on gauze or tea bag, and come to the office in the morning at 8 am.

The patient was still bleeding when he arrived at the office. 4 × 4 gauze was changed every ½ hour for two hours with no improvement. The patient was referred to the local emergency room and was later admitted to the hospital to conduct bleeding tests. The patient was diagnosed with Von Willebrand's disease, an abnormality of the coagulation cascade. Von Willebrand's factor (vWF) promotes normal platelet function and stabilizes factor VIII.

It was later discovered that the patient had a history of hematoma in his thigh sustained while playing soccer. This was unreported on his medical history and preoperative assessment. This case clearly illustrates the importance of a thorough preoperative medical history and assessment to rule out bleeding disorders. Patients with coagulation disorders may be identified by questions regarding

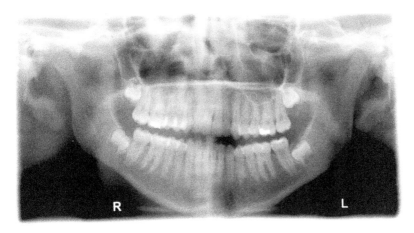

Figure 14.3 Full bony impacted third molars.

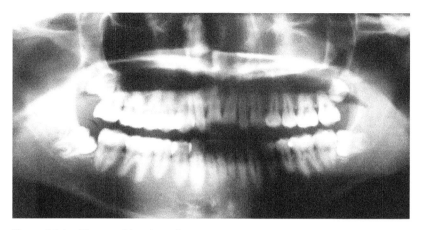

Figure 14.4   25-year-old male patient.

personal or familial history of bleeding and bruising. Preoperative assessment of intrinsic coagulation disorders and the use of anticoagulant and antiplatelet medications (Coumadin, Plavix) is essential.[1]

Lesson learned: Interview patients regarding any history of bleeding or bruising

Bleeding during Surgery

A 25-year-old male was scheduled for the removal of 4 third molars. See Figure 14.4

Some bleeding during the surgical removal of third molars is normal. This patient developed uncontrollable bleeding during the removal of #17, the lower left third molar. I follow a seven-step surgical protocol for impacted third molars. The first step, the soft tissue flap, was uneventful. The patient started heavy bleeding after troughing. The bleeding was severe enough that I couldn't continue. Pressure didn't help. My assistant was suctioning to keep the patient's airway dry. The patient was sedated and unaware of the bleeding issue.

After 10 minutes I considered calling EMS. This is when my assistant, Diego, suggested using epinephrine 1:50,000. We infiltrated the soft tissue around the surgical site. The bleeding stopped immediately.

Lesson learned: Epinephrine 1:50,000 can stop bleeding; listen to your assistant.

BMI

The patient was a 16-year-old female scheduled for the removal of 4 third molars with sedation. See Figure 14.5

Her panoramic X-ray and medical history were reviewed prior to scheduling. Her BMI was not included on her medical or dental history.

I had not met this patient prior to the day of surgery. Six patients were scheduled; this patient was number three. My assistant gave the patient 0. 5 mg triazolam sublingual while we were treating the second patient.

This is what I saw when she was moved to the surgical operatory. See Figures 14.5a and 14.5b Her BMI was 66.1.

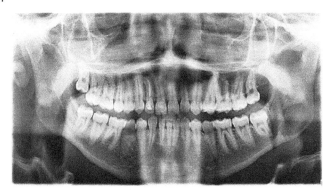

Figure 14.5   16-year-old female patient.

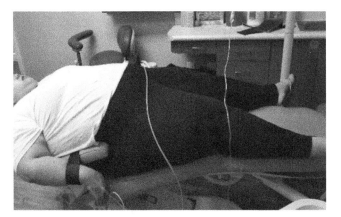

Figure 14.5a   BMI 66.1.

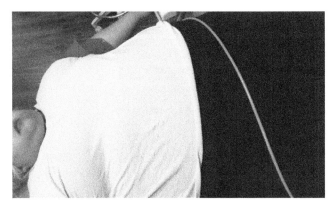

Figure 14.5b   5'1" 350 lbs.

Patients with this BMI should be seen in the hospital with an anesthesiologist. She is an ASA III patient per her BMI. I normally don't see ASA III patients. However, she was orally sedated earlier and her parents missed work to be with her. The third molar removal on her panoramic X-ray looked very easy and predictable. She was completely relaxed with no signs of anxiety. I told her that she would be lightly sedated during the procedure due to her weight. She would be able to talk to us and cough if needed.

We started an IV (very difficult venipuncture) and added 2 mg of Versed. The procedure was very simple and predictable. We were finished in less than 10 minutes. Height and weight plus BMI are now on each patient's medical and dental record.

Lesson learned: Include height and weight on the medical/dental record.

Airway

This lesson was learned while teaching an IV sedation course. The patient was a 48-year-old Hispanic female. Her chief complaint was pain lower left and right. The panoramic X-ray shows the third molars located in the ramus. This is an indication of a small mouth and poor access. Clinically, all of her molars were covered by her tongue. Surgical access was very poor. See See Figure 14.6

Coughing is a reflex behavior that protects the airway from aspiration of blood, tissue, and debris. Sedated patients experience some degree of central nervous system depression and a reduced coughing reflex. A throat pack with gauze is used in oral surgery to protect against aspiration when patients are sedated.[2] A Weider retractor and oven, filled 4 × 4 gauze were used with this patient. See Figure 14.7.

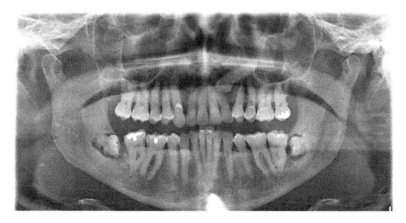

Figure 14.6   Pain lower left and right.

Figure 14.7   Weider retractor and 4 × 4 filled gauze pharyngeal screen (throat pack).

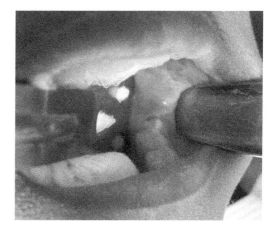

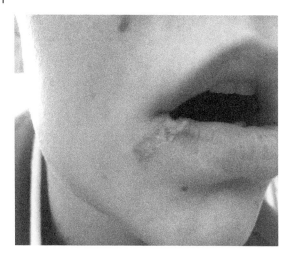

Figure 14.8   Laceration of lip from rotating bur and heat.

The patient was moderately sedated with fentanyl and midazolam. During the procedure class participants asked many questions. The patient began moving and appeared agitated. Capnography showed breathing impairment.

The patient had partially aspirated the throat pack gauze and was gagging. Fortunately, a corner of the large gauze is always available as a "handle" if needed. See Figure 14.7 The gauze was easily removed and the patient's breathing returned to normal. If left unattended, this could have been fatal.

Lesson learned: Difficult airway. Focus on the patient. Don't be distracted.

Surgical Drills

Burns and abrasions are caused in dentistry by rotary drills. Careful attention is a must when using them to avoid catching soft tissue with the shank of the bur and creating a laceration. This usually occurs with the buccal mucosa and the corner of the mouth. This is especially true when using a surgical drill for third molars. Access is limited and the corner of the mouth is usually stretched when using the drill.

This complication can usually be prevented by careful attention of the assistant to the location of the bur shank when the surgeon is cutting. In this case, the assistant and instructor notified the participating dentist that the handpiece and bur were touching the patient's lip and chin. See Figure 14.8.

In 2010 the FDA issued an alert to dentists warning them about the danger of patient injury from electric handpieces overheating. If a surgical drill is worn, damaged, or clogged, the electric motor may overheat. Patients have been severely burned when surgical drills have overheated. Surgeons often continue to use these drills because the handpiece housing and surgical gloves insulate the surgeon and the anesthetized patient cannot feel pain.

Lesson learned: keep surgical drills away from soft tissue.

Infratemporal Fossa

The accidental displacement of a maxillary third molar into the infratemporal fossa is a rare complication that can occur even with experienced surgeons.[3]

The author has had one third molar displaced into the infratemporal fossa. The patient was a 12-year-old, healthy, male referred to me by his orthodontist. See Figure 14.9

Several things contributed to this complication:

1) Small mouth with lower third molars in the ramus
2) Orthodontic brackets, and arch wires
3) The right maxillary third molar was lingually positioned close to the infratemporal fossa
4) Poor patient selection

Unlike the maxillary sinus, the infratemporal fossa is not an empty space. It contains many vital structures including motor nerves, arteries, and veins. A third molar displaced into the infratemporal fossa is considered a major complication. See Figures 14.10a and 14.10b.

Figure 14.9 Maxillary third molar in the infratemporal fossa.

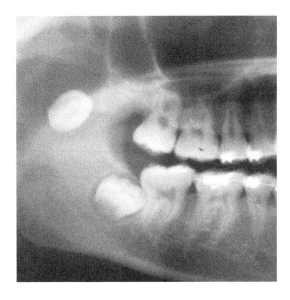

Figure 14.10a Infratemporal fossa in red (Reproduced with permission from Joanna Culley BA(hons) IMI, MMAA, RMIP).

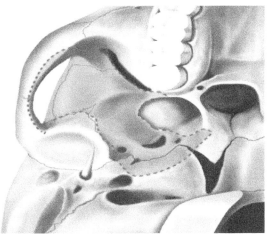

Figure 14.10b Infratemporal fossa boundaries.

Anterior: posterior maxilla

Posterior: tympanic plate and temporal bone

Medial: lateral pterygoid plate

Lateral: ramus of the mandible

Superior: greater wing of the sphenoid bone

Inferior: medial pterygoid muscle

The patient was referred to the Department of Maxillofacial Surgery at UCSF School of Dentistry in San Francisco. Several department instructors evaluated the patient with CBCT scans. He was seen by UCSF 3 times over a period of 3 months. The patient had no symptoms, and there was no sign of infection. The department chair recommended no treatment.

Lesson learned: Waiting a few years would have avoided this complication. Refer or wait.

References

1 Susarla SM, et al. Third molar surgery and associated complications. *Oral Maxillofacial Surg Clin N Am*. 2003;15:177–86.

2 Gupta A, Sarma R, Gupta N, Kumar R. Current practices and beliefs regarding the use of oro throat packs in India: a nationwide survey. *Indian J Anaesth*. 2021 Mar;65(3):241–7.

3 Lutz JC, Cazzato R, Le Roux MK, et al. Retrieving a displaced third molar from the infratemporal fossa: case report of a minimally invasive procedure. *BMC Oral Health*. 2019;19:149.

15

Insurance and Third Molars

Dental offices have a fee schedule for dental services they offer. Dental insurance companies also have fee schedules which are generally based on average fees in an area. The insurance company list of average fees is used to determine payment.

Dental insurance is designed to pay a portion of the costs associated with dental care. There are several different types of insurance plans grouped into three primary categories: Indemnity, Preferred Provider Network (PPO), and Dental Health Managed Organizations (DHMO).[1]

Indemnity dental plans generally pay a percentage of the cost of services. Restrictions usually include a waiting period, deductibles, annual maximum paid, and the length of time that the policy has been owned.

A Preferred Provider Organization (PPO) has an agreement with an insurer to provide health insurance at reduced or low rates. Patients can be seen by any dentist. The dentist does not need to be "In-Network." Any difference between office fees and insurance fees is paid by the patient. Many PPO plans have an annual maximum limit.

Dental Health Maintenance Organization (DHMO) plans require dentists to be an In-Network Provider. The office must charge their DHMO patients a reduced fee dictated by the provider. DHMO's rarely have an annual maximum limit.

Every dental procedure has an ADA code. The codes for removal of third molars and impactions begin with D7152 and end with D7250.

D7152 intentional partial tooth removal performed when a neurovascular complication is likely if the entire impacted tooth is removed.

D7210 surgical removal of erupted tooth requiring elevation of mucoperiosteal flap and removal of bone and/or section of tooth. Includes cutting of gingiva and bone, removal of tooth structure, minor smoothing of socket bone and closure.

D7220 removal of impacted tooth – soft tissue. Occlusal surface of tooth covered by soft tissue; requires mucoperiosteal flap elevation.

D7230 removal of impacted tooth – partially bony. Part of crown covered by bone; requires mucoperiosteal flap elevation and bone removal.

D7240 removal of impacted tooth – completely bony. Most or all of crown covered by bone; requires mucoperiosteal flap elevation and bone removal.

D7241 removal of impacted tooth – completely bony, with unusual surgical complications

D7250 surgical removal of residual tooth roots (cutting procedure). Includes cutting of soft tissue and bone, removal of tooth structure.

Impacted Third Molars, Second Edition. Edited by John Wayland.
© 2024 John Wiley & Sons, Inc. Published 2024 by John Wiley & Sons, Inc.

A dentist's clinical decisions determine what procedures are delivered to a patient. The full CDT Code entry, as published in the CDT manual, must be considered when determining which dental procedure code should be used to document services provided.[2]

Bony impactions can be completely bony (D7240) or partially bony (D7230). These insurance codes need clarification. The American Dental Association offers Guidance on Coding for Impacted Teeth.

The ADA's Glossary of Terms defines a crown as "that portion of a tooth normally covered by enamel." The "crown" referenced in partial and full bony codes is the portion of the tooth above the cemento-enamel junction. It follows that "part of the crown" should be interpreted as "less than 50% of the entire crown" and "most or all of the crown" should be interpreted as "at least or more than 50% of the entire crown". **An interpretation that some portion of the occlusal surface must reside below the bone in order for D7240 to apply is incorrect." (ADA quote)** The dentist who removes an impacted tooth should consider this guidance when determining the code, 7230 or D7240, that appropriately describes the service she or he delivered.[3]

Panoramic X-rays are distorted and not accurate when determining the correct code for bony impactions. However, when submitting X-rays to insurance for pre authorization, the panoramic

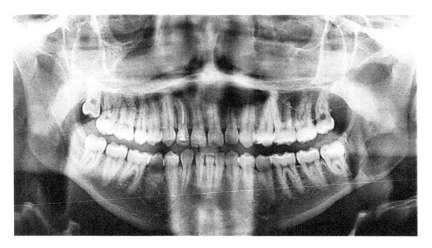

Figure 15.1   Full bony impactions (FBI) can look like erupted teeth.

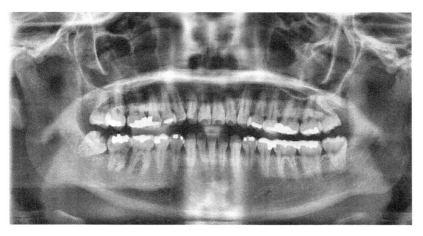

Figure 15.2   Third molars with 1% of crown covered be bone are partial bony impactions.

X-ray is the standard of care and must be used to determine the insurance code. Completely bony third molars, as seen on a panoramic X-ray can look like erupted teeth. See Figure 15.1.

Partial bony impactions, by ADA definition, include third molar crowns covered by less than 50% bone. See Figure 15.2.

The mandibular crowns shown in Figure 15.2 have bone above the third molar cemento-enamael junction. They are partial bony impactions.

Medical or Dental Insurance?

Dentists are responsible for diagnosis and must select the appropriate insurance code for claim submission. CPT codes report medical procedures to medical plans. CDT codes report dental procedures to dental plans. Different insurance codes and forms are used for medical and dental billing.

Medical claims are usually filed as primary insurance while dental claims are typically filed as secondary insurance. Dental insurance should be billed with a copy of the medical insurance Explanation of Benefits (EOB). When dental procedures qualify for medical insurance reimbursement, they must be reported with CPT codes. CPT stands for Current Procedural Terminology. These codes meet HIPAA requirements to report medical procedures to medical insurance plans. The codes describe the services provided and are reported to the medical carrier on a CMS 1500 claim form. Medical insurance claims often require a detailed clinical note describing the surgery. CPT codes are reviewed annually by the American Medical Association (AMA) and updated as needed.[4]

Dental insurance companies use CDT codes to determine what dental procedures are eligible for reimbursement. The dental code always starts with the letter D and is followed by 4 numbers. For example D7240. CDT codes are ADA intellectual property, maintained by the ADA Council on Dental Benefit Programs. The codes are reviewed and updated annually as dental technology changes. New codes are added and other codes are deleted.

Sedation is usually not covered by dental insurance. Most insurance companies consider sedation to be a "non-essential dental procedure," meaning sedation is more of a luxury than a need. However, IV sedation for bony impactions is sometimes covered. The American Dental Association updated sedation codes D9239 and D9243 were effective Jan. 1, 2018.

D9239 – for intravenous moderate (conscious) sedation/analgesia, initial 15 minutes. D9239 was a new procedure code in 2018.

D9243 – for intravenous moderate (conscious) sedation/analgesia, each subsequent 15 minute increment. This code was revised in 2018.[5]

Early Third Molar Removal and Insurance

The early removal of third molars benefits the patient clinically and financially.

Early third molar removal benefits the patient clinically by reducing complications. A study by Osborn evaluated the surgical and postoperative complications of 9,574 third molar patients. The study concluded that third molars should be removed during the teenage years, thereby decreasing complications.[6]

Teenage patients usually have bone covering their third molar clinical crowns. This benefits the patient financially since the insurance payment to remove bony impactions is more than the benefit for soft tissue or surgical extractions.

References

1 PPO dental insurance vs. DHMO – what's the difference? www.dentalplans.com.

2 www.ada.org/en/publications/cdt/coding.

3 D7230 and D7240 – guidance on coding for impacted teeth removal procedure. www.AmericanDentalAssociation.org.

4 Dental Claim Support. CDT codes vs CPT codes: what's the difference? 2022 Nov 2.

5 Reporting Guidelines for Dental Anesthesia. D9223 and D9243 Revised, the American Dental Association updated the description codes for IV conscious sedation on Jan. 1, 2018. https://content.highmarkprc.com/Files/Region/navinet/PlanCentral/pc-all-dental-anesthesia-112918.pdf.

6 Osborn TP, et al. A prospective study of complications related to mandibular third molar surgery. *J Oral Maxlllofac Surg*. 1965;43:767–9.

16

The Mobile Third Molar Practice

This chapter has been written in response to inquiries from dentists regarding my mobile third molar practice. These dentists are looking for an alternative to private practice. The typical private practice dentist wears many hats: CEO, business manager, negotiator, therapist, and politician. Several studies have reported a high prevalence of stress and burnout among dentists.[1–4]

The suicide rate of dentists is more than twice the rate of the general population and almost three times higher than that of other white-collar workers. Emotional illness ranks third in order of frequency of health problems among dentists, while in the general population it ranks tenth.[5]

Dr. Randy Lang sites nine causes of stress and burnout in dentistry.[5] Seven of these stressors are eliminated or reduced in the mobile third molar practice.

1) Confinement. "The average dentist spends most of his or her life confined to a small, sometimes windowless, 7ft. by 9ft. operatory, which is smaller than the cells in our penal institutions." The mobile third molar practice work space changes every day. The office atmosphere, staff, and patient demographics change every day. This promotes an atmosphere of openness and freedom.
2) Isolation. "Most dentists practice alone. Consequently, they do not have the opportunity to share and solve problems with their colleagues the way other professional groups do through peer support." The mobile third molar practice meets with a different colleague every day.
3) Stress of perfection. "The relentless pursuit of perfection and permanence in an inhospitable oral environment is a major cause of stress and frustration for dentists." Restorative dentistry requires a focus on intricate and meticulous detail. The removal of impacted third molars also requires attention to detail, but is less intense and prolonged.
4) Economic pressure. "Office overhead rises to meet income." Private practice begins with school and practice loans. Office overhead may increase as income increases. The mobile third molar practice has consistently low overhead; no lab bills, staff, rent, and minimal supplies.
5) Time pressure. "Attempting to stay on schedule in a busy dental practice is a chronic source of stress." The mobile third molar practice sees one patient at a time in one operatory. The schedule is predictable and flexible.
6) Compromised treatment. "Many patients, due to financial restraints, poor insurance plans or low appreciation of quality dental care, will not accept 'ideal' treatment plans." The removal of impacted third molars is an "all or none" treatment. No compromise on ideal treatment is necessary.
7) Patient anxiety. "There is now considerable evidence that dentists experience patterns of physiological stress responses (increased heart rate, high blood pressure, sweating, etc.) that parallel the patient's responses when performing dental procedures that evoke patient fear and

anxiety." Sedation is an integral part of the mobile third molar practice. Patient stress is controlled and there is little or no memory of the procedure.

A modification of life style may be the answer for the practitioner that is burned out in private practice. The reader of this book, who enjoys oral surgery and is looking for an alternative to private practice, might consider the mobile third molar practice. My mobile practice ended my emotional and physical burn out.

My dental journey and interest in minor oral surgery began at UCSF School of Dentistry in 1977. Most dentists receive minimal oral surgery training in dental school. All challenging procedures are referred to AEGD, GPR, and oral surgery residents. This was especially true when I was in dental school. My oral surgery rotation consisted of forceps removal of mobile erupted teeth.

Oral surgery continuing education courses were virtually non-existent when I graduated in 1981. Fortunately, Brånemark presented his research on osseointegration in 1982 and many implant continuing education courses became available. I began reading oral surgery books and attending implant continuing education courses. Attending implant lectures and live patient hands-on courses increased my surgical skill and confidence. I received my IV sedation training from Dr. Stanley Malamed at USC in 1983.

After associating for three years, I opened my first dental office in 1984 in the small San Francisco suburb of Hercules. The town of Hercules had no dentists and a population of about 7900 men, women, and children. My office was surrounded by empty land filled with fields of knee-high weeds. Hercules became a boomtown and my practice flourished and continued to grow to more than 5000 active patients. I opened a second satellite office in 1989.

By 1999 I was burned out and struggling to practice with a herniated disc in my lower back. I sold both dental practices and took a year off to let my back heal and reflect on my life in dentistry. A year later my back was better and I had a plan to practice without stress and trauma to my back. I would open a boutique, one operatory, office in an affluent suburb of San Francisco. I would limit my practice to large case reconstruction dentistry, work 3 days a week, and treat a handful of patients each day. This plan looked perfect on paper.

However, soon after opening my dream boutique office it became obvious that an occasional big case was not going to pay my bills. It has been said that "necessity is the mother of invention." I needed to do something. I picked up the phone and called my colleagues to offer my services removing impacted third molars. The fact that I had my IV sedation permit was a big selling point.

A few months later I was working 1 day a week in my mobile practice removing impacted third molars with IV sedation. My single day income removing impactions was more than 3 days in my office. I reached a tipping point after a busy day removing impactions. I was driving home with my mobile gear in the back of my SUV. I had a nice check in my pocket, my back was OK, and I wasn't stressed out. I sold my "dream" practice in 2005.

I now have independent contractor agreements with 37 offices in the San Francisco Bay Area. I have no office, employees, or insurance issues. My overhead is close to zero and I have unlimited scheduling flexibility. I've lived in Hawaii since 2007. I commute to California for work 10 days a month. My mobile practice has been limited to the removal of impacted third molars for 20 years.

Some of my contracted offices don't even know I live in Hawaii.

Mobile Practice Benefits

The dental industry is evolving at a monumental pace. Dentistry is increasingly competitive with the advent of corporate dentistry and DMOs.[6] New graduates are facing increasing school debt.[7] Specialists are receiving fewer referrals.[8]

The goal in a competitive market is to stand out, find a niche, or distinguish a practice in some way. One competitive niche is the mobile dental practice offering services that the general dentist would normally refer to a specialist. This alternative practice style benefits both the general dentistry practice owner and mobile practice contactor.

Benefits to the general dentistry practice owner:

1) Revenue stays in the office. In a competitive dental marketplace, the multispecialty practice makes sense.
2) Patients don't want to be referred. They prefer to stay with their trusted general dentist. They don't want to drive to a distant location to meet with a stranger. General dentists often have the following conversation. "Mary, you need a root canal. I'm going to refer you to Dr. X." Invariably, the patient's response is "Dr., are you sure you can't do it?"
3) Patient referrals increase. Difficult procedures that are not normally provided by the practice are completed in familiar surroundings. This enhances the practice image and increases patient referrals.
4) Communication is improved. The mobile dentist and practice owner can meet together with the patient.

Benefits to the mobile practice contractor:

1) Reduced stress
2) Overhead close to zero
3) No staff or insurance headaches
4) Unlimited scheduling flexibility

Once established, the mobile third molar practice has many benefits. Contracted offices provide staff and manage insurance. You control your schedule. Since you don't have a leased office space and staff, you are free to travel and spend time with your family.

There are also many challenges to consider. Building your client base is a major undertaking that can take years. Maintaining the client base requires constant nurturing. You must be willing to load, unload, and transport your surgical equipment and supplies every day. It is highly recommended that you are certified in IV sedation. Patient management issues are more easily controlled and your patients will have little or no memory of the procedure. You should be ACLS certified and able to handle sedation emergencies. Most importantly, there is not much point in pursuing this idea unless you can confidently, efficiently, and safely remove impacted third molars

Can you finish most partial and full bony impaction cases (four impactions) in 45 minutes or less without complications? Can you handle surgical complications when they occur? If you are a general dentist, you will be held to the same standard as an oral surgeon. The efficient, confident, and safe removal of impacted third molars leads to happy patients, parents, and contracted offices.

General Dentist or Specialist

Can a GP practice to the same standard as an oral surgeon when removing impacted third molars? The maxillofacial surgeon deserves respect. There is no question that the maxillofacial surgeon's training is extensive. A typical maxillofacial dual degree residency could include rotations in anesthesia, plastic surgery, surgical oncology, gastrointestinal surgery, thoracic surgery, cardiothoracic surgery, transplant surgery, trauma surgery, surgical intensive care, dentoalveolar surgery, salivary gland lesions, implants, TMJ surgery, orthognathic surgery, nerve repair, facial trauma, and more. However, exodontia represents a small part of the maxillofacial surgeon's training. A GP focused on extractions could have more exodontia experience than a maxillofacial surgeon who has just completed a residency.

Dr. Gordon Christensen has stated that if a GP "feels competent to accomplish a procedure and can do it to the level of a specialist, do not hesitate to incorporate that procedure into your practice."[9] The American Dental Association Principles of Ethics and Code of Professional Conduct states that "general dentists who wish to announce the services available in their practices are permitted to announce the availability of those services so long as they avoid any communications that express or imply specialization." The ADA advisory opinions, published in January 2009, state that nothing "prohibits a general dentist from truthfully informing the public that the dentist limits services to an area of dentistry not recognized as a specialty by the American Dental Association." Examples of areas of dentistry not recognized as specialties include cosmetic dentistry, temporomandibular disorders, implantology, and exodontia.

A GP with extensive experience and training in exodontia can practice in multiple offices as an independent contractor as long as he or she does not mislead the public regarding specialty status. The general dentist that limits his/her practice to the removal of impacted third molars should have extensive experience and many hours of continuing education in minor oral surgery. Alternatively, they should have completed Advanced Education in General Dentistry or General Practice residencies.

One could argue that the GP is held to a higher standard than the specialist. If a patient has inferior alveolar or lingual nerve paresthesia after a GP removes an impacted mandibular third molar, it may be assumed that the GP is incompetent or negligent. However, if a patient has paresthesia after the same procedure is completed by a maxillofacial surgeon, it may be assumed that it was a difficult procedure.

Mobile Practice Promotion

Building a viable third mobile practice is not easy, especially for a GP. Routine procedures are usually completed by general dentists. Challenging procedures and difficult patients are referred to specialists. Dentists who want to reduce referrals are usually looking for a contractor or specialist for their office. The GP mobile third molar dentist must convince potential offices that they are as competent removing impacted third molars as the maxillofacial surgeon who has credentials and years of formal training. Potential offices want someone who will enhance their office and increase new patient flow.

The typical office will resist working with a non-oral surgeon. Building this type of practice will take time, even for the oral surgeon. I recommend maintaining your existing practice or employment while building your mobile practice. No one is going to call you to request your services until you have established a good reputation within your community and have built a solid base of referrals. How do you get started?

Word of Mouth

Start marketing your practice by word of mouth. It doesn't cost anything and it can be very effective. Contact every dentist, classmate, and staff member that you know and offer your services. Consider offering a complimentary day of patient treatment to demonstrate your skills. This is a small concession in exchange for a relationship that could last years.

Community Service

Community service lets people know you can deliver quality third molar services. It's also a way to meet other dentists who might want to work with you. I have volunteered several times for Dentistry From The Heart (DFTH). DFTH is a worldwide nonprofit organization dedicated to providing free dental care to those in need. Every year, thousands of dentists, hygienists, and staff donate their time and resources at DFTH events. This type of community service represents a golden opportunity to interact with dental teams and showcase your skills and compassion.

Another example of community service is the free dental clinic. Many communities offer free medical and dental to low-income families. These clinics usually welcome volunteers, especially dentists with special skills.

Dental Meetings

What better venue than dental meetings to meet fellow dentists? Dentists love to talk about dentistry. Inevitably, the discussion turns to the economics of dentistry or where you practice. Most general dentists refer impacted third molars to specialists. Removal of impacted third molars is one of the most profitable services in dentistry. Take advantage of this opportunity to educate these dentists about your service.

Business Cards

Dental meetings and community service events are great venues to offer your business card. Never miss an opportunity to introduce yourself with a business card containing your website address. (See Box 16.1.) A business card portrays more than just a name, phone number, and web address. It can reflect a professional image or lack of it. A poor quality, dirty, or otherwise unimpressive business card will be quickly forgotten. Make your card stand out by using a professional printing service that offers high quality paper and a variety of patterns and colors to create visual appeal. Don't forget to include your logo.

Box 16.1 Offer your business card whenever possible.

Jane Doe, DDS – General Dentist
"Practice Limited To Impacted Third Molars."
www.thirdmolars.com
000-123-4567

Testimonials

A key part of promoting your service will be testimonials. Patient and dentist testimonials will add credibility to your mobile practice. Begin by collecting testimonials from your own patients. The patient testimonial is a powerful promotional device. Your mobile practice dentist testimonials should be added as your mobile practice grows. It's impossible to have too many testimonials. Testimonials can be written or video recorded.

Written testimonials are best used for direct mail to potential dental offices. They should contain the dentist's name and city where their office is located. This is much more meaningful than an anonymous testimonial. Video testimonials from patients work best on the internet and your website. Prospective offices need to know that their patients will be treated well.

Website

In today's business environment, a quality website is mandatory. Your website should communicate professionalism, organization, and precision. Every contact you make should link to your website through your business card. Your website should be both personal and professional. It should contain 6 elements. (See Box 16.2.)

Box 16.2 The mobile practice website should reflect professionalism, organization, and precision.

Video greeting and introduction	Dentist written testimonials
Your mobile practice story	Patient video testimonials
Biography and Curriculum Vitae	Personal interests – hobbies, family, etc

---

Social Media

Facebook, LinkedIn, and Twitter and other social media are essential marketing tools for the mobile third molar practice. Social media can have a big impact on your mobile practice success with very little cash invested. According to *Social Media Examiner*'s seventh annual Social Media Marketing Industry Report, 92% of marketers working with small businesses (between 2 and 10 employees) agree or strongly agree that social media is crucial to success.[10]

Social media posts are like virtual flyers or internet newspaper ads. Facebook groups can be private or public. These groups can help to build a community of like-minded dentists. LinkedIn and Twitter can help you stay in contact with dentists you know and dentists met at meetings or community service events. The ROI from social media can be impressive.

Making dentists aware of your mobile practice is good. Enticing them to visit your website is even better. Share blog posts, promote your services, and share important news about your mobile practice and third molar knowledge. When you share links on social networks, they should link to specific website pages or dedicated landing pages. Directing dentists to your homepage isn't as effective as sending them to pages containing patient video testimonials or surgical procedures.

Newsletter

In marketing, top-of-mind awareness (TOMA) refers to a brand or specific product being first in customers' minds when thinking of a particular industry or category.[11] A quarterly newsletter targeting offices in your area can help brand your services. In a survey of nearly 200 senior marketing managers, 50% responded that they found the "top-of-mind" metric very useful.[12] Your newsletter should contain valuable information related to the removal of impacted third molars. Case selection, complications, and surgical techniques are just a few topics available.

Direct Mail

Direct mail can be a very effective marketing tool. According to Direct Mail News, in 2012 the average response rate for direct mail was 4.4% for business-to-business mailing.[13]

The cost per lead of direct mail is in line with print and pay-per-click, and significantly less than telemarketing. Production costs are somewhat more than email, but the response rate is far better. Direct mail contacts, converted to long term relationships, generate many thousands of dollars in impacted third molar revenue. The value of these relationships must be weighed against the production costs of printing and mailing.

Post cards are the most cost effective direct mail method. The card should have a "sound bite" message on the front and detailed information and testimonials on the back. (See Figure 16.1a and 16.1b.)

(a)

WISDOM TEETH REMOVAL
...IN YOUR OFFICE!

(b)

www.IVwisdom.com
Impactions and Early Third Molar Removal

PRSRT STD
US POSTAGE PAID
PHOENIX, AZ
PERMIT # 5558

Don't Refer Third Molar Patients

Dr. Wayland will come to your office and remove impacted third molars and germectomies with IV sedation.

He has removed more than 25,000 third molars with IV sedation in more than 50 Bay Area offices.

Call 415-297-9046

Benefits for Your Office

• Your patients don't want to leave your office for third molar removal. They can stay in familiar surroundings where they are comfortable.

• Your patients sleep lightly and have no memory of the procedure.

• 30+ years of experience removing impacted third molars

• ACLS certified and a conscious sedation evaluator for the California Dental Board

• Master of the College of Sedation, American Dental Society of Anesthesiology

Testimonials

Dr. Wayland is exceptionally knowledgeable, talented, and above all, caring and considerate of patients and staff. –Frank Gontarski, DDS

My patients have been very satisfied with his surgery. –Yvonne Wong, DDS

Thank you so much Dr. Wayland for making my practice a success. –Linda Ridder, DDS

Dr. W is an excellent surgeon, my patients heal quickly without complications. Shital Kari, DDS

Dr. Wayland has made an astounding impact on my practice. –Cecelia Fetarang, DDS

My patients and their parents really appreciate that they can have their surgery performed in familiar surroundings. Without exception, the patients' experiences with Dr. Wayland have been positive. –Synneve Skeie, DDS

Figure 16.1a and 16.1b Direct mail should be used as an adjunct to other promotional efforts.

Imagine a typical day in your mobile third molar practice. A very relaxed schedule might be three patients in the morning, lunch, and three more in the afternoon. A reasonable fee for the removal of four impacted third molars with sedation should be at least $1500. We now have a $9000 production day. 50% compensation results in $4500 for the day with virtually no overhead. Now imagine repeating this day 10 times a month for many years. I think you get the point. Removal of third molars is profitable!

Everything you do to promote your mobile practice has one objective – an introductory meeting with the dentist and entire staff. The staff members need to be familiar with your practice philosophy and protocol. This is your chance to impress the office. A key element of the initial office meeting is the Procedure Manual. It is given to every office, as a reference, at the initial meeting. The manual is reviewed with the dentist and staff at the meeting. Using the manual and briefing guide allows you to control the meeting. The manual is reviewed and questions are answered.

Your procedure manual should be customized to fit your practice. It should be comprehensive, including everything the office should know about your practice and patient treatment. It should include information about instrument set up, consultation appointments, consent forms, insurance and fees, sedation, and anything you think will benefit the office and patients. A well organized and professional procedure manual will increase your credibility. My procedure manual is included in this chapter for reference.

Third Molar Procedure Manual

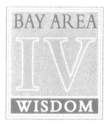

Early Third Molar Removal

JOHN B. WAYLAND, DDS, FAGD, MACSD
*Diplomate – American Dental Implant
Association*

123 Your Street
Anywhere, CA 00000

FAX: 000.000.0000
CELL: 000.000.0000
EMAIL: DDS@aol.com

Third Molar Removal with I.V. Sedation

Introduction

Welcome to your office manual on the selected removal of impacted third molars with IV sedation. This manual has been prepared to provide you with necessary information regarding the removal of third molars with IV sedation. It is divided into sections for easy reference and review.

Why Remove Third Molars?

A study published in the October 1985 issue of the *Journal of Oral and Maxillofacial Surgery* involved more than 16,000 impacted third molar extractions. This clinical study of more than 9,500 patients revealed that the optimum time for extraction is between the ages of 14 and 25 years. Results of the study show that as patients become older the incidence of post operative complications rise and become more significant and prolonged.

The American Association of Oral and Maxillofacial Surgeons also endorse the early removal of third molars. I personally have removed more than 25,000 impacted third molars without any significant complications. What I have learned is that case selection is critical to the success of third molar surgery. When specific guidelines are carefully observed third molars can be removed safely, comfortably, and predictably.

Why IV Sedation?

IV sedation is a safe and effective way to make patients comfortable during and after third molar surgery for the following reasons:

- Removing impacted third molars without some form of sedation is uncomfortable and patient management interferes with a quality surgery. This is not a practice builder. Conversely, virtually all of my patients have reported a comfortable experience with IV sedation.
- The degree of sedation can be controlled with IV sedation. Titration of the sedation drugs allows for complete control of the depth of sedation. Oral medication must be given in a bolus and the degree of sedation can vary from patient to patient.
- The IV route of drug administration provides a pathway for antagonistic drugs to reverse the effects of the sedation. This is not possible with oral sedation.

Guidelines for Third Molar Surgery

Preoperative Appointment

- Appointment 1–2 days before surgery
- Ages 14 to 25 years old
- Healthy ASA Category I and II patients
- Record preop vital signs on sedation record
- Good venipuncture site
- Pre op prescription given – Ibuprofen, Amoxicillin, Triazolam
- All consent forms reviewed with patient and/or parent, signed, and dated (3).

Patient selection is paramount to a successful outcome. Any patient scheduled for third molar surgery should be seen first for a preoperative appointment. Ideal patients are age 14 to 25. Patients in this age group are generally healthy, bone is relatively elastic, patients recover faster, and there is a lower incidence of dry socket. Vital signs are recorded at this appointment to provide a baseline measurement for the day of surgery.

All patients must be ASA category I or II patients to have oral or IV sedation. This means that they are healthy and without any known health risks.

Important

Medication Rx is given at the pre op appointment as follows:

Ibuprofen 800 mg three times a day x 15 tablets
Amoxicillin 500 mg three times a day x 15 tablets*
Triazolam .25 mg x 2 tablets

Take 800 mg ibuprofen and 500 mg amoxicillin one hour before surgery and continue, three times a day, until all medication is gone.

Bring triazolam (2 tablets) to appointment.

No food or liquids of any kind for 6 hours before appointment. A small amount of water may be used to take any medications prescribed for the appointment.

*(Amoxicillin allergy – Clindamycin (Cleocin) 300 mg, three times a day x 15 tablets)

Surgery Appointment

- Schedule 1 ½ hour appointments
- Set up operatory (see instruments Section 3)
- Dispense two .25 mg triazolam tablets (powder only) sublingual, without water, when patient arrives for their appointment. Ask them if they have had any food or liquids within the last 6 hours. Reschedule if not NPO for 6 hours.
- Wait ½ hour for oral sedative to reach peak concentration before seating patient
- Monoject 412 syringe dispensed to clean lower third molar surgical site

Patients ages 14 to 25 can be scheduled for one and a half hour appointments. Ideally, six patients would be scheduled in a given day. If six patients cannot be scheduled on a given day, it is recommended that a minimum of four appointments be scheduled for third molar surgery in the morning or afternoon. These guidelines will assure that these procedures are completed in an efficient and profitable way.

When the patient arrives at the office the assistant should question the patient to make sure that they are ready for surgery.

- Have they had any food or liquids six hours prior to appointment?
- Did they take their preoperative medication as prescribed?
- Are contact lenses removed?
- Are they wearing loose clothing?
- Do they have a ride home?
- Do they have any questions?

Postoperative Appointment

- Appointment scheduled one week following surgery
- Sutures removed
- Healing checked by dentist
- Review Monoject 412 socket irrigation

Postoperative appointments should be scheduled one week after the surgery. At one week most patients can open wide enough to comfortably remove sutures. Polyglycolic acid (PGA) sutures should dissolve completely in 7–10 days. Any remaining suture should be removed at this appointment.

A dentist should check for normal healing. Check for color, unusual pain, and exudate. Normal healing includes swelling, limited opening, and tenderness to palpation. Bruising is extremely unusual.

INSTRUMENTS / OPERATORY SETUP

Dr. Doe will provide instruments, monitors, and anesthesia supplies.
Contracted office will provide disposables listed below.

1 30 gauge needle
1 27 gauge needle
4 lidocaine 2% with epinephrine 1:100,000
2 Septocaine 4% with epinephrine 1:100,000
2 marcaine 5% with epinephrine 1:200,000
Vaseline
1 mask
1 medium latex glove box
1 protective eyewear
1 alcohol gauze
1 blanket
2 sterile monoject 412 syringes

#12 and #15 scalpel blades
2 sterile white surgical suction (101-2270) Schein
2 sterile green surgical suction (102-9023) Schein
1 ACE PGA 3.0 suture (003-3930) ACE Surgical
2×2 - filled gauze (100-8608) Schein
4×4 - 8 ply filled gauze (100-3725) Schein
Cool Jaw – T800C-4B (optional)

*Ace Surgical Supply 800-441-3100
*Henry Schein 800-372-4346
*Cool Jaw 877-411-7009

INSTRUMENTS / STERILIZATION

Weider retractor
Minnesota retractor
Hemostadt
Scissors
Needle holder
Bard parker handle (2)
Anesthetic syringes (2)
Cotton pliers
Periosteal elevator
Surgical currette
Root tip pick
46R elevator
Bite block
Metal dish

*15 instruments

Emergency Procedures

The state of California Board of Dental Examiners has mandated that all dentists using intravenous sedation must pass an evaluation and receive a permit to perform sedations. Knowledge of several emergencies must be demonstrated. Those emergencies and correct responses are listed below.

1) Airway Obstruction – high pitched "crowing" on inspiration, sternal retraction, thoraco-abdomial rocking, cyanosis
   - Head position with jaw thrust
   - Suction
   - Heimlich
   - Positive pressure oxygen with mask
2) Bronchospasm – impairment of respiratory exchange, <u>wheezing</u>, increased resistance to ventilation, cyanosis, desaturation
   - Patient in sitting position

- Positive pressure oxygen with mask
- Drugs: Isoprotenenol mist, epinephrine, steroids

3) Emesis and Aspiration – rales, dyspnea, tachycardia, partial airway obstruction, cyanosis, hypotension, desaturation
  - Patient positioning on right side, Trendelenburg position
  - Suction with large bore and Yankauer
  - Magill forceps
  - Positive pressure oxygen
  - Drugs for bronchospasm (Ventolin or Alupent), blood pressure

4) Angina Pectoris – chest pain lasting a few minutes, palpitations, faintness, dizziness, dyspnea
  - Recognize problem
  - Oxygen
  - Drugs – Nitroglycerin spray sublingually up to 3 doses

5) Myocardial Infarction – chest pain, dsypnea, anxiety, weakness, hypotension
  - Recognize problem-chest pain unresponsive to nitroglycerin
  - Oxygen
  - Drugs
    1) Pain – Morphine sulfate 3–4 mg IV and administer 1 aspirin orally, or Demerol or Nubain
    2) Heart rate – Atropine
    3) Blood Pressure
  - Hospital?

6) Hypotension – progressive reduction in blood pressure, impending loss of consciousness, nausea, weakness
  - Recognize problem and cause
  - Position patient – Trendelenburg position, open airway
  - IV fluids
  - Drugs – Ephedrine or epinephrine (Vasopressor) Consider Narcan and Flumazenil (Romazicon)
  - Sequential blood pressure

7) Hypertension – elevated blood pressure, headache, blurred vision
  - Preventive measures
  - Oxygen
  - Reassure patient
  - Blood pressure
  - Niphedipine (Procardia) 10 mg sublingual?
  - Hospital?

8) Cardiac Arrest
  - Basic CPR
  - Positive pressure oxygen
  - Start IV

9) Allergic Reaction – rash, edema, dyspnea/wheezing, salivation, tearing, rhiitis, pruritis, urticaria
  - Diagnosis: Mild (Diphenhydramine/Benadryl 50 mg) to Severe (Epinephrine 3-5cc 1:10,000)
  - Trendelenburg position
  - Oxygen
  - IV fluids
  - Drugs – Benadryl or Epinephrine
  - Hospital?

10) Convulsions – tonic-clonic convulsion, excessive salivation, poor air exchange, disorientation
    - Cause
    - Prevent injury – place patient on side with head extended, restrain patient, open airway
    - Oxygen
    - Monitor respiration
    - Drugs – Valium 10 mg
    - Hospital?
11) Hypoglycemia – sudden onset, history of insulin administration and inadequate intake of food, dizziness, weakness, nausea, possible loss of consciousness, low blood sugar
    - Diagnosis
    - Drugs- administer oral dextrose, oxygen, IV 50% dextrose
    - Hospital?
12) Syncope
    - Position patient
    - Oxygen
    - Check vital signs
13) Respiratory Depression – poor air exchange, decreased chest expansion, falling oxygen saturation, possible cyanosis
    - Correct anatomical airway
    - Positive pressure oxygen with mask
    - Drug antagonist – Narcan
    - Monitor vital signs

MEDICAL HISTORY

1) **Have you ever had any problems with:**

Heart _____

Diabetes _____

Lungs _____

Epilepsy _____

Kidney _____

High Blood Pressure _____

Liver _____

Low Blood Pressure _____

Asthma _____

Seizures _____

Allergies _____

Reaction to anesthetic _____
(General, Local, Sedation)

2) **Medications routinely used at home** _____

3) **Past surgeries:**

Dates   **Operation**   **Type of Anesthesia** (General, local, sedation)

_____

_____

4) **Do you smoke?** _____ **Packs / Day?** _____ **Number of years?** _____

5) **Do you drink alcohol?** _____ **How often?** _____

6) **Have you ever had any health problems we should know about?** _____

Patient Name _____

_____   _____
Patient's or Guardian's Signature   **Date**

_____   _____
Witness Signature   **Date**

_____   _____
Doctor's Signature   **Date**

PRE – SURGICAL INSTRUCTIONS

Patient Name: _____

Today's Date: _____ **Surgery Date & Time:** _____

It is extremely important that you follow these instructions prior to your appointment for surgery.

1) **No food or drink within six (6) hours of your appointment.**
   If your appointment is in the morning, do not have anything to eat or drink from midnight the night prior to your appointment day. If your appointment is in the afternoon, you should have a light breakfast in the morning, as long as you finish your meal six (6) hours prior to your appointment.

   *A small amount of water may be used to take any medications prescribed for your appointment.

2) **Pain and Infection Control – TAKE MEDICATIONS AS DIRECTED**
   Take ibuprofen and amoxicillin one hour prior to appointment. Bring triazolam (2 tablets) to your appointment.

   *If you are allergic to amoxicillin you will be given another antibiotic.

3) **Do not drive on the day of your appointment.**
   You will be sedated during your appointment. We will not be able to release you unless you have a responsible adult to drive you home.

4) **If you are not able to follow these instructions we cannot complete the planned treatment.**

I HAVE READ AND UNDERSTAND THE ABOVE ENTIRELY.

_____

Patient's or Guardian's Signature

POST – SURGICAL INSTRUCTIONS

1) **DO NOT CHEW FOOD, RINSE, BRUSH TEETH, OR SMOKE FOR TWO DAYS AFTER SURGERY.**
   Avoid all foods that require chewing for 2 days after surgery. Drink lots of liquids and eat soft foods that can be swallowed easily. Ginger Ale, Ensure, Jamba Juice (no straw), ice cream, yogurt, soups (broth only), and similar food is recommended.

2) **SWELLING**
   - **ICE (TODAY ONLY)** - Swelling normally increases for three to four days following surgery and then gradually decreases. Ice (or a bag of frozen peas) may be applied for 15 minutes and removed for 15 minutes, alternating on and off.
   - **WARM SALT WATER RINSE (AFTER 2 DAYS)** - RINSE YOUR MOUTH GENTLY WITH WARM SALT WATER. Use ½ teaspoon of salt per cup of warm water. Rinse for one minute 5-6 times per day for four days.

3) **TAKE MEDICATION THREE TIMES A DAY**
   Take ibuprofen and amoxicillin 3 times a day, "by the clock", until all medication is gone. For example, take both medications when you wake up, when you go to sleep, and once in between. You should do this even if you do not experience pain. Two Extra Strength Tylenol (500 mg) can be taken with ibuprofen 4 times a day if needed for pain. Do not exceed 8 Tylenol Extra Strength tablets per day.

4) **BLEEDING WILL CONTINUE THROUGHOUT THE FIRST DAY**
   - Sleep is recommended after surgery. Blood pressure is lowered when sleeping which helps to slow bleeding. Upon waking, clean any excess blood, begin using ice, eat something soft and drink liquids.
   - Cotton gauze should be removed when sleeping.
   - If bleeding is excessive, wipe away any old clots and place a moist tea bag on the surgical site. Any tea bag will work, but black tea is the most effective.
   - Talking and rinsing will increase bleeding

5) **PATIENTS SHOULD NOT BE LEFT ALONE THE DAY OF SURGERY**

6) **USE THE PLASTIC IRRIGATION SYRINGE AFTER 4 DAYS.**
   Fill the syringe with warm water. After each meal, place the syringe tip into the lower sockets and flush out food until clean. Continue using until the socket is closed, usually about one month.

NOTE: If you have any reason or believe that you are not recovering satisfactorily, please call Dr. Wayland at (000) 123-4567.

PROGRESS NOTES

Patient_____ Date_____

SUBJECTI3VE

Asymptomatic   Orthodontics   Pain   LL   LR   UL   UR

OBJECTIVE

Roots   0-1/3   1/3-1/2   1/2-2/3   2/3-1/1   1/1

Access   Good   Large tongue   Small mouth   Limited opening

Ramus proximity to third molar   0   0 – 1/2   1/2 - 1

Tissue distal   1_____ 16_____17_____32_____None_____

Angulation   1_____ 16_____17_____32_____

Malampatti class   I   II   III   IV

ASSESSMENT

Impaction Pericornitis GP Class   I   II   III   Orthodontics

PROCEDURE - See IV record

Risk, alternatives, benefits   PT   MO   FA   B   S   FR   GFR   BFR   W   H

● 1	Flap	RBODB		Section		ED		BF	I	1x3.0 PGA
● 16	Flap	RBODB		Section		ED		BF	I	1x3.0 PGA
● 17	Flap	RBODB		Section		ED		BF	I	1x3.0 PGA
● 32	Flap	RBODB		Section		ED		BF	I	1x3.0 PGA

Post-op written and oral   MO   FA   B   S   FR   GFR   BFR   W   H

Complications_____

Signature_____

PROGRESS NOTES KEY

SUBJECTIVE: LL, lower left; LR, lower right: UL, upper left; UR, upper right

OBJECTIVE:

Roots = root development

Access = surgical access

Ramus proximity to third molar   0 = room for eruption

0 – 1/2 = some of the third molar is in the ramus

1/2 – 1 = most or all of the third molar is in the ramus

Tissue distal = tissue covering distal of third molar

Angulation = Mesioangular, distoangular, vertical, horizontal, transverse

ASSESSMENT: Diagnosis. GP class is Gregory Pell position class I, II, or III

PLAN / PROCEDURE:
Risk, alternatives, benefits given to patient, mother, father, brother, sister, friend, girlfriend boyfriend, wife, or husband

RBODB = remove buccal, occlusal, distal bone

ED = elevator delivery

BF = bone file

I = irrigation

1x3.0 PGA = one 3.0 polyglycolic suture

Post operative instructions given to mother, father, brother, sister, friend, girlfriend boyfriend, wife, or husband

SEDATION RECORD

Patient Name: _____**Surgery Date:** _____

Pre-op: Height: _____Weight_____ B.P _____ Pulse _____Date: _____

Verifications: NPO6hr ____ Consent _____ Rx _____ ASA _____ Airway _____ Rationale _____ M / F

I.V. Infusion: Started: _____ a.m. / p.m. with a _____ gauge Catheter in_____

Time (1 box = 10 min)																			
B.P.																			
Pulse																			
Resp																			
O2																			
ETCO2																			
2% Lidocaine **1:100,000**																			
5% Marcaine **1:200,000**																			
4% Septocaine **1:100,000**																			
Fentanyl **(50 mcg/ml)**																			
Midazolam **(1 mg/ml)**																			
Dexamethasone **(4 mg/ml)**																			
Triazolam **(.5 mg)**																			
Zolpidem **(10 mg)**																			

The procedure lasted _____ hrs _____ minutes and the patient received _____ ml of D5W / NS. The patient tolerated the procedure well and was discharged at _____ a.m. / p.m. in good condition to the custody of_____ _____ . Written and verbal postoperative instructions were given.

AMBULATORY   **ALERT**   **CONVERSATIONAL**

Complications: _____

_____   _____

DENTIST   ANESTHETIST

Third Molar Impaction Consent

What Is an Impacted Tooth?

An impacted tooth is a tooth that has not erupted normally. It may be covered by bone as well as gum tissue. Impacted teeth that press against other teeth may cause damage to those teeth. They may also cause crowding, infections, swelling, pain, cysts, earaches, headaches, generalized head and neck pain, and even tumors.

What Is a Surgical Extraction?

Since impacted teeth are partially or completely beneath the surface of the gum tissue or bone, their removal is a surgical procedure. A surgical extraction requires the removal of bone, soft tissue incisions, or sectioning of teeth. Pain medication and instructions will control post-operative pain, swelling, bleeding, and discomfort.

Discomfort, Swelling, Limited Opening, and Bleeding are Normal Following
Surgical Extractions

Slight bleeding may continue until the morning following surgery. The corners of the mouth may be irritated. Curved and thin root tips can fracture during extraction. They are usually removed, but may be left in place if they are near vital structures. Post-operative infections occasionally occur and are treated with antibiotics. Because of the close proximity of impacted teeth to adjacent teeth, occasionally a tooth or dental restoration may be damaged. VERY RARELY, post-operative complications include sinus opening, displacement of a tooth into the sinus or infra temporal fossa, lip or tongue numbness which can be temporary or permanent, damage to other oral structures, severe infections, jaw joint problems and broken jaws. In extremely rare circumstances even death may occur. A CT scan radiograph (xray) may be recommended when a wisdom tooth is near a nerve.

We will do our very best to make this a comfortable experience. If you have any questions please ask for clarification.

I UNDERSTAND THAT DR. WAYLAND IS **NOT** *AN ORAL SURGEON. I HAVE READ AND UNDERSTAND THE ABOVE ENTIRELY AND HEREBY CONSENT TO THE PERFORMANCE OF SURGERY AS PRESENTED TO ME.*

_____

Patient's or Guardian's Signature   **Date**

_____

Witness Signature   **Date**

_____

Doctor's Signature   **Date**

IV SEDATION AND WISDOM TEETH BRIEFING*

Why is early removal of wisdom teeth recommended?
- 5 year study
- How to explain to parents that wisdom teeth need early removal. Big oak tree vs. little oak tree.

Case selection
- Age – 14 to 25 with some exceptions
- Good health, ASA 1-2
- Partial root development

Preop vist – day before surgery
- Amoxicillin 500mg, 15, one hour before appointment and then one three times a day until gone. For infection.
- Ibuprofen 800mg, 15, one hour before appointment and one three times a day until gone. For inflammation and pain.
- Triazolam .25mg, 2, bring medication to appointment
- Review forms and consents and have them signed. Take BP and pulse and record on IV record.
- Give patient Pre-Surgical Instructions to take home

Surgery day
- Schedule 1 ½ hour per patient. Actual surgery averages about 30 minutes
- Consents, medication, no food or drink for 6 hours
- Triazolam .5 mg, in office, 1/2 hour before appointment. For anxiety
- Post op instructions in writing
- Cool Jaw Ice and Compression

Post op visit
- Expect tenderness, normal color, and limited opening
- Check for color, exudates, and unusual pain
- Remove sutures

IV Sedation / Oral Sedation
- Safety
- Patient and clinical expectations

Scheduling
- Schedule target date in advance
- Use letters to communicate with patient and parent

Insurance and fees
- Most are billed as completely bony impactions
- Use your office fee schedule – IV fee can be adjusted

*This form is for the initial office meeting. Please refer to the Guidelines section of the procedure manual for pre-op, surgery, and post-op details.

Third Molar Research

This section contains third molar research articles and studies. My manual has 13 articles including the 2007 AAOMS white paper on third molars.

CONTRACTUAL AGREEMENT FOR DENTAL SERVICES

This agreement is entered into on this 1st day of January 2016 by John Doe, DDS, *(hereinafter termed Lessor),* and John B. Wayland, DDS, FAGD, MaCSD *(hereinafter termed Lessee).*

RECITALS

A) Lessor owns and possesses a leasehold interest in the dental office located at 1234 Dental Avenue, Anywhere, CA 12345. Lessor and Lessee are both licensed dentists, duly licensed to practice their respective professions by the state of California.

B) Lessee desires to perform and deliver oral surgery services and other associated procedures at the aforementioned premises to numbers of the general public (hereinafter termed "Patients"), subject to the terms and conditions as set forth herein.

C) In consideration for the mutual promises herein contained, and other valuable consideration, the Lessor and Lessee agree to the following terms and conditionsas set forth herein.

   I **STATUS of the PARTIES**
1) Lessee is an independent dental contractor.
2) All patients referred to Lessee by Lessor for said treatment shall remain the responsibility of the Lessee for that respective treatment until that treatment has been completed, suspended either because of termination of this agreement as provided in Section X (2) or otherwise interrupted due to unforeseeable circumstances.

  II **TERMS of the CONTRACTUAL AGREEMENT**
1) The terms of this agreement shall remain effective unless otherwise terminated by written notice from either respective party hereto at any time during any period thereof. Such termination notice shall be provided to other party with at least 30 days prior to date of expected termination.
2) Following receipt of the termination notice or expiration of that respective period, any extensions beyond the "pre-agreed" deadline will not be allowed, unless superseded by a new written agreement memorialized by both parties prior to that deadline.
3) The terms of this agreement shall remain effective for an initial period of *one year*, unless otherwise terminated in accordance with provisions designated in Section II (1), or Section II (2).
4) Following the completion of the initial period, the terms of this agreement shall continue in full force for additional periods of *one year*, unless otherwise terminated in accordance with provisions designated in Section II (1), or Section II (2).
5) The terms of this agreement may be extended for additional *one year* periods provided that both parties mutually agree and abide with the provisions of this agreement.

 III **DENTAL SERVICES**
1) Lessee shall engage in the performance and delivery of oral surgery treatment aforementioned at the said premises. Said services shall be rendered in compliance with the provisions of the **Dental Practice Act** of the State of California, Rules and Regulations.
2) Lessee shall record and maintain accurate records of all treatment provided to all patients treated at the premises. Lessor shall maintain possession of the original charts, radiographs, and related materials for said services performed by Lessee on patients at the premises.
3) Lessee shall have the right to an audit of all records related to said services provided by Lessee to patients at the premises.

4) Upon request made by Lessee to Lessor, Lessor shall provide Lessee, within a reasonable time not to exceed 14 days, up-to-date copies of those materials requested by Lessee related to said services performed by Lessee.

IV FURNISHINGS, FURNITURE, and EQUIPMENT

1) Lessor hereby agrees to provide to Lessee and Lessee hires from Lessor nonexclusive use of the clinical and administrative equipment, furniture, and furnishings within the premise. The use of this equipment, furniture, and furnishings shall be subject to the following conditions:

   a) Title to the Lessor's equipment, furniture, and furnishings will remain the Lessor's at all times, unless otherwise stipulated by mutual consent of both parties hereto, title to equipment, furniture, and materials provided by Lessee shall remain the Lessee's, unless otherwise stipulated by mutual consent of both parties hereto.

   b) Maintenance and repair of the respective equipment, furniture, and furnishings shall be the responsibility of the respective party.

V SUPPLIES

1) Lessor agrees to provide for Lessee all administrative and clinical materials to reasonably enable Lessee to carry out the professional day-to day delivery of said services at the premises and shall be subject to the following conditions:

   a) Lessor and Lessee agree to be responsible for providing all personal surgical instrumentation and materials used in the delivery of said services at the premises, for providing an emergency number service made available to all patients seen by Lessee. In addition, Lessee agrees to maintain malpractice insurance to cover the delivery of said services at the premises.

VI PERSONNEL

1) Lessor agrees to provide all the necessary personnel to handle all patient scheduling, clerical, bookkeeping, billing, coordination and sequencing of treatment with Lessor or other doctors, maintenance of patient records.

2) Lessor agrees to provide competent staff to assist Lessee in the delivery of the said services for patients at the premises.

VII DISBURSEMENT for LESSEE'S SAID SERVICES

1) Lessor agrees to pay Lessee, **on the day services are delivered**, a fee equal to **fifty percent (50 %) of Lessee's production** for the delivery of services at the premises.

2) The term **"production for delivery of said services"** means the actual fees charged for delivery of said services, services designated by procedure code, and which reflect actual services provided by Lessee at the premises.

3) At the end of each tax year, Lessor will provide Lessee with a copy of **IRS form 1099-MISC.**

VIII INSURANCE

1) Lessee agrees to provide, keep, and maintain malpractice insurance coverage of at least $1,000,000 per claim and $3,000,000 in aggregate throughout the entire term of this agreement to cover the delivery of said services at the premises.

2) Lessor agrees to provide, keep, and maintain general liability of insurance for the premises for the same said period.

IX INDEPENDENT CONTRACTUAL RELATIONSHIP

1) Lessor and Lessee shall indemnify, defend, and hold each other harmless from and against any liability, loss, cost, expense, demand or claim asserted by or in behalf of any patient arising from the delivery of said services rendered to said patient by either party.

X **TERMINATION**

1) Lessor and Lessee agree that the clinical materials and records of patient's treated by Lessee at the premises during initial period or any following periods are the property of Lessor. Said patients will always remain as Lessor's patients of records. It is further agreed and understood that ongoing professional care of those patients of record, other than the delivery of said services provided by Lessee noted herein, will remain the responsibility of Lessor.

This instrument as construed is in accordance with the laws of the State of California, and represents the complete and total agreement of both parties. Any additions, deletions or modification to this agreement will require a new written agreement endorsed by both parties in order to become effective.

Dated this 1st day of January, 2017

_____   _____
John Doe, DDS, Lessor   John Wayland, DDS, FAGD, MaCSD Lessee

DOCUMENTS

This section should include all legal documents pertaining to your practice. My dental license, sedation permit, DEA permit, and insurance declaration are included in this section of my procedure manual.

SCHEDULING LETTER

The letter below has been helpful when initially scheduling patients. Your office can send this letter to the parents of all teenagers between the ages of 13 and 19. It is a good idea to check the charts of patients slightly older as well. You can modify the letter as necessary for any patient.

This letter can also be used after a recall exam to introduce the procedure to your patients.

Mr. And Mrs. Guardian of Patient   January 1, 2016
1234 Main Street
Your City, CA 94010

Dear John and Jane,

The ideal time to remove wisdom teeth is before the roots are fully developed. Removing wisdom teeth early has been shown to decrease future pathology and surgical complications. Furthermore, most orthodontists recommend the removal of wisdom teeth to prevent crowding of the remaining teeth. Jill's dental record indicates that it may be time to remove her wisdom teeth.

Dr. John Wayland, limits his practice to wisdom teeth removal, and is available to do the procedure in our office with IV sedation. Jill will be comfortable during the procedure and will typically have little or no memory of the event. I've enclosed Dr. Wayland's biography for your review.

An updated panographic xray is needed to evaluate the status of Jill's wisdom teeth. Please call our office at (000) 123-4567 to schedule an appointment for this xray.

Sincerely,

Your Name, DDS

Scheduling Protocol

All offices have a tentative date scheduled with Dr. Wayland in their appointment book. Patient panoramic radiograph, age, and a general statement of health are sent to Dr. Wayland at IVwisdom@aol.com prior to scheduling and financial arrangements. Panos should be included in the email as an attachment. Dr. Wayland will approve panos and recommend insurance codes for each case.

Examples of email sent to Dr. Wayland .

1) John Doe, age 18, no medical problems.
2) Mary Doe, age 16, asthma, tetracycline for acne
3) Justin Doe, age 38, recent heart bypass surgery, taking several medications.

Examples of Dr. Wayland response.

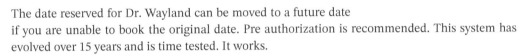

1) OK to schedule, 4 FBI
2) OK to schedule, 1+16 STI, 17+32 FBI
3) Recommend referral

The date reserved for Dr. Wayland can be moved to a future date
if you are unable to book the original date. Pre authorization is recommended. This system has evolved over 15 years and is time tested. It works.

Scheduling Tips

Scheduling dental patients is a challenge for any dental procedure, but this is especially true for removing wisdom teeth. People may have friends that have had a very bad experience removing wisdom teeth leaving them nervous about the procedure. The best way to handle this situation is to educate the patient.

Since our patients of choice will be between the age of 14 and 20, you will be scheduling the surgery with the parent or guardian of the patient. Parents will often be extremely protective of their child and rightfully so since they are the parents and you are trying to schedule surgery for their child. Please be aware and sensitive to the issues that concern the parents. The bottom line is, you are asking a parent to approve and allow you to schedule surgery for their child.

Get all their questions and attempt to answer them. If you cannot answer any of the questions, please insure them that you would get the answer for them as soon as you get a chance to call Dr. Wayland. Make sure they know that you will call them back later the same day to give them answers. While you may not be able to give them all the answers they need, you will need to make the parents feel comfortable, or less nervous, about the procedure by giving them information as well as answering their questions.

Explain to the patient and the parents why wisdom teeth should be removed while the patient is a teenager and how their child can benefit from early removal:

1) Teenagers typically do not have fully developed roots on their wisdom teeth. After the teenage years, wisdom teeth, if not removed, will have developed roots with hooks on them. These can break and cause damage to nerves or openings into their sinus.
2) Teenagers typically heal faster than older patients.
3) The procedure is much more predictable in teenagers than older patients. Because of this, the chances of complications for teenagers are reduced to a minimum.

The patients and the parents should be informed that every patient might respond differently to any procedure. If they have friends who had a bad experience, it does not mean they will experience the same. Try to find out what "bad experience" they are concerned about. You will need to determine what the real issues are based on the information you get from your patient and their parents. Once you understand the concerns, you are on your way to putting the patient and their parents at ease by addressing their concerns as well as giving some basic information about the early third molar removals and IV sedation.

The word "surgery" may get the parent upset. It makes removing wisdom more scary and risky than it really is. Try using the word "procedure" in place of "surgery" when you talk to the patient or their parents. This will leave a different and hopefully more positive impression of the procedure in their minds.

IV sedation is not general anesthesia. Sedation is used to make the patient as comfortable as possible during the procedure. Most patients will be asleep during the procedure and, although they can respond to commands, will not remember the procedure. To the patient, it will seem as if it only took ten minutes to remove their wisdom teeth when it really took 45 minutes. Sometimes it really does only take ten minutes to remove four teeth, but each patient will have different experiences.

If you find that the patient and/or their parents continue to have concerns about the procedure after giving them all the information you have, let them know that Dr. Wayland can call them and speak with them on the phone to address their concerns and address any questions they may have on the procedure. If this is necessary, please call and give Dr. Wayland a summary of the situation and what you think the primary concerns are, along with the patient's name, parent's names, and a number to contact them on. Dr. Wayland will call as soon as he possibly can.

Insurance

The recommended sedation fee is $500. However, insurance may not pay for IV sedation. Only a few offices get paid from Delta. Other companies are more likely to pay.

The average fee accepted by insurance companies for a completely bony impaction is $425. The highest Delta fee that I have seen is $550. The minimum fee for four full bony impactions, with IV sedation, should not be lower than $1,900.

You can use the sedation fee to reach this minimum. For example, a patient with four completely bony impactions is covered at $250 for each impaction. The patient would be responsible for their co-payment for the surgery plus $900 for the sedation. This would reach the $1,900 minimum.

The other situation would be an office that has a high surgery fee and the patient does not want to pay for the sedation fee. For example, the same patient is covered at $475 or more for each impaction. You have reached the minimum of $1,900 with the surgery alone. The IV sedation fee can be used as a scheduling tool. If you feel a patient may not schedule because they do not want the out of pocket cost of the sedation fee, you could adjust the IV sedation fee to the satisfaction of the patient. If necessary, you could waive the sedation fee, especially if you feel this is the only thing keeping them from scheduling the appointment. Keep in mind that the fee for four completely bony impactions, with IV sedation, should not be lower than $1,900.

I believe the $500 IV sedation fee is reasonable and should not be waived except in special cases.

PROCEDURE CODES

09243 IV Sedation per 15 minutes

07210 Surgical removal of erupted tooth
07220 Soft tissue impaction (STI)
07230 Partial bony impaction (PBI)
07240 Completely bony impaction (FBI)

Summary

The mobile third molar practice is not going to be a good fit for everyone. However, this niche might be the answer if you love to remove third molars and have the necessary skills. Creating a viable mobile third molar practice is challenging, but the rewards are many. Reduced stress, scheduling flexibility, low overhead, and financial freedom are just are few of the benefits awaiting you.

Contributing authors, Mathew Diercks and Jamieson Brady, share their mobile third molar stories in the following chapters.

References

1 Felton JS. Burnout as a clinical entity – its importance in healthcare workers. *Occup Med*. 1998;48: 237–250.

2 Osborne D, Croucher R. Levels of burnout in general dental practitioners in the south-east of England. *Brit Dent J*. 1994;177:372–7.

3 Gorter RC, Freeman F. Burnout and engagement in relation with job demands and resources among dental staff in Northern Ireland. *J Affect Disord*. 2011;9: 87–95.

4 Divaris K, Polychronopoulou A, Taoufik K, Katsaros C, Eliades T. Stress and burnout in postgraduate dental education. *Eur J Dent Educ*. 2012;16: 35–42.

5 Lang R. Stress in dentistry — it could kill you! Oral Health, 2007 Sept 1.

6 Solomon E. The future of dental practice: demographics dental economics. 2015 Apr 10.

7 Diringer J, Phipps K, Carsel B. Critical trends affecting the future of dentistry: assessing the shifting landscape. Prepared for the American Dental Association, 2013 May.

8 Weston J. The multispecialty practice: a unique practice model for challenging times. *Dent Econ*. 2016 Oct 26;106(10).

9 Christensen GJ. Interaction between GPs and specialists. *Dent Econ*. 2016 Oct 26;106(10).

10 Olenski S. Social media for small business: how it's different from how big brands do it. CMO Network, 2015 Oct 29.

11 7 publicity myths that can hurt your business by Pam Lontos, published in exchange magazine. 2012.

12 Farris P, et al. *Marketing metrics: the definitive guide to measuring marketing performance*. Upper Saddle River, NJ: Pearson Education, Inc., 2010.

13 Beasley L. Why direct mail still yields the lowest cost-per-lead and highest conversion rate. On Line Marketing Institute, 2013 Jun 13.

17

My Mobile Practice

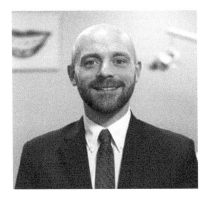

Jamieson Brady, DDS

A Different Way to Practice

My career could be considered non-traditional because while I am a general dentist, I've never practiced general dentistry. After graduation I entered an Oral Surgery internship at Cook County Hospital in Chicago where I worked in a fast-paced extraction clinic, treating low-income patients of all ages. After leaving the internship, I took over for a retiring oral surgeon at a group practice and continued to focus my practice exclusively on extractions.

Getting Started

Only repetition and training can increase speed and efficiency. This is not provided in dental school. The job I took was a great opportunity to increase my speed because the office was extremely high volume. I would see anywhere from 20 to 30 patients a day for extractions under local anesthesia. I was able to hone my skills, gain confidence and clinical proficiency, and increase my speed. I was also able to encounter complications that undoubtably occur to any doctor who does enough surgery. I was able to see my follow-ups, learn from mistakes, and perfect my technique.

However, since this office mostly treated public aid patients, the production numbers were bleak considering the amount of work I was doing. After just 3 years of practice, I was already starting to

Impacted Third Molars, Second Edition. Edited by John Wayland.
© 2024 John Wiley & Sons, Inc. Published 2024 by John Wiley & Sons, Inc.

experience major burnout. My hands were blistered, and I was developing pain in my shoulders and hands.

I learned about Dr. John Wayland on a post he made on Dentaltown.com, where he described how he successfully maintained a "mobile practice" where he works as a traveling dentist, providing third molar extraction services with IV sedation to many different dental offices. I realized that Dr. Wayland was teaching IV sedation in California, and I immediately signed up for his course. After training under Dr. Wayland and spending time shadowing him in his practice, I decided conclusively that this model of practice was something I wanted to pursue.

The Benefits of Mobile Practice

I was intrigued by the flexibility offered by this model. You can make your own schedule – work as much or as little as you want. You are not burdened by managing large numbers of staff or maintaining a physical location where your office is housed. Insurance claims are not a concern since they are handled by the host office. Assuming you love surgery more than other aspects of dentistry (which I do), it allows you to focus your practice on providing a procedure you enjoy doing.

On top of the freedom offered by a mobile practice, the model also makes sense financially, assuming you are able to fill your schedule. There are not many procedures in dentistry that offer higher production per hour than removing impacted third molars under IV sedation. The overhead is extremely low so you get to keep more of what you produce compared to most dental procedures. I split the collectable production with offices 50/50, and go home with a check at the end of each day.

One of the most memorable days of my career was the first time I had a completely full schedule of impacted third molars. After doing 9 surgeries back-to-back, I still felt energized. Compared to the 30 patients I was seeing in my public aid position; this was an easy day. I worked out of one operatory instead of three or four. And when I received my paycheck for the day I could not stop smiling. In just one day I was able to make more money than I had made in a week of hustling in my associateship. I immediately called Dr. Wayland to share my success and thank him for guiding me down this path.

My Process and Techniques

As of this writing I am fully employed in my mobile practice. My typical day consists of 4–8 extraction patients under IV sedation. My patients are referred to me by the host office in advance – I am able to review the panoramic radiographs and age of patient remotely, provide the office with the correct codes and amount of time I need for the procedure in advance. The host office then gives the patient an appointment on the day I am scheduled to be there and makes the financial arrangements.

When I arrive to the office, my assistant and I unload my car and convert the operatory into a surgical suite. I meet the patient (and usually their parents) for the first time, introduce myself, and consult them the same day as their planned procedure. Medical and surgical history is reviewed in detail. I discuss the risks, benefits, and alternatives with them, discuss the procedure, and provide after-care instructions. All questions are answered. Since the treatment plan and payment arrangements were completed in advance, it makes for a simple day.

After completion of the consultation, parents are dismissed to the waiting room and we begin with the surgery. I place the IV catheter, typically in the antecubital fossa or dorsal surface of the hand. Sedative medications are titrated slowly to achieve a state of moderate sedation. Local anesthesia is then achieved, which is arguably the most important step of the entire procedure. Without adequate local, the sedation will fail.

I approach every third molar extraction with the same technique. The first step is establishment of the flap. I create an envelops flap starting mesially at the mid-buccal of the first molar with a distal-buccal release distal to the second molar. If the tooth is a horizontal impaction, I may extend my envelope mesially by an additional tooth. It is critical not to stretch or tear the flap, as treatment of the soft tissue will greatly impact the postoperative course of healing for the patient.

After establishing access by creating a proper flap, the next step is bone removal. I use a #1703L bur on a straight handpiece to "trough" the buccal of the tooth until the CEJ of the crown is visualized. The purpose of creating a trough is to allow space for the tooth to move, and to create room to gain purchase with your elevator.

Before I section any tooth, I like to elevate the tooth gently to obtain "primary mobility." While I know the tooth will not come out without sectioning, I place elevator with a good purchase until the tooth starts to "rock in the socket." Engage the elevator point and elevate. In the case a root fractures, recovering the tooth fragments is much easier when they are mobile.

The next step is sectioning of the tooth. For mesioangular and vertical impactions, I hemisection the tooth, cutting through middle of the crown down to the furcation. For horizontal impactions, I also hemisection the tooth, but often times an additional section is required to remove the crown before removing the roots. The key with horizontal impactions is to remove the entire crown. For distoangular impactions, I remove the distal 2/3 of the crown to create space for the remaining tooth to move distally.

After sectioning is complete the tooth pieces are removed from the socket, I degranulate, irrigate copiously, and suture. Once the patient has recovered satisfactorily, they are dismissed and the process is repeated.

Getting Started

For those who may be interested in transitioning into a mobile practice I thought it would be useful to describe my path and how I was able to transition to full-time mobile practice quite quickly:

The first step to starting a mobile extraction practice is obviously to become clinically proficient in extractions. You will not be able to be successful unless you are able to provide high-quality treatment. Host offices will not ask you to return if you are not providing their patients with the highest level of care. You must be experienced in case selection, and know when to refer patients out of the office to avoid complications. And if complications arise, you should be well versed in handling them.

Reading oral surgery texts, continuing education, and shadowing experienced surgeons will get you started – but the only way to truly become a good surgeon is to do A LOT of surgery. You need repetitions. As I wrote, I was able to do this by working in a high-volume extraction clinic.

In my opinion, this model will not work unless you are certified to provide IV sedation. Being sedation certified sets you apart as a general dentist. While most general dentists can perform extractions, only a very small percentage are certified to provide IV sedation. This service is what makes your mobile practice extremely easy to market.

Once you are completely confident in your surgical skills, the next step is to acquire all of your own instrumentation. My setup includes 6 "trays" which are identical. You will also need an electric surgical motor with straight handpieces, vital signs monitors, anesthesia supplies, and a "crash cart" with emergency response equipment. Check your state laws to ensure that you are completely compliant. I prefer to bring everything I need with me to safely provide extraction and sedation services. The host office is in charge of providing disposables. Controlled substances are also ordered to the host office, not carried outside the office, and logged in compliance with DEA standards.

While starting a traditional dental office can cost anywhere from half a million to a million dollars, the mobile extraction practice can be started for significantly less. To purchase the equipment and instruments I would estimate I spent somewhere between $10,000 and $20,000. In a matter of a few good days you will be able to recoup your startup costs.

Personally, I also hired my own assistant who is experienced and certified in IV sedation. Some doctors rely on the office to provide staff, but for me bringing my own assistant is critical. I also ask the host office to provide me with an additional dedicated assistant who is BLS certified assistant to help with monitoring, sterilization, and patient flow.

After you have purchased the instrumentation necessary to provide extractions and IV sedation it is time to market your talents to potential offices who are in need of your services. Depending on your market, this could be the most difficult step. Ironically, my model works better in larger metro areas that are more saturated with general dentists. In smaller metro areas this practice model may not even be viable. If you work in a small town where every general dentist has a close relationship with their specialist, they not may be interested in bringing in an outside dentist.

Building Your Practice

Over the years I have identified key factors when determining whether or not a host office would be a good fit for a mobile exodontist. The busier an office is, the better it seems to work out. A good sign is when an office has several general dentists working in the same office. If they have an orthodontist or pediatric dentist, even better. And if they have extended hours – evenings and weekends – this is another good sign. The key is patient flow. If there are multiple dentists and specialists under one roof this typically means they have a high flow of patients.

In the beginning of my mobile practice journey, I worked in many single-doc offices on an as needed basis. What I found is that when there is only one doctor in the practice, they do not have the patient volume to consistently fill your schedule. Some days are very good, and other days there are no patients. Sometimes offices would cancel the day last minute, leaving me with an unexpected day off. There are exceptions to this rule, of course.

As time has gone on, I have concentrated my mobile practice into a small handful of group practices. These offices are much more consistent in providing a good schedule. I am able to come to these offices on a weekly basis, rather than just "as needed." This has resulted in a smaller logistical load when making my work schedule. And I have noticed that larger offices tend to be more organized, have better systems in place, and even communicate better with patients when it comes to giving preoperative instructions and making financial arrangements.

Building your practice takes considerable time and patience. I grew my practice through the use of a combination of techniques including classified ads, cold calling/cold emailing, and word of mouth.

Classified Ads

Classified ads on local dental society websites, indeed.com, and similar job post websites can be a valuable tool for locating host offices. I found my first position in my mobile practice by responding to a classified ad on the internet looking for a surgeon twice a month. This particular general dentist owns 2 offices and was looking to replace her itinerant oral surgeon because he was relocating out of state. I was able to secure an interview and confidently presented myself as a general dentist who only performs extractions. I got the job, cut back 2 days a month from my high-volume associateship, and worked for "myself" for the first time. My first day in mobile practice was the most I had ever produced at that point in my career and was a huge confidence booster.

Cold Calling/Cold Emailing

I have been able to source several opportunities by simply calling offices and making a pitch. In preparation for these calls, I Google search dental offices in the area I am interested in and check out their website. If the information on their website passes the initial filters (large office, multiple doctors, office appears busy, etc.) then I call the office and ask to speak with the hiring manager. Typically, the office manager or the doctor will come to the phone. I then introduce myself and describe my practice.

"Hi, this is Dr. Jamieson Brady. The reason I am calling is to ask how your office handles its third molar and IV sedation case referrals. I have a travelling surgery practice and I am available to come to your office on an as-needed basis to remove impacted third molars with IV sedation. I have my own assistant who comes to the office with me and bring all supplies necessary to provide extractions and IV sedation in your office. Is this something you might be interested in?"

This simple script is surprisingly successful. Sometimes the office is not interested and they let you know immediately, in which case you lost 5 minutes of your time and it cost you nothing. Many times, they are intrigued and want more details. Answer their questions with confidence and set up a time to come meet them in person to describe your operation in greater detail and make sure the office is a good fit for all parties involved.

You can also cold email a written version of this script to host offices, although I have not found much success in getting responses with that approach.

Word of Mouth

While not probable early in your journey, as time goes on word of mouth is an extremely powerful practice builder. Assuming you are providing excellent service, your name will make its way through the community quickly. Doctors you work with will speak highly of you to their colleagues and share your information. Often I find myself with voicemails from doctors I have never met inquiring about my services. Some of these have turned out to be my best offices and presently word of mouth is my only marketing tool.

Other Promotion Techniques

Other techniques which I don't personally use would be development of a website and promoting yourself online, networking at dental meetings or through local dental society, direct mail campaigns. You could also drive your prospective area and stop by promising offices to introduce yourself and offer your services directly. No one technique will work for everybody, so my advice is to try everything and see what works best for you. Most of all, have patience and persistence, and understand that while the process takes time in the end it is totally worth it.

Living the Dream

Although there is a lot to love about having a mobile practice, the model is not without its downsides. Certainly, this way of practicing is not for everybody. Working as a travelling dentist means you do not have a "home base" which at times can be frustrating. You need to dedicate part of your home to storing certain supplies which you plan to carry with you. Depending on the size of your home, this could be a burden. You must be willing to spend a lot of time in the car as it is unlikely that your host offices will all be located close to where you live. My offices are located within a

90-minute radius of my house, which means I drive roughly 2000 miles per month. The schedule can be unpredictable, especially in the beginning when you are building your practice. Lastly, you must make yourself available for postoperative issues. This means you will spend a lot of time communicating with patients on phone, triaging their issues, and on rare occasions traveling very far out of your way to handle follow-ups.

All in all I am so grateful to have found this path. The flexibility to make my own schedule, be free from the headaches of practice management, and low overhead combined with the freedom to practice how I want have made me more fulfilled than I could have imagined. Limiting my scope of practice to procedures I love allows me to enjoy my job while offering a higher quality of care to my patients. I would not have it any other way.

18

My Third Molar Journey

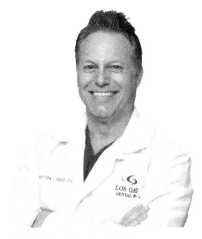

Dr. Matthew Diercks, DDS

The first time I met John Wayland was as a student taking his IV conscious sedation course. I had about 15 years of dental practice experience under my belt, and I was getting tired of referring third molar patients out to the oral surgeon because they wanted to be sedated. Removing third molars was always one of my favorite procedures and I wanted to do more of it and getting my IV sedation license was the missing puzzle piece that I needed to keep growing my skills. During the course John explained to me and the other students how his mobile third molar practice worked and I remember thinking to myself that it sounded kind of awful – driving around dealing with traffic, hauling equipment around, multiple offices, different operatories. It made me think of my early days in dentistry when I worked in several offices and was even doing some temp work just to fill my schedule. John and I became fast friends and it was maybe a year or so later that he asked me if I would be interested in taking over some of his mobile business as he cut back his workload. My first reaction was "thanks, but no thanks." I was a 50% owner in a very successful practice that my partner, our office manager and I had worked very hard to get to where it was and I had just finished paying off my business loan. We had a beautiful office with twelve operatories, three hygienists, and around ten supportive staff members. It was everything I had always dreamed of in dental school – I had finally reached what I thought was the pinnacle of my dental career so why would I want to leave all this for a mobile practice? John's offer kept spinning around in my brain and the more I thought about it the more interested I became in trying it out. I met with one of John's offices and started doing one day a month there removing wisdom teeth under IV sedation.

That one day a month quickly became my favorite day. I found that my days became much more enjoyable and easier when I was doing the same procedure all day. I was seeing five to ten patients per day, and my ability to provide safe, predictable IV sedation and third molar removal grew exponentially. My arrangement with offices that I work with is a 50-50 split of the collections, payable the day of service. See Figure 18.1.

Impacted Third Molars, Second Edition. Edited by John Wayland.
© 2024 John Wiley & Sons, Inc. Published 2024 by John Wiley & Sons, Inc.

There is no better feeling than having a full schedule doing the procedure you enjoy the most and then going home with a check for five to ten thousand dollars. I decided that this was something I wanted to do more of, I just had to figure out how to make it happen.

I have found that having options in life and work is always a good thing. I am in my early fifties and I want to have the option of retiring in ten to fifteen years. After thinking things through I decided that the best thing for me would be to split my time between my primary practice and the mobile third molar business. I can grow both businesses over the next ten years or so and eventually sell the primary business and scale back the mobile third molar business to whatever schedule suits my needs. Over

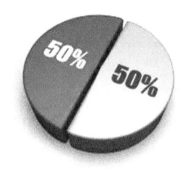

Figure 18.1 50% of collections. Photo from Berman, Fink, Van Horn.

time I cut my days in my primary office to three days a week (Monday through Wednesday) leaving Thursday, Friday, and Saturday available for the mobile third molar business. My partner and I brought in an associate to my primary office so we can each focus on the procedures we want to do which for me is third molars, implants, and endodontics. I rarely end up working all six days a week but I will gladly do it when needed because my third molar days are so profitable. Some days there are only three to five patients; I can be done by 2pm and still come home with a check for several thousand dollars.

When John was getting ready to write the second edition of this book he asked me to contribute a chapter detailing my experiences with the mobile third molar practice model and sharing insights that I have learned over the five years or so I have been doing it. I'll divide it into three sections: (1) what you need before you can start a mobile third molar business, (2) equipment and the day-to-day stuff, (3) the pros, cons, and insights I have learned that may be of use to you.

What You Need

Before getting into a mobile third business you have to decide if it is for you. Just like dentistry, it isn't for everyone. You have to be able to balance flexibility with structure and be able to live with a degree of chaos at times. Organization is supercritical and you have to build redundancy into your equipment. The transition from being the boss and business owner to being an associate employee can take some getting used to. Some offices may not hold themselves to the same standards you have enforced at your own office. My primary business is a fee for service practice in an affluent area; we are out of network for all insurance companies. Many of the offices I go to are PPO offices with a different clientele and run much differently than my own business. Some offices are a little rough around the edges, run-down or their cleanliness is not always up to my standards. Sometimes I have to keep my mouth shut when I see things in an office that I don't agree with; I have to remind myself that I'm not the boss here. Every office has its own personality and work culture which may or may not be compatible with you. If you are a person who is very set in their ways and has a hard time going with the flow then a mobile third molar practice may not be for you. Some offices are very organized and have minimal no-shows, patients have had consent forms read and signed, preop and postop instructions given, and your days run smoothly. Other offices can be poorly organized, have a difficult time following my instructions, and have problems keeping the schedule full. Offices like these are generally not a good fit if you cannot turn them around.

How you manage your schedule and make sure that you are at the right place on the right day is something that needs to be done to perfection. There is nothing worse than an office calling you at 8am wondering where you are when you are somewhere else, not a good business builder either. You have to assume the role of your own front desk scheduling coordinator and develop a system that works consistently.

The Day-to-day Stuff

If all of the above works for you then the most important thing is your ability to provide sedation and third molar removal predictably, efficiently and safely. You should have the ability to remove 4 full bony impaction third molars with IV conscious sedation in 45 minutes and the experience to identify cases which are going to be problematic in one way or another and should be referred out to an oral surgeon's office. Most of this is obtained by experience and repetition. There are many CE courses out there that teach third molar removal techniques but you really need to take out at least a couple hundred third molars until you really know what you are doing so starting off in a low-cost clinic setting may be a good way to get exposure to a lot of cases quickly. If a case is going to take you longer than an hour, has significant paresthesia risk based on your assessment of the preop panoramic, or the patient has medical issues I would recommend passing on the case and referring it out. Complications are going to happen no matter what but you want to weed out the obvious ones as much as possible. Once the patient has taken time off and is in the chair it is really bad form to bail out on the case because you failed to notice something in the pre-op workup. For each patient I see I require a current health history, a list of all medications being taken, a panoramic radiograph less than six months old, and a height and weight. Taking the time to explain to each office what cases you will and will not see and why is something that can save you from some of these scenarios, but it has to be reinforced every year or so. I choose my cases carefully and am able to finish them quickly with minimal complications which gives the staff the impression that I can do anything, at which point they can get pushy and try to schedule cases that are not appropriate, which is why I have learned to remind them every year or so what an ideal case looks like and what we are referring out. Obesity, developmental disorders (autism, Down's syndrome, etc.), behavioral issues, drug addiction and patients on multiple depression or ADHD drugs are all referred out because they need to be sedated by an anesthesiologist. Sometimes the patient is not the problem but the parents are difficult, another reason for referral. Most offices will also want you to do other things besides third molars such as place implants, bone grafts, expose and bond unerupted teeth for ortho, or remove deeply impacted supernumerary teeth so it is up to you to be clear about what services you are willing to provide and how to factor in the cost of implant parts or regenerative materials into your compensation structure. I only do extractions when I am at my mobile offices. I have placed implants for other offices in the past, but if something fails all the fingers usually get pointed at the guy who placed the implant even if the prosthetics were done poorly, or if someone breaks a screw or strips the internal implant threads. I like to keep things simple which is why I have limited my mobile practice to extractions only.

Pros, Cons, and Insights

The only thing left to start a mobile third molar business is finding offices that are willing to hire you and can provide enough patients to book you one or two days a month. I have found that larger, multi-practitioner offices are better able to provide a consistent flow of patients. Pediatric and orthodontic dental offices can also be a great place to look. Being specialty offices, their fees are usually higher than those of a GP office and their teenage patient demographic is perfectly suited to third molar extraction. Some offices are leery of having a general practitioner (like myself) doing third molars extractions – they are of the opinion that only a certified oral surgeon should do these cases. I explain to these (and all) offices that I am not here to replace the oral surgeon they are currently referring to but just to keep the predictable 90% of the cases in-office and continue to refer the unpredictable 10% to the oral surgeon. It is a win-win situation for both me and the office that I work with, most offices can easily generate an additional $100,000 in yearly collections after paying me my 50%. The first day in a new office is critical; I make sure I will be seeing good cases and I get there extra early to get setup and have time to do some assistant training. Once they see how smoothly the day goes they are usually sold on having you there on a regular basis so it is imperative that your surgical skills and preop selection are rock solid. You are not responsible for setting the fees that are being charged so you need to ask how much they are for each office and establish a bottom fee limit for how much you are willing to get paid for your services. In the beginning you will probably take whatever you can get but that will change as you pick up more offices. In my area (San Francisco Bay Area) my minimum for a third molar case (four teeth with iv sedation) is $2000 of which I get 50% of; I am comfortable passing on offices that are charging less than that but most offices are generally charging well above the $2000, especially pedo and ortho offices. Finding offices that want your services is best done through word of mouth or a mail campaign but I have found that a good start can be made by contacting some of your local dentist friends and describing what you can do for them. Coming into their office once a month is a great way to add some income to both you and your friend's office and will usually lead to referrals to other offices in need of your services.

I recommend setting up some kind of lunch and learn with your new offices to help educate the staff and dentist exactly how you do things and what needs to be done before any appointments are made. Most general dentistry offices will have no idea what you are doing or how to evaluate a pano for third molar removal. They need to be taught how to discuss conscious sedation with patients and set the proper expectation as well as screen the patients for you to make sure you do not end up with a patient in your chair who you are not comfortable sedating or is just not a good candidate for conscious sedation. They are your first line of patient screening and need to be educated by you.

Equipment and Instruments

The instruments and equipment I use for my mobile third molar business are completely separate from my primary practice which makes forgetting to bring something more difficult to do. Everything I need to sedate and remove third molars is organized and stored in rolling tool boxes that I got from Home Depot, and is sterilized and ready to go at all times. I keep my sedation medications and surgical handpieces in a small case that can be brought with me for safekeeping and warm days when the inside of the car can get hot enough to ruin my sedation meds. Most offices will not have a lot of the things I need. If something breaks down I need to be prepared with a backup. I always bring a backup patient monitor, electric motor, and multiple handpieces as well as extra fuses for every piece or equipment that has a fuse. A portable suction unit is a smart investment as well. See Figure 18.2.

There was a day when the office vacuum went down and my unit saved the fully scheduled day. I bring my own oxygen tanks and ensure that they are full and the regulator is functioning properly. I keep an extension cord with my gear because some offices won't have an electrical outlet close

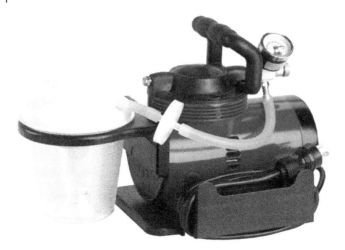

Figure 18.2 Portable suction unit (Medical Depot, Inc.).

enough to where I want to put my surgical motor or patient monitor. Do not count on the office having something that you forgot to bring. I have ten identical surgical instrument setups that have everything I need for third molar removal. I am a big fan of buying instruments on eBay, mostly due to the fact that putting together ten instrument sets would be prohibitively expensive if I was purchasing everything from Karl Schumacher, Hu-Friedy or one of the other surgical instrument companies. I rarely pay more than 20 dollars for an elevator or forceps on eBay so I do not get upset if something disappears from time to time which will happen when you are busy with multiple offices. There is absolutely no uniformity to instruments on eBay so I have had to find the ones I like through trial and error. You can order a 46R elevator from different sellers on eBay and none of them will be the same but you will eventually find one that works well for you. I always purchase more than I need so I have back stock on hand for when something goes missing or breaks because I never know if I am going to be able to get the same instrument again since things are always changing on eBay. I have found that oral surgery instruments are like golf clubs; you can go out and buy the best ones that money can buy and still get terrible results if you do not know how to use them properly. Spend your time and money on learning how to use the instruments properly and you will find that you can get excellent results with the cheap eBay stuff like I do. As time goes by and your skills evolve you will probably start using different instruments as well so sticking with the inexpensive stuff is the way to go to avoid having a box full of expensive instruments that you are no longer using sitting around collecting dust. You will also find that the number of instruments you need will go down as your skills increase. The first time I saw Dr. Wayland's instrument setup I had to ask him where the rest of his stuff was because I could not believe that he was able to remove teeth with so few instruments but as time went by I ended up shrinking my instrument set up to what it is today. My core instruments are Molt 9 periosteal elevator, 46R elevator, 190/191 elevators and the Cogswell B. I use a Saeshin X-Cube implant motor with a BienAir 1:2 straight surgical handpiece for sectioning and bone removal. See Figure 18.3.

I also carry some specialized instruments (Stieglitz forceps, proximators, periotomes, etc.) for special circumstances but if you are choosing ideal cases there should be minimal need for these types of instruments and one set of each is plenty.

At every office I work with I try to find one employee who will be my main contact person and will be responsible for all scheduling and communicating with me. I have found that assigning my needs

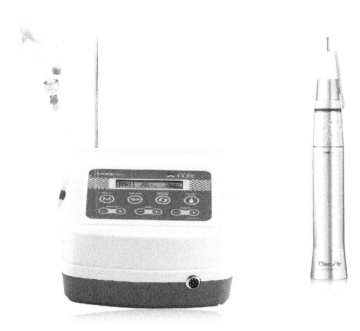

Figure 18.3   X Cube motor and surgical handpiece.

to a single person will reduce mistakes and make for a better overall experience for everyone involved. I do not bring an assistant with me so I have to train one or two assistants at each office exactly what I need from them and go over emergency protocols. The assistants are always super excited to work with me because they get to assist and observe a procedure that is not done at their office, but as we all know employees come and go so it is really helpful to have more than one assistant trained to assist you. How and when you get paid from the offices you go to needs to be laid out and agreed upon in no uncertain terms from day one. Having a lawyer draw up a contract that you present to each office and is signed by both you and the practice owner is something you have to do. My contract states that I am to be paid on the day of service and most offices are fine with that. There are a few offices that do their payroll electronically every two weeks and have talked me into receiving payment electronically at the end of the pay period which is fine, but it does require me to keep an eye out for the deposit and make sure it is accurate. I have had slow paying offices that I have to continually hound to get paid for my services, there is always an excuse or a sob story as to why they are taking so long to pay. My best advice is to cease doing business with offices like this; I have found that they never get it together and the resentment and displeasure I begin to associate with these businesses is just not good for my well being and I am better off without them in my life. I want to keep my mobile third molar days as low stress as possible.

Sedation, Third Molars, and Mentors

The best advice or insight I can share would be the fact that if I could go back in time and do things again I would have started down this path sooner. Learning how to provide conscious sedation for patients is a great way to grow your practice even if you are not removing third molars yet. There is a big group of people out there who will not go to the dentist because of fear and once you can

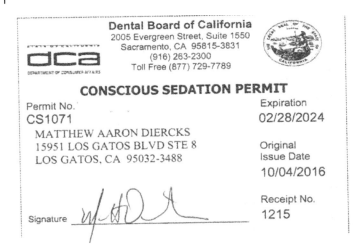

Dental Board of California
2005 Evergreen Street, Suite 1550
Sacramento, CA 95815-3831
(916) 263-2300
Toll Free (877) 729-7789

CONSCIOUS SEDATION PERMIT

Permit No.
CS1071

MATTHEW AARON DIERCKS
15951 LOS GATOS BLVD STE 8
LOS GATOS, CA 95032-3488

Expiration
02/28/2024

Original
Issue Date
10/04/2016

Receipt No.
1215

Signature

Figure 18.4 Sedation permit.

provide them with sedation it can really add a lot of new patients to your business. Having a sedation license also enabled me to expand my third molar surgical skills because I could do something that just was not possible on most patients with local anesthetic and nitrous oxide. See Figure 18.4

Sedated patients have a very good experience and tend to refer other patients to you. My other piece of advice is that if I can do this then so can you. Sedation and impacted third molars can be scary and intimidating at first but it is really just like anything else in life; the more you do it the better you get at it. Pick your cases and patients carefully and make these procedures your favorite thing to do as I have. I consider myself very fortunate in that I met Dr. Wayland and found not only a great friend but a mentor who guided me through the bumpy early stages of sedation and third molar removal. I was also fortunate that I had a dental partner at the time who was really good at placing IV lines when I was not. There are many great courses and people out there who can teach you a lot about these procedures, their expertise and advice is invaluable so reach out and see if you can find yourself a Dr. Wayland too.

Index

Page locators in **bold** indicate tables. Page locators in *italics* indicate figures. This index uses letter-by-letter alphabetization.

Impacted Third Molars, Second Edition. Edited by John Wayland.
© 2024 John Wiley & Sons, Inc. Published 2024 by John Wiley & Sons, Inc.